NOVEL DESIGNS OF EARLY PHASE TRIALS FOR CANCER THERAPEUTICS

NOVEL DESIGNS OF EARLY PHASE TRIALS FOR CANCER THERAPEUTICS

Edited by

SHIVAANI KUMMAR
Stanford University, Stanford, CA, United States

CHRIS TAKIMOTO
Forty Seven Inc., Menlo Park, CA, United States

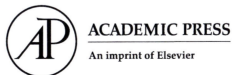

ACADEMIC PRESS

An imprint of Elsevier

Academic Press is an imprint of Elsevier
125 London Wall, London EC2Y 5AS, United Kingdom
525 B Street, Suite 1800, San Diego, CA 92101-4495, United States
50 Hampshire Street, 5th Floor, Cambridge, MA 02139, United States
The Boulevard, Langford Lane, Kidlington, Oxford OX5 1GB, United Kingdom

Notices
Knowledge and best practice in this field are constantly changing. As new research and experience broaden our understanding, changes in research methods, professional practices, or medical treatment may become necessary.

Practitioners and researchers must always rely on their own experience and knowledge in evaluating and using any information, methods, compounds, or experiments described herein. In using such information or methods they should be mindful of their own safety and the safety of others, including parties for whom they have a professional responsibility.

To the fullest extent of the law, neither the Publisher nor the authors, contributors, or editors, assume any liability for any injury and/or damage to persons or property as a matter of products liability, negligence or otherwise, or from any use or operation of any methods, products, instructions, or ideas contained in the material herein.

British Library Cataloguing-in-Publication Data
A catalogue record for this book is available from the British Library

Library of Congress Cataloging-in-Publication Data
A catalog record for this book is available from the Library of Congress

ISBN: **978-0-12-812512-0**

For Information on all Academic Press publications
visit our website at https://www.elsevier.com/books-and-journals

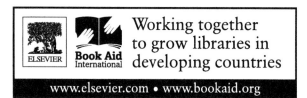

Working together
to grow libraries in
developing countries

www.elsevier.com • www.bookaid.org

Publisher: John Fedor
Acquisition Editor: Rafael E. Teixeira
Editorial Project Manager: Timothy Bennett
Production Project Manager: Mohanapriyan Rajendran
Cover Designer: Mark Limbert

Typeset by MPS Limited, Chennai, India

To my parents
Surendra Nath Kumar and Archana Mukherji Kumar

To my parents
Hideyo H. Takimoto and Mitzi M. Takimoto

Contents

List of Contributors

Pedro C. Barata Cleveland Clinic Foundation, Cleveland, OH, United States

Lucia Baratto Stanford University, Stanford, CA, United States

Brian Booth U.S. Food and Drug Administration, Silver Spring, MD, United States

Jessica S. Brown Royal Marsden Hospital, London, United Kingdom; The Institute of Cancer Research, London, United Kingdom

Alice P. Chen National Cancer Institute, Bethesda, MD, United States

Johann S. De Bono Royal Marsden Hospital, London, United Kingdom; The Institute of Cancer Research, London, United Kingdom

Khanh Do Dana-Farber Cancer Institute, Boston, MA, United States

James H. Doroshow National Cancer Institute, Bethesda, MD, United States

Katherine V. Ferry-Galow Leidos Biomedical Research, Inc., Frederick National Laboratory for Cancer Research, Frederick, MD, United States

Terry J. Fry National Institutes of Health, Bethesda, MD, United States

Sanjiv S. Gambhir Stanford University, Stanford, CA, United States

Elizabeth Garrett-Mayer Medical University of South Carolina, Charleston, SC, United States

Lacey Greene Stanford University, Stanford, CA, United States

Bahru A. Habtemariam Alnylam Pharmaceuticals, Cambridge, MA, United States

Negin Hatami Stanford University, Stanford, CA, United States

David Hong The University of Texas MD Anderson Cancer Center, Houston, TX, United States

Susan P. Ivy National Institutes of Health, Bethesda, MD, United States

John Janik Incyte Corporation, Chadds Ford, PA, United States

Patricia Keegan U.S. Food and Drug Administration, Silver Spring, MD, United States

Samir N. Khleif Georgetown University Medical School, Washington, DC, United States

Hahn Khuu National Institutes of Health, Bethesda, MD, United States

Shivaani Kummar Stanford University, Palo Alto, CA, United States

Joline S.J. Lim Royal Marsden Hospital, London, United Kingdom; National University Cancer Institute of Singapore, Singapore, Singapore

Lian Ma U.S. Food and Drug Administration, Silver Spring, MD, United States

Nitin Mehrotra Merck and Co, Kenilworth, NJ, United States

Lori M. Minasian National Cancer Institute, Bethesda, MD, United States

R. Rita Misra National Cancer Institute, Frederick, MD, United States

Sandra A. Mitchell National Cancer Institute, Bethesda, MD, United States

Abhilasha Nair U.S. Food and Drug Administration, Silver Spring, MD, United States

Tomomi Nobashi Stanford University, Stanford, CA, United States

Nathaniel O'Connell Medical University of South Carolina, Charleston, SC, United States

Olanrewaju O. Okusanya U.S. Food and Drug Administration, Silver Spring, MD, United States

Christy Osgood U.S. Food and Drug Administration, Silver Spring, MD, United States

Lee Pai-Scherf U.S. Food and Drug Administration, Silver Spring, MD, United States

Ralph E. Parchment Leidos Biomedical Research, Inc., Frederick National Laboratory for Cancer Research, Frederick, MD, United States

Sonya Park Stanford University, Stanford, CA, United States

Bhanumati Ramineni National Institutes of Health, Rockville, MD, United States

Houssein A. Sater National Cancer Institute, Bethesda, MD, United States; Johns Hopkins Medicine, Bethesda, MD, United States

Nirali N. Shah National Institutes of Health, Bethesda, MD, United States

Haneen Shalabi National Institutes of Health, Bethesda, MD, United States

Shyam Srinivas Stanford University, Stanford, CA, United States

Diane C. St. Germain National Cancer Institute, Bethesda, MD, United States

Chris H. Takimoto Forty Seven, Inc., Menlo Park, CA, United States

Marc R. Theoret U.S. Food and Drug Administration, Silver Spring, MD, United States

Akira Toriihara Stanford University, Stanford, CA, United States

Timothy A. Yap The University of Texas MD Anderson Cancer Center, Houston, TX, United States

Preface

Impressive advances in the field of cancer therapeutics beginning at the turn of the last century have yielded a rapidly growing number of effective anticancer therapies with novel mechanisms of action. For example, the advent of targeted molecular therapeutics designed to selectively impact specific tumor types, and, more recently, immunotherapies that harness the power of the body's own immune system to attack malignant cells have dramatically altered the therapeutic landscape. These changes have directly impacted our approach to early-phase clinical trials and, to a large extent, have upended many traditional strategies in drug development that were executed unchanged for many decades.

Nowhere is this tectonic shift in strategic thinking felt more acutely than in the arena of first-in-human and first-in-cancer patient clinical trials. The infusion of scientific thinking and translational research that now permeates early-phase clinical trial designs in oncology is a welcome step forward. Clinicians and other early-phase clinical trial stakeholders must be well versed in molecularly profiling, biomarkers, and translational research, and they can no long rely upon simplistic, algorithmic, study designs that dominated the field of oncology drug development for so many decades.

In the modern era the early-phase oncology clinical trialist must now design and implement studies of greater complexity than in yesteryear, but the potential payoffs in terms of speed and efficiency are huge. In the following 13 chapters, leading experts in the field of early-phase clinical trials provide a clear and distinct road map for navigating these shifting paradigms. Included are biostatistical, operational and regulatory perspectives as well as discussions on dose selection, precision medicine, molecular profiling, and on the rational integration of biomarkers into early-phase studies. Additional perspectives on specific classes of new cancer therapies of growing importance in cancer drug development include overviews of immuno-oncology agents and cell-based therapies, and the impact these are having on early-phase clinical trials. Finally, the role of imaging, drug combinations, and patient reported outcomes are discussed.

Although the range and scope of this book are broad, we, nonetheless, hope that the careful reader will be well prepared to meet the considerable challenges of bringing the next wave of transformational therapies to cancer patients everywhere.

Changing Landscape of Early Phase Clinical Trials: Beyond the Horizon

Khanh Do[1], Chris H. Takimoto[2] and Shivaani Kummar[3]

[1]Dana-Farber Cancer Institute, Boston, MA, United States [2]Forty Seven, Inc., Menlo Park, CA, United States [3]Stanford University, Palo Alto, CA, United States

1.1 HISTORICAL PERSPECTIVE

The field of drug development has evolved dramatically over the past 60 years, beginning with the first law put in place to protect against misbranding and adulteration of foods, drinks, and drugs—the 1906 Pure Food and Drugs Act. It would take an additional 30 years before the 1938 Food, Drug and Cosmetic Act was passed, which required premarket proof of safety before a drug could go on the market. This was enacted in response to several deaths that occurred when the elixir sulfanilamide, which contained a solvent analog of antifreeze, was marketed as an antiinfective. More recently, 2012 marked the 50-year anniversary of the 1962 Kefauver-Harris Amendment to the Food, Drug and Cosmetic Act that required drug manufacturers to provide proof of efficacy and safety before a drug application could be approved. This landmark piece of legislation was enacted in response to birth defects arising from the use of thalidomide, which at the time was marketed as a sedative and

widely prescribed in Europe and Canada. Shortly after this, the FDA formalized the drug review process, delineating each step and phase in the development of investigational agents. Informed consent would now be required of participants in clinical trials and reporting of adverse drug reactions to the FDA would be mandated. Together with increasing legislative hurdles came longer review processes before a drug could come to market. Currently, in the field of oncology, the likelihood of FDA approval for drugs entering clinical development in Phase 1 studies is estimated at 6.7%, the lowest of all investigational drugs reviewed by the FDA during the period of January 1, 2003 to December 31, 2011 [1]. In response to increasing pressure from patients, patient advocates, and Congress to improve patient access to investigational drugs, the FDA Safety and Innovation Act of 2012 (FDASIA) was passed, which established two modifications to the Food, Drug and Cosmetic Act. First, this Act allowed for a new "breakthrough therapy" designation for

Novel Designs of Early Phase Trials for Cancer Therapeutics
DOI: https://doi.org/10.1016/B978-0-12-812512-0.00001-4

1

investigational drugs. Second, in an effort to expedite the development and review of drugs intended to treat a "serious condition" and have "preliminary clinical evidence indicating that the drug demonstrates substantial improvement over available therapy on a clinically significant endpoint" it allowed for expansion of the statute regarding accelerated approval of investigational agents [2].

Historically, the majority of oncology drugs in development prior to the 1990s were cytotoxic agents. The principles of early drug development initially focused on defining the highest tolerable dose based on observations of direct correlation between dose and cell killing of cytotoxic agents [3]. Phase 1 trials accordingly serve as the cornerstone of drug development, shepherding the transition from the preclinical to clinical stage, testing the safe and maximum tolerable dose (MTD) of a drug in order to define the recommended dose to be carried forward in Phase 2 trials. Rule-based designs have traditionally been the most accepted and widely used of early phase clinical trial designs [4]. In particular, the 3 + 3 design remains the prevailing method used in Phase 1 clinical trial design. The structure of this design assumes that toxicity increases with dose and involves enrollment of three-patient cohorts in escalating preestablished dose levels with the starting dose extrapolated from animal toxicology data. Escalation proceeds until two patients experience dose-limiting toxicities (DLT) in a cohort of three to six patients, whereupon the dose level below this toxic dose level is designated the recommended dose for Phase 2 trials (RP2D). While this design is simple to implement and allows for gathering of data to establish PK-toxicity curves, critics have argued that it requires an excessive number of escalation steps, which prolongs the time required to reach MTD. This also increases the exposure of a disproportionate number of patients to subtherapeutic doses [5–7].

Over the past decade and a half, evolving knowledge of the human genome and molecular pathways has resulted in an exponential growth in the development of molecularly targeted agents (MTAs). Unlike cytotoxic agents, MTAs can demonstrate delayed or cumulative low-grade toxicities that may not be captured within a predefined DLT-assessment window. Additionally, dose may not directly correlate with toxicity or efficacy, depending on the mechanism of action of the agent and the exposures required for target engagement. In response to these challenges, newer strategies for dose escalation have included accelerated titration designs and model-based designs. Accelerated titration designs have the advantage of allowing for rapid dose escalation in single patient cohorts, as well as intrapatient dose escalation, thereby minimizing the proportion of patients potentially treated at subtherapeutic doses [8]. An analysis of 270 published Phase 1 studies from 1997 to 2008 showed that studies using accelerated titration designs resulted in the evaluation of a greater number of dose levels (7 vs 5, $P = 0.0001$) and reduced numbers of patients treated at doses below the RP2D (46% vs 56%, $P = 0.0001$) [9]. In accelerated titration designs, dose escalations occur in increments of either 40% or 100% until a DLT or two moderate toxicities are observed, whereupon the dose escalation and stopping rules revert to the 3 + 3 design. Some of these accelerated design have the drawback of allowing for intrapatient dose escalation with regard to delineating toxicity data. Specifically, a single patient may contribute data for more than one dose level and delayed toxicities may be masked by presumed cumulative toxicities. Additionally, analyses comparing 3 + 3 design and accelerated titration designs have not shown convincing data that accelerated titration designs shorten the overall accrual time nor increase the efficacy of Phase 1 trials [9]. Other rule-based designs have been proposed, including the isotonic regression model [10], improvements on the original up-and-down design [11], accelerated biased coin up-and-down design [12], and the "rolling six" design [13]. Attempts have also been made to propose the use of pharmacologic data to guide dose escalation, however, the logistical practicality of this model, requiring real-time patient pharmacokinetic (PK) data and variability in the PKs between patients and challenges in extrapolation of plasma exposure data from one patient to the next, has limited the widespread acceptance of this model [14].

Alternatively, model-based designs use mathematical modeling based on Bayesian probability statistics to predict a dose level, which would produce a prespecified probability of DLT using real-time cumulative toxicity data from all enrolled patients, thereby producing a dose-toxicity probability curve that allows for computation of the optimal safe dose for the next cohort of patients. The continual reassessment method (CRM) was the first Bayesian model-based method to be adopted in Phase 1 trial designs [15]. In this design, the estimation of probability of encountering a DLT is updated for each new patient entering the study, allowing for multiple dose escalations and de-escalations, until the prespecified probability of DLT at the estimated MTD level is achieved. Multiple modifications of the original CRM design have been developed with the aim of enhancing safety, including restricting dose escalation to one level at a time [16], allowing for treatment of several patients at the same dose level [17], expanding the cohort of patients at the RP2D [18,19], and implementing overdose control in an effort to limit exposing patients to potentially higher toxic doses [20,21]. More recently, additional modifications of the CRM model have been proposed to account for low-grade chronic toxicities often seen with MTAs, e.g., using ordinal toxicity outcomes [22−26] and late-onset or cumulative toxicities using a time-to-event continual reassessment method (TITE-CRM) [27]. A practical challenge with the implementation of model-based approaches is the need for real-time biostatistical support, which may not be readily available at all institutions.

1.2 CURRENT TRENDS

With evolving selectivity of each generation of MTAs, the biologic effective dose has emerged as the more relevant endpoint in early phase clinical trials. While toxicity remains an important endpoint, the highly selective nature of MTAs results in widening of the dose-toxicity curves and a RP2D that may be well below the MTD. Increasingly, more trials are now incorporating mandated biopsies to further explore the pharmacodynamic (PD) effects of receptor occupancy and target inhibition in tumors in an effort to characterize the biologically active dose. A greater emphasis is also being placed on characterization of the PK−PD relationship to guide the decision on the declaration of the RP2D. In line with this shift in paradigm in oncology drug development, various novel approaches including the TriCRM method have been proposed, to address the incorporation of toxicity and efficacy data into the estimation of the biologically effective dose [28]. In response to the complexity of incorporating PD endpoints in early clinical trial modeling, the Task Force on Methodology for the Development of Innovative Cancer Therapies was developed to provide guidance on dose escalation methods specific for molecularly targeted compounds [29]. The Task Force acknowledged the importance of establishing the "biologically active" dose range for future development of targeted agent combinations where overlapping toxicities have the potential to limit the tolerability of administering both agents in full doses. With increasing emphasis on PD-driven trials, more attention has been drawn to the challenges of tissue acquisition and assay performance. In an effort to address the call for development of more sensitive and specific biomarkers and enhance the efficiency of investigational drug development, the National Cancer Institute Investigational Drug Steering Committee and Biomarker Task Force was charged with the development of guidelines for the incorporation of biomarker studies in early clinical trials of novel agents and set the standards for assay performance [30]. Although the evaluation of safety remains the primary goal of early clinical trials, assessment of efficacy and PK/PD parameters are emerging as the key objectives in the new era of drug development where advances in next-generation sequencing can provide rapid genomic mutation profiles of tumors.

Phase 1 trials are increasingly being used as a platform to explore predictive biomarkers and to enable early evaluation of antitumor efficacy by enriching subsets of patients selected according to molecular criteria who are expected to most likely respond to a particular MTA, focusing on ever smaller subsets of patients. This paradigm shift in oncology drug development has culminated in the "precision-medicine" based approach where the selection of patients is limited to certain mutations of interest or presence of target, based on the mechanism of action of the agent being studied. The ability to identify and treat specific subsets of patients based on presence of a molecular target has increased the complexity of early phase trials and has necessitated multi-center collaborations.

These "patient enrichment" strategies have been utilized in order to enroll fewer patients, demonstrate larger treatment effects, and expedite the drug development process. However, apart from identifying the mutations of interest and designing agents that effectively target these alterations; this approach presents the logistical challenge of

patient selection and timely enrollment. The clinical trial demonstrating high response rate and clinical benefit for crizotinib in patients with nonsmall cell lung cancer carrying the EML4-ALK rearrangement screened approximately 1500 tumor samples to enroll the required 82 patients [31]. The need to obtain archival or fresh tumor tissue for screening, laboratory infrastructure to perform adequately qualified assays in a clinically relevant time frame for patient selection, and treatment of selected patients requires an infrastructure that allows the study to be conducted in multiple centers with adequate oversight. To aid in overcoming potential barriers to fulfilling these requirements, the Moonshot Initiative was announced and tasked with the mission of accelerating cancer discovery by breaking down administrative and financial barriers, increasing data sharing across research sectors, and enhancing collaboration between the public and private sectors [32].

Together, the advent of MTAs and concept of precision medicine has resulted in Phase 1 trials evolving from relatively simple safety and dose finding studies to larger trials with proof-of-mechanism, proof-of-concept, and recently, registration intent. The desire to expedite development of promising anticancer therapeutics has resulted in the so-called "seamless Phase 1 design" with an initial dose escalation phase followed by multi-arm expansion cohorts exploring dose, schedule, and efficacy in various histologies. Phase 1 trials have therefore transformed from small 20 to 30 patient trials, to trials enrolling a few hundred to over a 1000 patients. This is exemplified by the Phase 1 trial of pembrolizumab, an anti-programmed cell death protein-1 antibody. The initial dose escalation phase of this trial enrolled a total of 10 patients, with 13 patients participating in the intrapatient dose escalation portion of the first-in-human (FIH) trial [33]. Over 2.5 years and after multiple amendments, the patient number treated on this FIH trial expanded to >1100 enrolled in nine distinct expansion cohorts [34].

The growing complexity of clinical trials presents a number of logistical challenges. In an effort to expedite patient accrual, industry-sponsored studies now commonly utilize multiple participating centers in order to fill slots on a competitive basis and often depend on contract research organizations to oversee conduct of the trial across multiple sites and meet timelines. Additionally, as trials become more PD-centric, the costs of supporting these assays are major financial considerations for the conduct of trials. Currently, the median number of procedures performed per trial has increased by 57% (105.9 procedures in the period between 2000 and 2003 to 166.6 procedures between 2008 and 2011), with a 211% increase in the median number of case report forms per protocol comparing the same time periods [35]. The increasing complexity and larger size of clinical trials has also contributed to the escalating costs of drug development, going from 1 billion dollars in the decade of the 1990s to 2.6 billion dollars over the past decade. As trial designs evolve to meet the pace of early drug development, these financial considerations need to be taken into account during the initial stages of development. It is therefore likely that we can expect increasing legislation in the years to come, to maintain oversight of multi-center trials in a continuing effort to monitor safety and efficacy.

References

[1] Hay M, et al. Clinical development success rates for investigational drugs. Nat Biotechnol 2014;32 (1):40–51.
[2] FDA. Fast track, breakthrough therapy, accelerated approval, and priority review—breakthrough therapy. <http://www.fda.gov/forpatients/approvals/fast/ucm405397.htm>; 2016.
[3] Skipper HE, Schabel Jr. FM, Wilcox WS. Experimental evaluation of potential anticancer agents. Xiii. On the criteria and kinetics associated with "curability" of experimental leukemia. Cancer Chemother Rep 1964;35:1–111.
[4] Storer BE. Design and analysis of phase I clinical trials. Biometrics 1989;45(3):925–37.
[5] Le Tourneau C, Lee JJ, Siu LL. Dose escalation methods in phase I cancer clinical trials. J Natl Cancer Inst 2009;101(10):708–20.
[6] LoRusso PM, Boerner SA, Seymour L. An overview of the optimal planning, design, and conduct of phase I studies of new therapeutics. Clin Cancer Res 2010;16 (6):1710–18.
[7] Eisenhauer EA, et al. Phase I clinical trial design in cancer drug development. J Clin Oncol 2000;18 (3):684–92.
[8] Simon R, et al. Accelerated titration designs for phase I clinical trials in oncology. J Natl Cancer Inst 1997;89 (15):1138–47.
[9] Penel N, et al. "Classical 3 + 3 design" versus "accelerated titration designs": analysis of 270 phase 1 trials investigating anti-cancer agents. Invest New Drugs 2009;27(6):552–6.
[10] Leung DH, Wang Y. Isotonic designs for phase I trials. Control Clin Trials 2001;22(2):126–38.
[11] Ivanova A, et al. Improved up-and-down designs for phase I trials. Stat Med 2003;22(1):69–82.
[12] Stylianou M, Follmann DA. The accelerated biased coin up-and-down design in phase I trials. J Biopharm Stat 2004;14(1):249–60.
[13] Skolnik JM, et al. Shortening the timeline of pediatric phase I trials: the rolling six design. J Clin Oncol 2008;26(2):190–5.
[14] Collins JM, Grieshaber CK, Chabner BA. Pharmacologically guided phase I clinical trials based upon preclinical drug development. J Natl Cancer Inst 1990;82(16):1321–6.
[15] O'Quigley J, Pepe M, Fisher L. Continual reassessment method: a practical design for phase 1 clinical trials in cancer. Biometrics 1990;46(1):33–48.
[16] Goodman SN, Zahurak ML, Piantadosi S. Some practical improvements in the continual reassessment method for phase I studies. Stat Med 1995;14 (11):1149–61.
[17] Piantadosi S, Fisher JD, Grossman S. Practical implementation of a modified continual reassessment method for dose-finding trials. Cancer Chemother Pharmacol 1998;41(6):429–36.
[18] Faries D. Practical modifications of the continual reassessment method for phase I cancer clinical trials. J Biopharm Stat 1994;4(2):147–64.

[19] Heyd JM, Carlin BP. Adaptive design improvements in the continual reassessment method for phase I studies. Stat Med 1999;18(11):1307–21.

[20] Babb J, Rogatko A, Zacks S. Cancer phase I clinical trials: efficient dose escalation with overdose control. Stat Med 1998;17(10):1103–20.

[21] Rogatko A, et al. New paradigm in dose-finding trials: patient-specific dosing and beyond phase I. Clin Cancer Res 2005;11(15):5342–6.

[22] Iasonos A, Zohar S, O'Quigley J. Incorporating lower grade toxicity information into dose finding designs. Clin Trials 2011;8(4):370–9.

[23] Yuan Z, Chappell R, Bailey H. The continual reassessment method for multiple toxicity grades: a Bayesian quasi-likelihood approach. Biometrics 2007;63(1):173–9.

[24] Ezzalfani M, et al. Dose-finding designs using a novel quasi-continuous endpoint for multiple toxicities. Stat Med 2013;32(16):2728–46.

[25] Van Meter EM, Garrett-Mayer E, Bandyopadhyay D. Proportional odds model for dose-finding clinical trial designs with ordinal toxicity grading. Stat Med 2011;30(17):2070–80.

[26] Van Meter EM, Garrett-Mayer E, Bandyopadhyay D. Dose-finding clinical trial design for ordinal toxicity grades using the continuation ratio model: an extension of the continual reassessment method. Clin Trials 2012;9(3):303–13.

[27] Cheung YK, Chappell R. Sequential designs for phase I clinical trials with late-onset toxicities. Biometrics 2000;56(4):1177–82.

[28] Zhang W, Sargent DJ, Mandrekar S. An adaptive dose-finding design incorporating both toxicity and efficacy. Stat Med 2006;25(14):2365–83.

[29] Booth CM, et al. Endpoints and other considerations in phase I studies of targeted anticancer therapy: recommendations from the task force on Methodology for the Development of Innovative Cancer Therapies (MDICT). Eur J Cancer 2008;44(1):19–24.

[30] Dancey JE, et al. Guidelines for the development and incorporation of biomarker studies in early clinical trials of novel agents. Clin Cancer Res 2010;16(6):1745–55.

[31] Kwak EL, et al. Anaplastic lymphoma kinase inhibition in non-small-cell lung cancer. N Engl J Med 2010;363(18):1693–703.

[32] National Cancer Institute. Cancer Moonshot. <https://www.cancer.gov/research/key-initiatives/moonshot-cancer-initiative>; 2016.

[33] Patnaik A, et al. Phase I study of pembrolizumab (MK-3475; anti-PD-1 monoclonal antibody) in patients with advanced solid tumors. Clin Cancer Res 2015;21(19):4286–93.

[34] Theoret MR, et al. Expansion cohorts in first-in-human solid tumor oncology trials. Clin Cancer Res 2015;21(20):4545–51.

[35] PhRMA Chart Packs. The complexity of clinical trials has increased. <http://chartpack.phrma.org/2016-perspective/chapter-2/the-complexity-of-clinical-trials-has-increased>; 2016.

2

Requirements for Filing an Investigational New Drug Application

R. Rita Misra[1] and Bhanumati Ramineni[2]

[1]National Cancer Institute, Frederick, MD, United States [2]National Institutes of Health, Rockville, MD, United States

In the United States, Federal law requires that a drug or biologic product be the subject of an approved marketing application before it is transported across state lines. Before the sponsor (the individual or entity that is responsible) for the clinical investigation of a drug ships the drug to investigators in another state, they must seek exemption from that legal requirement. An Investigational New Drug (IND) application, filed with the US Food and Drug Administration (FDA) is the means through which the sponsor obtains such an exemption.

As defined in Title 21, Part 312 of the Code of Federal Regulations (CFR),[1] an IND application is synonymous with a "Notice of Claimed Investigational Exemption for a New Drug." An "investigational new drug" is a new drug[2,3] that is used in a clinical investigation, and an "investigator" is an individual who conducts a clinical investigation (i.e., under whose immediate direction the drug is administered or dispensed to a subject). When a clinical investigation is conducted by a team of individuals, the investigator is the responsible

---

[1] https://www.accessdata.fda.gov/scripts/cdrh/cfdocs/cfcfr/CFRSearch.cfm?CFRPart=312&showFR=1&subpartNode=21:5.0.1.1.3.1

[2] The Federal Food Drug and Cosmetic Act defines drugs as "articles intended for use in the diagnosis, cure, mitigation, treatment, or prevention of disease" and "articles (other than food) intended to affect the structure or any function of the body of man or other animals." [FD&C Act, sec. 201(g)(1)]

[3] The US Code defines a biological product as "...a virus, therapeutic serum, toxin, antitoxin, vaccine, blood, blood component or derivative, allergenic product, protein (except any chemically synthesized polypeptide), or analogous product, or arsphenamine or derivative of arsphenamine (or any other trivalent organic arsenic compound), applicable to the prevention, treatment, or cure of a disease or condition of human beings." [42 U.S.C, sec. 262(i)]

leader of the team and a "sub-investigator" is any other member of the team.

The IND sponsor may be an individual or pharmaceutical company, governmental agency, academic institution, or private organization. A "sponsor-investigator" is defined as an individual who initiates and conducts a clinical investigation, and under whose immediate direction the investigational drug is administered or dispensed. The requirements applicable to a sponsor-investigator under 21 CFR 312 include those that are applicable to an investigator or a sponsor.

Per 21 CFR 312, a sponsor or investigator (or any person acting on behalf of a sponsor or investigator), is prohibited from "promoting" the investigational drug by suggesting that it is safe or effective for the purposes for which it is under investigation. Sponsors must also obtain FDA authorization before charging patients for an investigational drug.

2.1 EXEMPTIONS TO FILING AN IND

A clinical investigation may be exempted from the IND application requirement if the study meets all the criteria for exemption under 21 CFR 312.2(b)[4]:

1. The drug is lawfully marketed in the United States.
2. The investigation is not intended to be reported as a well-controlled study in support of a new indication, or to support any other significant change in the labeling of the drug.
3. In the case of a prescription drug, the investigation is not intended to support a significant change in advertising of the drug.
4. The investigation does not involve a route of administration, dose, patient population, or other factor that significantly increases the

risk associated with the use of the drug product.
5. The investigation is conducted in compliance with the requirements for review by an Institutional Review Board (IRB) (21 CFR 56), and informed consent (21 CFR 50).
6. The investigation is not intended to promote or commercialize the drug (21 CFR 312.7).

The IND exemption provision provides flexibility regarding the "marketed product"; the provision allows the investigator to use drug product in a different dosage form, dose level, and patient population, as long as the risk to study participants is no greater than the risk described on the FDA-approved product label.

The sponsor or sponsor-investigator of a planned clinical investigation using a marketed drug is ultimately responsible for determining whether the investigation meets the criteria for an IND exemption. If there is uncertainty about whether the IND exemption criteria are met, the sponsor or sponsor-investigator can seek advice from the FDA.

2.2 TYPES OF IND APPLICATIONS

There are three types of IND applications:

- An *Investigator IND* application supports studies conducted by physicians under whose immediate direction the investigational drug is administered or dispensed. Investigator IND applications may support studies of an unapproved product, or an approved product for a new indication, or a new patient population (21 CFR 312.22).
- An *Emergency Use IND* application is used to treat a single-patient with an investigational drug in an emergency situation. It is also used for patients who do not meet the

---

[4] https://www.fda.gov/downloads/Drugs/GuidanceComplianceRegulatoryInformation/Guidances/UCM229175.pdf

criteria of an existing study protocol, or if an approved study protocol does not exist (21 CFR 312.36).

- A *Treatment IND* application is submitted for nonemergency use of an investigational drug that shows promise for serious or immediately life-threatening conditions while the final clinical work is conducted and FDA review for drug approval is taking place. Large numbers of patients can be treated under a treatment IND (21 CFR 312.35).

Emergency Use and Treatment IND applications allow for "expanded access" or "compassionate use" of investigational drugs outside of a clinical trial when all of the following criteria apply[5]:

1. Patient(s) have a serious or immediately life-threatening condition and there is no comparable or satisfactory alternative treatment for the condition.
2. The potential for patient benefit justifies the potential risks of treatment and the potential risks are not unreasonable in the context of the condition to be treated.
3. Expanded use of the investigational drug will not interfere with the initiation, conduct, or completion of clinical investigations that may support marketing approval of the drug.

The three IND application types fall into two categories:

- A *Commercial IND* is one for which the sponsor is usually a corporate entity or one of the institutes of the National Institutes of Health (NIH).
- A *Research (noncommercial) IND* is one for which the sponsor is usually an individual investigator or academic institution.

The FDA may designate any IND application as commercial if the sponsor intends to market the product in the future.

2.3 REGULATORY AND ADMINISTRATIVE COMPONENTS OF AN IND APPLICATION

An IND application includes[6]:

- Information pertaining to the composition, manufacturer, stability, and controls used for manufacturing the drug substance and drug product (this information will be assessed to ensure that the manufacturer can adequately produce similar batches of the drug).
- Detailed clinical study plans/protocols (these will be assessed to ensure that the proposed studies will not expose subjects to unnecessary harm).
- Information about the investigator and sub-investigators who will oversee drug administration (to assess whether they are qualified to fulfill their responsibilities to obtain informed consent from research subjects, to obtain review of the study by an IRB, and to adhere to investigational drug regulations).
- Data from studies of the drug in animals.
- Data from studies of the drug in humans.

Before conducting a clinical investigation, the IND sponsor must have pharmacological and toxicological evidence demonstrating that it is "reasonably safe" to administer the drug in people. Preclinical efficacy and safety studies may be conducted in vitro (in a test tube or cell culture) or in vivo (in laboratory animals), and used to estimate the drug's potential for benefit and harm. The types of

[5] https://www.fda.gov/Drugs/DevelopmentApprovalProcess/HowDrugsareDevelopedandApproved/ApprovalApplications/InvestigationalNewDrugINDApplication/ucm351748.htm

[6] https://www.fda.gov/downloads/Drugs/GuidanceComplianceRegulatoryInformation/Guidances/UCM074980.pdf

preclinical studies required varies with the nature of the drug and the proposed clinical investigation. Preclinical studies of the drug should help determine:

- How it is absorbed, distributed, metabolized, and excreted
- Its mechanism of action
- The most effective dose
- The most effective route of administration
- Its side effects/toxicity
- How it affects different groups of people (e.g., different genders, races, or ethnicities)
- How it interacts with other drugs
- Its effectiveness compared to similar drugs.

As drug development proceeds, additional nonclinical efficacy and safety information may be required by the FDA.[7]

The FDA requires researchers to use good laboratory practices (GLP) for nonclinical laboratory studies as described in 21 CFR Part 58.1.[8] These regulations set the minimum requirements for study conduct, personnel, facilities, equipment, operating procedures, reports, and oversight. Preclinical studies are not usually very large however, they should be designed to provide useful information on drug dosing and toxicity.

While preclinical research may answer basic questions about a drug's efficacy and safety, it is not a substitute for clinical research. Investigators should include a brief explanation of what they want to accomplish in clinical studies (i.e., in Phase 1, 2, and 3 trials), in an IND application "Introductory Statement and General Investigational Plan."

An IND application can be submitted to the FDA using a nonstandard format, or the standard, Common Technical Document (CTD)

format. The IND application can be submitted on paper through an FDA document control room, or electronically through the FDA Electronic Submission Gateway (ESG).[9] Once an initial IND or IND amendment is submitted electronically all future submissions to that IND must be submitted electronically.

In 1990, the International Council for Harmonisation of Technical Requirements for Pharmaceuticals for Human Use (ICH) brought international regulatory authorities and the pharmaceutical industry together to begin the process of developing guidelines to assemble drug quality, safety, and efficacy information in a common format (the CTD format), eliminating the need to reformat most of the information necessary to meet specific requirements for regulatory submissions in different countries. Since 2003 the CTD format has been mandatory in the European Union (EU) and Japan, and has been strongly recommended in the United States and Canada.

A CTD application is organized into five modules (Fig. 2.1).[10] Module 1 is region specific, and Modules 2, 3, 4, and 5 are common for all regions.

Module 1 for a US IND application typically contains FDA forms 1571, 3674, and 1572, a cover letter, draft labeling, letters of authorization to reference supporting applications, an environmental assessment or request for exclusion, key FDA correspondence (e.g., FDA meeting minutes), the introductory statement and general investigational plan, and the Investigator's Brochure (IB).

- Form 1571 is the cover sheet for all IND submissions. It indicates what is included in the submission and must be signed by the

[7] https://www.fda.gov/Drugs/GuidanceComplianceRegulatoryInformation/Guidances/ucm065014.htm

[8] https://www.accessdata.fda.gov/scripts/cdrh/cfdocs/cfcfr/CFRSearch.cfm?CFRPart=58

[9] https://www.fda.gov/downloads/Drugs/GuidanceComplianceRegulatoryInformation/Guidances/UCM333969.pdf

[10] http://www.ich.org/products/ctd

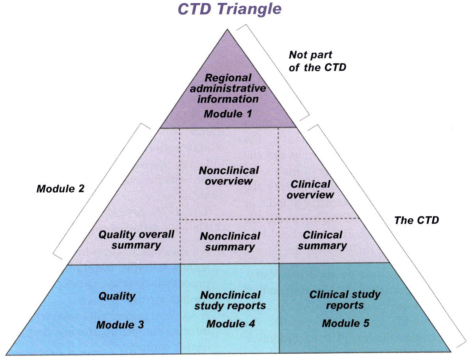

CTD Triangle

FIGURE 2.1   The Common Technical Document (CTD) triangle. The CTD is organized into five modules. Module 1 is region specific and Modules 2, 3, 4, and 5 are intended to be common for all regions.

sponsor or sponsor's authorized representative.[11]

- Form 3674 is a certification of compliance with registration and reporting requirements of the ClinicalTrials.gov databank for applicable drugs and devices.[12]
- Form 1572 Statement of Investigator is an agreement by the investigator to provide certain information about their own qualifications, study sub-investigators and laboratory sites, and to and comply with FDA regulations related to the conduct of a clinical investigation of an investigational drug. Some of the required information

(such as the investigator's Curriculum Vitae) is provided as an attachment to the form.[13]

- The IB is usually prepared by the product manufacturer and is updated as new information becomes available. The IB should contain: a brief description of the drug substance and the formulation; a summary of the pharmacological and toxicological effects of the drug in animals and humans; a summary of the pharmacokinetics and biological disposition of the drug in animals and human; a summary of information relating to safety and effectiveness in humans obtained from

[11] https://www.fda.gov/downloads/AboutFDA/ReportsManualsForms/Forms/UCM182850.pdf

[12] https://www.fda.gov/downloads/AboutFDA/ReportsManualsForms/Forms/UCM354618.pdf

[13] https://www.fda.gov/downloads/RegulatoryInformation/Guidances/UCM214282.pdf

prior clinical studies; a description of possible risks and side effects to be anticipated on the basis of prior experience with the drug under investigation or with related drugs; and a description of precautions or special monitoring to be done as part of the clinical investigation.[14]

Module 2 includes summaries of drug quality, nonclinical, and clinical, information. For IND applications where the sponsor is not the drug manufacturer, a letter may be provided by the manufacturer authorizing the FDA to reference the manufacturer's IND or Master File[15] for detailed information about the drug. These letters of authorization should be included in Module 1 of the IND application.

Module 3 should include detailed chemistry, manufacturing, and control (CMC) information for the drug substance and drug product.

Module 4 should include the reports for nonclinical pharmacology, pharmacokinetics, and toxicology studies.

Module 5 should include a tabular listing of all clinical studies conducted under the IND, detailed clinical protocols and informed consent forms, and clinical study reports.

2.4 FDA IND REVIEW

After receipt, the FDA will assign an IND number to the initial IND application; the sponsor must wait 30 calendar days before initiating any clinical trials. During this 30-day period, the FDA will determine whether the information in the IND application is sufficient to support the safety of subjects in the proposed clinical investigation. If the FDA is satisfied that the risks to subjects are

acceptable the investigator may proceed with the proposed clinical study.

If the FDA determines that the risks to subjects are unacceptable because the investigators are not qualified, information provided to the subjects is misleading, or information in the IND is insufficient to support safety, then the FDA will issue a "clinical hold" of studies under the IND. During or after the initial 30-day review period, FDA reviewers may provide the sponsor with "hold" and "nonhold" comments intended to improve the quality of a clinical trial.

The FDA review team consists of individuals with different scientific expertise:

- A project manager who coordinates the team's activities throughout the review process and serves as the primary FDA contact for the sponsor.
- A medical officer who reviews clinical study information before, during, and after the trial is complete.
- A statistician who reviews and helps interpret the design and results of the clinical study.
- A toxicologist who reviews the preclinical study data to assess safety.
- A pharmacologist who reviews absorption, distribution, metabolism, and excretion data to assess drug dosage and administration schedules.
- A chemist who evaluates the drug composition, how it was made, quality control, stability, presence of impurities, etc.

Amendments to the IND application that contain new or revised protocols should build logically on previous submissions and should be supported by submission of additional information, including results of animal or human studies, as appropriate. In general, new

[14] https://www.fda.gov/downloads/Drugs/GuidanceComplianceRegulatoryInformation/Guidances/UCM073122.pdf

[15] https://www.fda.gov/Drugs/DevelopmentApprovalProcess/FormsSubmissionRequirements/DrugMasterFilesDMFs/UCM2007046

protocols for a specific drug in related or similar diseases/indications may be submitted to an existing IND.

The FDA's primary objective, in all phases of the drug investigation, is to protect the rights and safety of subjects. The FDA's objective in Phase 2 and 3, is to help ensure that the clinical studies will yield data capable of meeting statutory standards for evaluating drug safety and efficacy.[16]

2.5 IND REPORTING REQUIREMENTS

2.5.1 Expedited Safety Reporting

Sponsors are required to notify the FDA and all participating investigators, in writing, of any new findings that suggest a significant risk to human subjects receiving the investigational drug. Any serious, unexpected, suspected, adverse reaction (SUSAR) to the investigational drug that is experienced by a subject in a clinical study must be reported in a timely manner.[17]

An investigator is required to "immediately" report all serious adverse events (AEs) to the sponsor regardless of whether they are drug related, including those AEs that are "expected" in the study population, independent of drug exposure. In the case of clinical trials using oncologic drugs associated with frequent, expected serious hematologic AEs, sponsors may request an FDA waiver for immediate reporting. The investigator must include an assessment of causality (i.e., whether there is a reasonable possibility that the drug caused the event) in their report to the sponsor however, the sponsor is ultimately responsible for determining whether the AE is a SUSAR.

An AE must be reported to the FDA as an "IND Safety Report" (typically, on an FDA MedWatch Form 3500A) within 15 days if the sponsor determines the AE is a SUSAR, and within 7 days if the sponsor determines the AE is a fatal or immediately life-threatening SUSAR. The day the investigator notifies the sponsor of a serious AE is considered "day 0." Additional information that may be pertinent to a previously submitted IND safety report must be submitted to the FDA as a "Follow Up IND Safety Report" as soon as the information is available.

2.5.2 Annual Reporting

Sponsors are required to submit annual reports on the progress of their investigations no more than 60 days after the anniversary of IND activation.[18] The IND annual report should include:

- Brief summaries of each active study and each study that was completed during the previous year, including: the study title, status, patient population, total number of subjects planned, enrolled, and withdrawn, tabulated by age, gender, race; a description of any significant protocol modifications made during the past year; and a description of any study results.
- Narrative or tabular summaries of the most frequent and serious AEs experienced in clinical and nonclinical studies conducted under the IND, by body system.

[16] https://www.fda.gov/Drugs/DevelopmentApprovalProcess/HowDrugsareDevelopedandApproved/ApprovalApplications/InvestigationalNewDrugINDApplication/ucm343349.htm

[17] https://www.fda.gov/downloads/Drugs/GuidanceComplianceRegulatoryInformation/Guidances/UCM227351.pdf

[18] https://www.fda.gov/Drugs/DevelopmentApprovalProcess/HowDrugsareDevelopedandApproved/ApprovalApplications/InvestigationalNewDrugINDApplication/ucm362663.htm

- A summary of any significant manufacturing or microbiological changes made during the past year.
- A brief description of any other information obtained during the past year, pertinent to the drug's mechanism of action, dose-response, bioavailability, efficacy, or safety.
- Any updates to the general investigational plan.
- Any updated versions of the IB.
- A summary of any significant foreign marketing developments during the past year.
- A log of any outstanding business with the FDA.

Sponsors may satisfy the annual safety reporting requirement by submitting a Development Safety Update Report (DSUR).[19] The DSUR sets a common standard for periodic reporting among the ICH regions and replaces the IND annual report with a comprehensive, harmonized summary of pertinent safety information, ongoing individual investigations, manufacturing changes, and overall development status and plans, related to the drug under investigation. When there is more than one sponsor of a drug development program, all sponsors should work together to prepare a single DSUR for the drug.

2.6 FDA MEETINGS

Sponsors may ask for guidance from the FDA at any point in the drug development process. The FDA has established procedures to ensure that meetings with sponsors are scheduled within a reasonable time frame, conducted efficiently, and documented appropriately.[20]

There are three types of FDA meetings:

- *Type A* meetings to help otherwise stalled product development proceed (e.g., for dispute resolution, to discuss a clinical hold), and are usually scheduled within 30 days of the sponsor request.
- *Type B* meetings which include Pre-IND meetings, End-of-Phase 1 meetings, and End-of-Phase 2 meetings, and are usually scheduled to occur within 60 days of the sponsor request.
- *Type C* meetings are any meeting other than Type A or B, and are usually scheduled to occur within 75 days of the sponsor request.

All meeting requests must be submitted formally by the sponsor, and should include:

1. The IND number
2. Product name
3. Chemical name and structure
4. Proposed indication
5. Type of meeting
6. Purpose of the meeting (list of specific objectives and brief background)
7. Proposed agenda
8. List of specific questions
9. List of participants from the sponsor's organization (including titles and affiliations)
10. List of FDA staff asked to participate
11. Proposed dates/times for the meeting (morning or afternoon)
12. The format of the meeting (face to face, teleconference or videoconference).

Once the meeting is granted a complete meeting package should be submitted to the FDA in accordance with the following time frames: 2 weeks before a Type A meeting, 4 weeks before a Type B meeting, and 4 weeks before a Type C meeting. Complete meeting packages should include the information outlined in the meeting request as well as any

[19] https://www.fda.gov/downloads/Drugs/GuidanceComplianceRegulatoryInformation/Guidances/ucm073109.pdf

[20] https://www.fda.gov/downloads/Drugs/.../Guidances/ucm153222.pdf

additional information to support discussion of the questions provided by the sponsor to the FDA. The FDA typically allows an hour for the meeting and provides written feedback to the sponsor prior to the meeting date. Questions and presentations during the meeting should be concise. The FDA will issue meeting minutes within 30 days, to serve as the official record of the meeting.

2.7 IND APPLICATIONS FOR COMBINATION THERAPIES

Combination therapies are important in many disease settings, including cancer. Because codevelopment generally provides less information about the safety, efficacy, and dose-response of the individual investigational drugs used in combination than would be provided if the individual drugs were developed alone, it may present greater risks to study subjects. Given this concern, the FDA recommends that codevelopment be reserved for situations that meet all the following criteria:

• The combination is intended to treat a serious disease or condition.
• There is a strong biological rationale for use of the combination.
• A full nonclinical characterization of the activity of the combination and the individual new investigational drugs, or a short-term clinical study of an established biomarker, suggests that the combination may provide a significant therapeutic advantage over available therapy and is superior to the individual agents alone.
• A nonclinical model demonstrates that the combination has substantial activity and provides greater activity, a more durable response (e.g., delayed resistance), or a

better toxicity profile, than the individual agents alone.
• There is a compelling reason why the investigational drugs cannot be developed independently (e.g., monotherapy for the disease leads to resistance, one or both agents would be expected to have very limited activity when used alone).

The FDA recommends that sponsors consult with FDA on the appropriateness of codevelopment before initiating clinical studies of a combination.

2.8 APPLICATIONS FOR COMPANION DIAGNOSTIC DEVICES

A laboratory developed test (LDT) is a test that is designed, manufactured and used within a single laboratory. Per 21 CFR 809.3, in vitro diagnostic (IVD) products are defined as "reagents, instruments, and systems intended for use in diagnosis of disease or other conditions" that are designed or manufactured completely, or partly, outside of the laboratory where they are used. IVD assays are defined as medical devices in section 210(h) of the FD&C Act and like other medical devices, IVD assays are subject to premarket and postmarket regulations. IVD assays are also subject to the Clinical Laboratory Improvement Amendments of 1988 (CLIA).[21] An FDA-approved investigational device exemption (IDE) permits a device to be shipped lawfully for clinical investigations.

Clinical evaluation of devices that have not been cleared for marketing requires:

• An investigational plan approved by an IRB. If the study involves a "significant risk

[21] https://www.fda.gov/downloads/MedicalDevices/DeviceRegulationandGuidance/GuidanceDocuments/UCM510824.pdf

device" an IDE must also be approved by the FDA.

- Informed consent from subjects.
- Labeling indicating that the device is for "investigational use only."
- Study reporting and monitoring.

A companion diagnostic device (often an IVD assay) provides information that is essential for safe and effective use of a specific drug. When results from an IVD assay are essential for patient treatment, inadequate performance of the test could have serious consequences; erroneous results could lead to withholding appropriate therapy or unnecessary exposure to toxic drugs.

On July 15, 2016, the FDA released a draft guidance intended to assist sponsors in identifying the need for companion diagnostic devices at an earlier stage of drug development to facilitate codevelopment of the drug and device where FDA review can be carried out collaboratively among the relevant FDA Centers (the Center for Devices and Radiological Health [CDRH] and the Center for Drug Evaluation and Research [CDER] or Center for Biologics Evaluation and Research [CBER]). During its review the FDA must determine whether the companion diagnostic

device has been properly validated to meet the applicable standard for safety and effectiveness for use as indicated in the drug product's labeling.

The FDA uses a risk-based approach to determine the regulatory pathway for companion diagnostic devices, i.e., the regulatory pathway will depend on the level of risk to patients based on the intended use of the device. A diagnostic device used to make critical treatment decisions is generally considered a "significant risk device."

A drug and companion diagnostic device can be used in the same clinical investigation if the studies meet the requirements of IDE (21 CFR 812) and IND regulations (21 CFR 312). Depending on the investigational plan, a sponsor may submit an IND alone, or an IND and an IDE, to support the clinical studies. For IND applications containing information about an investigational device, CDER or CBER will engage appropriate expertise from CDRH during the review process. The FDA recommends that the sponsor of the drug and the sponsor of the companion diagnostic device work together to solicit early FDA feedback regarding validation of the device via the CDRH "pre-submission" process.[22]

[22] https://www.fda.gov/downloads/MedicalDevices/DeviceRegulationandGuidance/GuidanceDocuments/UCM311176.pdf

The Evolution of Phase I Trials, Past, Present, and Future: A Biostatistical Perspective

Elizabeth Garrett-Mayer and Nathaniel O'Connell

Medical University of South Carolina, Charleston, SC, United States

Phase I trial designs for anticancer therapeutics have evolved substantially over recent decades. Some of the evolution is due to marked improvements in statistical methodology, such as designs that are more efficient and accurate in identifying an optimal dose or combination of doses, but a large part of the evolution is still occurring as targeted agents and immunotherapies are developed that do not conform to the assumptions of traditional dose finding. A standard Phase I dose-finding trial of a single cytotoxic agent performed a decade ago may have included no more than 21 patients and yet it allowed reasonable confidence at the end of the trial that a safe dose was identified to take forward to the next phase of drug development. In recent years, studies which began as relatively simple dose-finding trials have grown to samples sizes of more than 500 patients based on remarkable efficacy signals in the first few patients, and the new challenges we face with defining and then finding the optimal dose.

3.1 TRADITIONAL DOSE FINDING: TOXICITY-BASED DESIGNS

The primary objective in the vast majority of Phase I trials in oncology research is dose finding. That is, the identification of an optimal dose of the agent that is both safe and efficacious. For many decades, anticancer agents were primarily chemotherapeutics and dose finding relied upon two assumptions: (1) as dose increases, toxicity increases, and (2) as dose increases, efficacy increases. Under these assumptions, which are illustrated in Fig. 3.1, the objective of a dose-finding trial can be more simply stated: to identify the highest dose which can be safely administered. That is, if efficacy increases as dose increases, we want to maximize the dose, subject to a toxicity constraint. As shown in Fig. 3.1, where hypothetical dose-response and dose-toxicity curves are shown, an optimal dose would be dose level 4, where the probability of a clinical

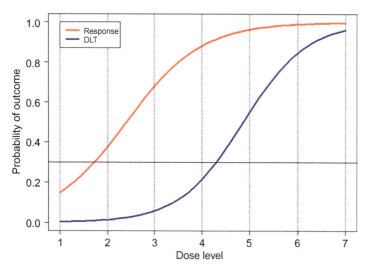

FIGURE 3.1   Hypothetical dose-response and dose-toxicity (DLT) curves.

response is greater than 0.80, and the probability of a dose-limiting toxicity (DLT) is only about 0.20. Thus, historically, dose-finding trials in oncology have not been designed to consider efficacy as part of dose finding based on the premise that the more of the agent the patient can tolerate, the more likely the patient is to experience a clinical response. The goal is then to find the maximum-tolerated dose (MTD).

The primary endpoint for toxicity-based dose-finding trials has most often been a "DLT." The definition of what constitutes a DLT varies across trials, but it will tend to include several types of Grade 3 or 4 adverse events (AEs) as defined by the NCI defined CTCAE (Common Toxicity Criteria for Adverse Events [1]), and possibly Grade 2 AEs, depending on the duration and intensity of the treatment, and the reversibility of the toxicity. The list of AEs to be included in the definition may be quite broad, or it may be narrow, depending on the context of the trial (including whether or not it is given in combination with another agent, and whether it is has been studied in other patient populations).

3.1.1 Common Trial Designs for Toxicity-Based Dose Finding of Single Agents

There is no contest for the most utilized dose-finding design in anticancer therapeutics: it is undoubtedly the "3 + 3" design, which falls under the broader class of "A + B" designs [2]. The design is algorithmic and can be simply implemented: no statistical calculations are required in advance of the trial, or even after the trial has been completed. The rules of the design are shown in Fig. 3.2. Three or six patients are treated per dose level, and dose levels of the agent to be explored must be prespecified. This design has been criticized for its poor operating characteristics, including treating too many patients at low (inefficacious) dose levels, and doing a poor job of selecting the optimal dose [3–7]. Specific criticisms that lead to poor performance include treating too few patients, inability to revisit doses, and lack of consideration of a target DLT rate. Many users of the "3 + 3" design assume it has a target DLT rate of about

Treat three patients at dose K:

• If 0 patients experience a DLT, escalate to dose K+1

• If 2 or more patients experience DLT, de-escalate to level K−1

• If 1 patient experiences DLT, treat three more patients at dose level K

    • If 1 of 6 experiences DLT, escalate to dose level K+1

    • If 2 or more of 6 experiences DLT, de-escalate to level K−1

If de-escalation occurs to a dose at which only three patients have been treated, enroll an additional three patients at that dose.

FIGURE 3.2   The "3 + 3" design dose escalation and de-escalation rules. The maximum-tolerated dose is defined as the highest dose at which 0 or 1 patient out of 6 enrolled at the dose have a DLT.

15%−30%. However, it has been shown that it does not target any dose level and the selected dose has much to do with the spacing of the doses and the shape of the dose-toxicity curve, neither of which is considered when identifying the MTD in this approach.

In 1990, a novel approach to dose finding was introduced: the Continual Reassessment Method (CRM) [8]. It is a model-based Bayesian adaptive design that uses information from patients treated in the trial to determine the optimal dose for the next patient to be treated. Briefly, a statistical model representing the relationship between dose and toxicity is assumed, such as the dose-toxicity curve shown in Fig. 3.1. Based on the assumed relationship, the optimal dose is selected as the starting dose (e.g., if 30% is the target DLT rate, then dose level 4 would be chosen as it is closest to a 30% DLT rate). A patient is treated at dose level 4 and observed for occurrence of a DLT. The data collected (1 = DLT; 0 = No DLT) is then used to update the model. If the first patient had a DLT, then the curve would shift to the left, suggesting that a lower dose would achieve a DLT rate of 30%. But, if the patient did not experience a DLT, the curve would shift to the right, suggesting that a higher dose may lead to a DLT rate of 30%. Patients are accrued and after each patient's DLT status

is observed, the model is updated to identify the optimal dose for the next patient until a predefined stopping rule is met (e.g., maximum sample size is achieved).

The CRM had several characteristics that set it apart from the "3 + 3" design, including: (1) the trial design team could identify a target DLT rate, such a 20% or 30%, (2) it quickly "honed in on" doses with DLT rates near the MTD, (3) it allowed more rapid escalation to therapeutic dose levels, and (4) the model-based design incorporated all of the data observed in the trial to estimate the MTD. After its introduction, a number of modifications to the initial design were proposed, which included the avoidance of skipping dose levels (which was allowed in the original CRM), using cohorts of size 2 or 3 (cohorts of size 1 were deemed too small in many settings), and using several different non-Bayesian approaches [9−12].

Another notable model-based design was developed shortly after, the Escalation with Overdose Control (EWOC) design [13]. The major difference between the CRM and the EWOC designs is that the EWOC includes constraints to ensure that there is a relatively small probability that a patient will receive a dose that is significantly toxic. Unlike the CRM, the EWOC acknowledges that overdosing is a more serious error in dosing than underdosing. In 2007, one of the authors of EWOC evaluated the uptake of these new designs, to see if the "3 + 3" designs were being phased out, given the noted superiority of the model-based designs. Specifically, Rogatko et al. [14] evaluated the all 1235 Phase I cancer trials in the Science Citation Index between 1991 and 2006 and found that only 1.6% of these trials (17 CRM and 3 EWOC) utilized a novel model-based design while the remaining 98.4% utilized up-and-down type methods, like the "3 + 3."

It has been 10 years between Rogatko et al.'s investigation and this publication and yet not much has changed. The algorithmic designs (specifically the "3 + 3") remains the favored choice of design for dose finding in oncology trials. Some reasons for this include its ease of implementation, its acceptability to review panels (such as Institutional Review Board (IRBs)), and the general comfort level with the approach given its broad use.

3.1.2 Toxicity-Based Dose-Finding Designs for Combinations

Combination trials, in which two or more drugs or treatments are given simultaneously to a patient, are becoming increasingly common in cancer trials. In a 3 year span from January 1, 2011 to December 31, 2013, Riviere identified 162 Phase I drug combination therapies in the literature [15]. Administering multiple treatments allows for potential synergistic effects and increased efficacy with or without an increase in toxicity, however, such trials pose unique challenges in certain contexts. In trials where multiple doses are considered for two or more agents, the number of possible combinations to explore can be unwieldy. With two or more agents, the relative severity of combined drug dose levels is not inherently known for all possible combinations. For example, even if one can assume that toxicity increases as dose increases for each agent, one cannot discern if Agent A dose level 2 + Agent B dose level 1 is more, the same or less toxic than Agent A dose level 1 + Agent B dose level 2 before performing the trial. In other words, no assumption can be made regarding the relative increase in severity when escalating doses in each drug and decreasing the dose of the other. For conventional methodology, this requires preselection of "true" combined drug dose ordering in terms of severity. Ad hoc selection of a subset of dose combinations may occur and algorithmic designs may be selected for determining dose combination levels to be too toxic, or acceptable. Alternatively, several model-based approaches have also been developed to efficiently explore two or more agents with multiple dose levels [16,17]. If toxicity information is available for treatments individually, a toxicity equivalence contour can be estimated yielding three "best" acceptable doses—one consisting predominately of drug A, one consisting predominately of drug B, and one being a mix of both agents [13]. In some instances, a second drug is included as an additional parameter in a dose-finding model and dose escalation follows procedure similar to the original CRM or EWOC [18–20]. The partial order CRM, established by Wages et al., takes into account the uncertainty regarding "true" dose ordering; it first estimates the probability for each of several possible monotonically increasing drug combination orders, and then assuming the estimated order with the highest probability, reduces to updating a dose-toxicity curve using conventional CRM methodology [14]. These designs exemplify only a few of many in the literature [21–23].

3.1.3 Other Toxicity-Based Dose-Finding Designs

There have been many other improvements to the "3 + 3" designs proposed in recent years and this section is not intended to be comprehensive. Thus just a few additional designs are noted here. The modified toxicity probability interval design (mTPI) [24] lends itself to simple implementation, where a desired DLT rate is established at the onset, and a spreadsheet is generated that trial investigators reference during the trial to determine if, based on the number of DLTs at a certain dose and the number of patients treated, the dose should be escalated, de-escalated, or maintained for the next cohort. This might be considered a hybrid, as there is some statistical modeling, but the mTPI does not utilize all of the observed information at all doses to make its decisions on the best dose for the next cohort. A comparison of the mTPI, the CRM and the Bayesian Optimal Interval Design (BOIN) demonstrate relative performance [25,26].

A major challenge of treatments with delayed toxicities is that common toxicity-based dose-finding designs require that DLTs related to the dose-finding design be observed within a relatively short timeframe from the initiation of treatment. This DLT observation period is usually specified to be one cycle (i.e., 21−28 days). For designs that restrict the observation period to one cycle but include treatments whose toxicities occur outside this window, the MTD will tend to be biased toward doses that are too high. Alternatively, designs which extend the DLT observation period to be longer may more accurately identify the MTD, but these designs may be slow to accrue because all patients in a cohort must be treated and observed for the full DLT observation window before the next cohort can be enrolled. This is particularly problematic in radiation and chemo-radiation trials where late effects of radiation may not be observed for several months. This problem motivated Cheung and Chappell to develop the time to event CRM (TiTE-CRM) design [27], which allows for delayed toxicities, and downweights observations for patients who have

been followed a relatively short amount of time. Like the CRM, it uses all of the available information to choose a dose for the next cohort of patients. The rapid enrollment design (RED) is similar, but chooses different weights for partial follow-up time information [28].

3.1.4 (Re)defining Toxicity Endpoints

Conventional dose-finding methodology simplifies the CTCAE defined AEs into a binary outcome. AEs of non-DLT grades are ignored such that they are treated equally to no toxicity at all, and potentially harmful combinations of AEs occurring together are ignored when none individually constitute a DLT. With the shifting paradigm of cancer therapeutics to immunotherapies and targeted agents, comes more diverse toxicity profiles, consisting of fewer hematological toxicities and more system specific toxicities [29,30]. Further, administration frequency also differs from cytotoxic agents; whereas chemotherapy maybe given every few weeks with AEs experienced intermittently, targeted agents and immunotherapies are often administered daily, leading to chronic AEs experienced continuously for months and potentially years. This highlights the idea that the relative severity of AEs are dependent on treatment. While a Grade 2 AE may be seen as acceptable when endured a couple days every few weeks, that same Grade 2 may be unacceptable when experienced every day for months on end.

Several model-based designs extending beyond the binary endpoint, taking into account multiple toxicity grades, have been proposed. Van Meter et al. extend the CRM to accommodate the range of ordinal grades for AEs (Grades 1−4) through a proportional odds model, improving MTD estimation in many scenarios [31]. Alternatively, methodology has been proposed around toxicity scores, a comprehensive toxicity endpoint based on entire patient toxicity profiles. The central idea is that each grade of each AE contributes some degree of burden weight to a patient, and all observed AEs combined yield an overall toxicity burden based on relative burden weights, which manifests as a toxicity score on continuous scale. Several model-based dose-finding methods utilizing toxicity scores exist in the literature, and generally yield increased performance in identifying the MTD more accurately and with fewer patients [32—36]. Rather than targeting a certain percentage of patients expected to experience a DLT, instead these methods target a maximum toxicity score deemed acceptable. For example, Bekele and Thall utilize toxicity scores in a soft tissue sarcoma trial to quantify patient burden for six unique AEs that may be endured [32]. A Grade 2 liver toxicity corresponded to a toxicity burden weight of 2.0, and a Grade 3 nausea/vomiting corresponded to a toxicity burden weight of 1.5; The "target" score was determined to be 3.04. If only a Grade 2 liver toxicity or Grade 3 nausea/vomiting was observed, neither would be too toxic since their burden scores are each less than 3.04. However, if observed together, their combined burden is the sum of 2 and 1.5 yielding a toxicity burden score of 3.5, which is greater than the target score of 3.04, deeming the dose resulting in this combination of toxicities too toxic.

3.2 EFFICACY AND TOXICITY-BASED DOSE-FINDING DESIGNS

After the introduction of the CRM, designs were developed to identify doses based on both efficacy and toxicity. As above, toxicity is generally defined in the context of DLTs. Efficacy has been incorporated as a categorical variable, usually a clinical outcome (e.g., clinical response), but could be based on a correlative outcome measure (e.g., PK parameter, immunologic response). The "Efftox"

approach uses efficacy-toxicity trade-offs to find optimal doses such that the relative benefit is constant [37]. Wages et al. propose an approach to identify dose(s) defined by low toxicity and high immune response for an immunotherapy dose-finding trial in melanoma patients where immune response is binary [38]. Chiuzan et al. develop a trial design for defining a set of promising doses which yield high immune response with an acceptable toxicity threshold, recognizing that an optimal immune response threshold may not be known and with the intent of further dose-ranging studies [39]. Riviere et al. propose a Bayesian design for combination of a cytotoxic agent with a molecularly targeted agent, modeling toxicity via logistic regression, while accounting for a possible "plateau" in efficacy for a targeted agent by modeling efficacy as a time to event outcome via survival analysis. Accounting for both toxicity and efficacy endpoints will remain a point of emphasis in a new era of cancer drug development [40]. Lee et al. extend the joint toxicity-efficacy outcome over multiple cycles of treatment for additional improvements [41]. Other designs have been proposed that consider both clinical efficacy and toxicity using model-based approaches [42—44].

3.3 EXPANSION COHORTS AND PHASE I/II TRIALS

It has been common for many decades to incorporate an *expansion cohort* upon identification of the MTD. In some designs (such as CRM designs), the expansion cohort occurs naturally, as the dose showing the most promise ends up with more patients than other doses. However, in "3 + 3" and similar designs for which no more than six patients will be treated at the MTD, at least one expansion cohort may be incorporated into the design. Historically, these expansion cohort have added 6—12 additional patients to further characterize toxicity and ensure that the MTD is reasonably safe to move into Phase II designs, or to combine with other agents. More rigorous evaluation of expansions can be performed to re-evaluate the MTD at the end of the expansion phase [45].

Additionally, the concept of combining Phase I and Phase II goals in a single protocol is not new: it has been a standard and accepted practice for many years. Trials can be designed with both Phase I and II in one protocol so that upon identification of the MTD, a Phase II portion of trial may begin without a pause in accrual that would occur if Phase I and Phase II were in two separate protocols (necessitating two rounds of approvals from IRBs and scientific review committees). In most trials, there are one or two Phase II cohorts in the study and the Phase II trial design is based on a hypothesis test, and appropriately powered to detect a clinically meaningful improvement relative to a control treatment.

3.4 RECENT TRENDS IN PHASE I TRIAL DESIGNS

3.4.1 Breakthrough Therapy Designation and Its Impact on Trial Designs

A new trend has emerged in recent years, at least in part due to the introduction of the United States FDA's "Breakthrough Therapy Designation" for experimental treatments, which was established as part of the FDA's Safety and Innovation Act (FDASIA), signed in July 2012. A breakthrough therapy is defined as "one which is intended alone or in combination to treat a serious or life-threatening disease or condition, and for which preliminary clinical evidence indicates the drug may demonstrate substantial improvement over existing therapies on one or more clinically significant endpoints" [46,47]. If an agent is designated to

be a breakthrough therapy by the FDA, the FDA will expedite the development and review of the agent. This effectively means that the FDA will have frequent interactions with the sponsor and ensure that the agent is expeditiously developed while maintaining acceptable standards for patient safety and scientific rigor, as overseen by the FDA.

Since FDASIA was signed, there are two remarkable breakthrough therapy examples in oncology drug development: nivolumab and pembrolizumab, both of which are novel immunotherapies that work by blocking a protein called programmed cell death 1 (PD-1) and freeing the immune system around the cancer by helping T-cells to attack cancer. In the case of pembrolizumab, breakthrough designation was achieved (in addition to priority review and orphan product designation) and, through successive protocol amendments, a relatively modest Phase I study (KEYNOTE-001), with a planned sample size of 32 patients in a variety of solid tumors in version 1, dated 2010 ballooned to a total sample size of 1235, with 11 dose expansion cohorts in advanced melanoma ($n = 655$) and nine in advanced non-small cell lung cancer ($n = 345$) including randomized assignments to dose levels by the end of the Phase I trial [48,49]. The results from the Phase I trial led to approval in September 2014 for patients with advanced or unresectable melanoma not responding to other treatments. Pembrolizumab as a single agent has been approved for metastatic melanoma, non-small cell lung cancer, head and neck squamous cell carcinoma, refractory classical Hodgkin lymphoma, urothelial carcinoma, and microsatellite instability-high or mismatch repair deficient solid tumors, and is currently being evaluated as a single agent and in combination with other agents in other malignancies.

Nivolumab had a similar experience, yet a smaller sample size at the end of the trial. In the first version of the protocol in July 2008, three dose levels were to be explored (1, 3, and 10 mg/kg) with a "3 + 3" dose-escalation design with 12 patients, followed by four dose expansion cohorts (defined by cancer subtypes) with up to 16 patients per cohort. This would yield a total maximum sample size of 76. The early clinical activity allowed the sponsor to receive breakthrough designation for nivolumab and expedited development. By the fifth version of the protocol (July 2012), several new dose levels had been added (0.1 and 0.3 mg/kg) and up to 14 expansion cohorts (defined by disease type and dose level) were included, with enrollment to seven cohorts already completed at that point. By the time the trial ended, 296 patients had been enrolled in five cancer subtypes [50]. Based on these results and additional randomized trials, nivolumab has been approved for metastatic melanoma, nonsmall cell lung cancer, advanced renal cell carcinoma, classical Hodgkin lymphoma, squamous cell carcinoma of the head and neck, urothelial carcinoma, microsatellite instability-high or mismatch repair deficient metastatic colorectal cancer, and hepatocellular carcinoma. Like pembrolizumab, it is being tested as a single agent and in combination with other agents in numerous other cancers.

The approval of these immunotherapies demonstrates success in two areas: improving clinical outcomes in patients who had few treatment options, and in expediting the development and approval process for treatments with strong early evidence of efficacy. The initial trials of nivolumab and pembrolizumab were unusual: the trials were designed as modest dose-finding designs, with reasonably small expansion cohorts in a small number of disease-defined subgroups at the MTD only to be dramatically expanded due to breakthrough designation.

However, in the wake of these successes and approvals, the proposed designs of Phase I trials for immunotherapeutics changed dramatically. Other companies initiated trials of their own checkpoint inhibitors, and

initiated trials of combinations of novel agents with nivolumab, pembrolizumab or another PD-1 blockade agent. These trials were not designed as typical dose-escalation studies, followed by 50 or so patients in expansion cohorts. Instead, many investigators used the final trial designs for pembrolizumab and nivolumab as blueprints for designing their Phase I trials (see supplemental information in references where protocols are provided demonstrating initial and amended protocols for nivolumab [51] and pembrolizumab [52]). Thus cancer centers and institutional review boards around the country saw a dramatic shift in the proposed design of Phase I trials in oncology.

The trial designs were met, in many places, with resistance and questions as details were not included and the sample sizes proposed (sometimes as large as 500 or more patients) were not consistent with the primary objective of the trials and the design for the primary objective, usually a simple "3 + 3" MTD design approach (which included only a small fraction of the total proposed sample size). The large sample sizes were included to allow expansion within disease-specific subgroups, and then to further expand if promising efficacy was seen. Statisticians tasked with evaluating these trials found that many of these newer trials lacked scientific rigor in their designs and they did not adequately consider safety monitoring of patients. Harkening back to ethical expectations, Emanuel et al. list seven requirements that make clinical research ethical. The second of these is scientific validity ("the research must be methodologically rigorous"), and the seventh is respect for enrolled subjects ("subjects should have their privacy protected, the opportunity to withdraw, and their well-being monitored") [53]. Many of these trials did not meet these two requirements, with problems including the lack of statistical justification of sample sizes and thresholds for expansion, no formal process for safety monitoring across and within cohorts, including no independent oversight (or independent members of data monitoring committees), and in some of the more egregious cases, no clearly defined endpoints for making expansion decisions. Thus many of these protocols were more like general guidelines for developing a drug, with many "adaptive" decisions made without formal objective rules for adapting included in protocols. No doubt, the hope was that some of the proposed regimens in these trials would be able to use the data from these large Phase I trials to achieve FDA approval and keeping trial designs flexible could facilitate rapid approval. However, the degree of flexibility was so great in some instances that scientific rigor was sacrificed.

As a result of the shift from traditional Phase I trials with 15–40 patients to trials that were orders of magnitude larger, the FDA addressed the expectations for drug development in the new age of promising novel therapeutics [54,55]. The term "Seamless Oncology Drug Development" implies a drug development model in which there is one evolving clinical trial that begins with Phase I, and (if the drug is successful) ends with regulatory approval. Given that pembrolizumab and nivolumab have achieved seamless development, several authors have addressed considerations for going down this road (with or without breakthrough designation) which requires clear attention to scientific validity of trial design to ensure that the inferences are unbiased and reasonably precise, and that patients are protected. Prowell et al. specifically list the following criteria to be considered when designing (or reviewing) large Phase I trials with the long term intent of seamless drug development [55]:

- Is there a compelling rationale for including multiple expansion cohorts?
- Is the sample-size range consistent with the stated objectives and endpoints?
- Is there an appropriate statistical analysis plan for all stated endpoints?

- Are the eligibility criteria appropriately tailored to the expansion cohorts?
- Is there a defined end to the trial, in terms of both efficacy and futility?
- Is there a system in place to communicate with all investigators in a timely fashion?
- Does the informed consent reflect the current knowledge of safety and efficacy of the investigational drug and other agents in the same class?
- If the trial may be used for regulatory approval, is there an independent oversight committee?
- If the trial may be used for regulatory approval, has there been communication with regulatory agencies?

Prowell et al. consider "first in human" trials, but many criteria in this list would also be applicable to combination trials, and other single agent Phase I trials in different contexts. If these criteria are considered, large Phase I trials with multiple expansion arms can be rigorously and ethically executed.

3.4.2 Statistical Challenges in Dose Finding Based in the Era of Immunotherapies and Targeted Agents

The first studies of nivolumab and pembrolizumab highlight a major departure in dose-finding trial designs in the new era of anticancer immunotherapies. Both studies began as relatively small dose-finding studies which employed "3 + 3" designs to identify an MTD. However, as is evidenced by the resulting study groups investigators considered quite a range of doses realizing that an MTD may not be the optimal dose, and the studies became dose-ranging studies (see especially [48], Fig. 3.1). This appears to be true for two reasons: (1) the dose-toxicity curve appears relatively flat, and (2) the dose-efficacy curve appears relatively flat. Note that the initial doses to be explored in the Phase I trial of nivolumab were 1, 3, and 10 mg/kg, all of which were deemed tolerable based on the "3 + 3" design. After seeing striking clinical responses with long duration of response in some patients, the trial was amended to add dose of 0.1 and 0.3 mg/kg, suggesting that investigators were considering doses that were a tiny fraction of the MTD, due to the observed flat dose response across the previously considered doses (1, 3, and 10 mg/kg) (see protocol amendments in supplemental materials [52]), leading to dose-ranging designs.

Immunotherapies have demonstrated that the standard assumption that dose finding for anticancer agents has been founded upon is not always valid: for immunotherapeutic and targeted agents, we cannot and should not assume that "more is better" in terms of efficacy, or even that "more is worse" in terms of toxicity. Nivolumab and pembrolizumab demonstrate relatively flat dose-toxicity curves for the range of doses studied which support this idea. Fig. 3.3 demonstrates three scenarios for anticancer agents that violate the assumption that the dose-response curve is monotonically increasing with dose. For each of these scenarios, a toxicity-based dose-finding design would identify an incorrect dose. In all three scenarios and assuming a target DLT rate of 20%, the MTD would be dose level 7. In Panel A, dose level 7 is unnecessarily high: all doses have the same efficacy, and by selecting dose level 7 (instead of dose level 1), the DLT rate is higher than it needs to be for the same level of efficacy at any of the lower doses. Panel B shows an agent that has decreasing efficacy beyond dose level 4. Thus choosing the MTD will result in a much less efficacious dose being taken forward. Lastly, Panel C demonstrates a plateau in efficacy where efficacy is approximately constant for dose levels 4 through 7. In Panels B and C, the optimal dose would be dose level 4 and yet toxicity-based dose finding would result in having a high probability of selecting dose level 7.

Some of the previously mentioned designs which account for both toxicity and efficacy can address the types of dose-toxicity and dose-efficacy relationships seen in Fig. 3.3, but those which target a specific DLT rate may fail to identify an appropriate dose. Several designs proposed in recent years specifically address immunotherapy trials, with the efficacy endpoint based on either a continuous or binary measure of immune response [38,39].

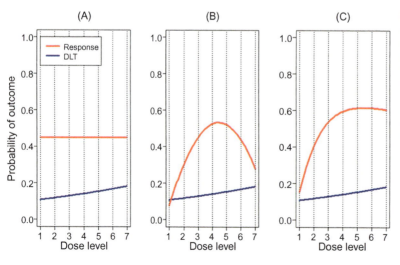

FIGURE 3.3 Theoretical dose-response and dose-toxicity curves for noncytotoxic agents. All three panels show agents with a relatively flat dose-toxicity curve, which ranges from about 10% at dose level 1 to 18% at dose level 7. (A) Flat dose-response curve; (B) Parabolic dose-response curve; (C) Plateau dose-response curve.

3.5 WHERE DO WE GO FROM HERE: RECOMMENDATIONS FOR OPTIMAL EARLY PHASE DOSE-FINDING TRIALS

Moving forward, Phase I trials (large and small) must be scientifically valid and protect patients. This is nothing new, but with the proposal of numerous large Phase I trials that have fallen short of these two criteria, it is important to be reminded that clinical trial designs must be developed to answer important scientific questions, and minimize harm. Additionally, the considerations set forth in Prowell et al. should be followed (see Section 3.4.1). Setting these more traditional statistical issues aside, there are numerous additional areas for exploration and consideration in novel dose-finding designs in this new era of anticancer drug development.

3.5.1 Windows of Time for Evaluation of Toxicities

Traditional dose-finding designs in oncology have focused on toxicities that occur in the first cycle, with escalation and de-escalation decisions based on these first cycle toxicities, and MTDs based on the highest-tolerated dose from cycle 1. Several authors have proposed utilizing information from later cycles to (re)define the MTD even if the design only incorporates cycle 1 toxicities for escalation and de-escalation decisions [45,56,57]. However, the toxicity profiles for novel agents are not like those for chemotherapeutics, and many patients stay on novel therapies in early phase trials for many months. To optimize dose, given that safety is still a concern, toxicity outcomes that occur in later cycles should be incorporated into final dose recommendations, and, if possible, into designs. Exemplifying this, across 14 individual bortezomib dose-finding trials with a cumulative total of 481

patients, the first DLT was observed after the first cycle of treatment in 46% of patients. By only considering DLTs occurring in the first cycle of treatment in the bortezomib trials, the approved dose was estimated to lead to a >50% cumulative incidence of DLT [56]. The TiTE-CRM and the RED allow incorporation of late toxicities [27,28]. These designs can be generally applied when toxicity-based dose finding is of interest, regardless of the expected time of onset of toxicities (i.e., whether they are delayed or not).

3.5.2 Intrapatient Dose Escalation

In traditional Phase I trial oncology trials, intrapatient dose escalation is not allowed, and is often discouraged in the design phase. (The accelerated titration design encouraged intrapatient dose escalation, but few others of the same era did so [58]). Some of the reason for this is the challenges intrapatient dose escalation creates in interpreting the resulting data (e.g., a late occurring toxicity in a patient who dose-escalated from their initial dose: to which dose level do you assign them when evaluating the MTD?). Another reason is that it is often assumed that patients will have decreasing tolerance to anticancer agents due to cumulative effects of treatment resulting in later cycle DLTs. For example, a patient who has been treated at dose level 2 for four cycles might be more likely to have a DLT at dose level 3 in her fifth cycle than patients treated at dose level 3 in the first cycle. While this may have been true in the era of chemotherapeutics, there is anecdotal evidence that for some patients treated with immunotherapies, there is tolerance to treatment that increases over time, suggesting intrapatient dose escalation may be safe and potentially more efficacious. Thus, as we move into this new era, consideration of intrapatient dose escalation may be a more viable and ethical option than in the past.

3.5.3 Delayed Clinical Responses, "Pseudo-Progression," and Duration of Response

Immunotherapies have demonstrated a delayed effect by common metrics of clinical outcome. The RECIST criteria measures antitumor effects by decreases in the largest dimension of target lesions based on standard imaging (such as CT-scans) [59]. Not only have effects from immunotherapies been delayed, but "pseudo-progression" may occur. Pseudo-progressions look like increases in the volume of tumor and thus tumor growth, but upon further inspection, the increase in size is due to something else altogether, such as an infiltration of T-cells at the tumor site. In traditional cancer trials, an increase in tumor size would lead to removing a patient from study. However, continuing treatment at this stage is likely the best option for the patients if the increase in size is due to pseudo-progression. Newer trials need to accommodate rules for continuing treatment and careful measurement of tumor viability in the case of pseudo-progression. This suggests that alternate measurement approaches, such as using irRECIST which has shown to be a more robust measurement approach than RECIST in cancer immunotherapy trials [60,61].

Lastly, in the trials of nivolumab and pembrolizumab, one of the striking results was the duration of responses (DOR) among responders. In the initial trials in patients who were relapsed or refractory, expected DORs were short, but observed DORs were greater than 6 months in many cases, and were a key criterion that the FDA considered in their approvals. Thus DOR has emerged as a popular endpoint. Trials planning to use DOR as a primary endpoint need to recognize that only a fraction of the patients enrolled in a trial will achieve a tumor response, and so trials need to include sufficient patients to adequately characterize DOR among responders.

3.5.4 Measures of Efficacy for Dose Finding: Clinical Versus Correlative Outcomes

Given that we can no longer proceed according to the paradigm demonstrated in Fig. 3.1 (as dose increases so do both toxicity and efficacy), dose-finding approaches need to identify an optimally efficacious dose while constraining the dose level due to toxicity. To do so requires an efficacy outcome, but in the Phase I setting, it may not be feasible to utilize an outcome that takes a long time to evaluate (like overall survival). Adaptive designs which incorporate both efficacy and toxicity outcome information should have a reasonable timeframe for measurement of both outcomes. If the goal is to adaptively assign patients to doses based on accumulating efficacy and toxicity information, then it may only be feasible to utilize correlative outcomes (e.g., change in an immunologic marker). However, the relationship between the correlative outcome and clinical outcome may not be robust.

As has been shown by several authors, regardless of the design used for determining which doses are visited and how many are allocated to each dose, utilizing a comprehensive analysis (incorporating information from multiple cycles beyond cycle 1, and/or by including additional patient data from expansion cohorts) is more accurate in selecting the correct dose [45,56,57]. This has been shown in the case of toxicity-based dose finding. It is also possible to take this approach for dose finding based on both toxicity and efficacy outcomes. As is discussed in the Section 3.2, combining the goals of Phase I and Phase II trials will allow better determination of the optimal dose based on clinical efficacy and toxicity by accruing enough patients at more than one dose level to accurately evaluate relative benefits of different doses.

3.5.5 Sample Size and Cohort Selection

As noted above, Phase I trials just a decade ago were designed with sample sizes in the range of 20–40 patients, but recent years have seen Phase I trials with hundreds of patients due to both an increase in the number of expansion cohorts per trial, and the sample size per expansion cohort. Dahlberg et al. demonstrate the trends in both the increase in the number of Phase I trials and the size of Phase I trials at the Dana Farber Cancer Institute between 1998 and 2012 [62]. The size of expansion cohorts is often selected without any statistical design considerations. For small cohorts, utilized to further characterize safety and numbering an additional 10 or so patients, this seems reasonable. However, when the number of patients in an expansion cohort exceeds 20, there should be both a clearly stated objective of what is to be learned from the expansion cohort, and a rationale for the sample size (such as a power calculation). Many trials plan to enroll a certain number in a cohort, and then, depending on the results after a fixed number of patients have been treated, further expand. The criteria for further expansion should be well justified (including the endpoint on which it is based) using statistical reasoning. Additionally, the cohorts to be expanded should be prespecified based on scientific rationale from preclinical data, or results from trials of agents with similar mechanisms of action. Allowing "to be determined" cohorts for expansion without defining the eligibility criteria leads to a weak protocol that should not be acceptable to IRBs and scientific review committees. Amendments can be made at a later date should data arise necessitating the need for new expansion cohorts.

3.5.6 Using Expansion Cohorts to Recalibrate Dose

The traditional designs with an escalation phase followed by an expansion phase presume that the dose from the escalation phase is correct and usually consider no opportunity within the expansion phase to redefine the MTD. Iasonos and O'Quigley demonstrate that one can relatively simply address this problem by fitting a model at the conclusion of the expansion phase [45]. Even so, moving forward, it should be recognized that doses found by small numbers of patients are inherently inaccurate and utilize all of the information available to recommend a "best dose."

3.5.7 Abandon the Terms "Phase I, II, and III"

Ratain posited that the current Phase I paradigm in oncology is illogical for targeted therapies [63]. In his view, a Phase I trial should not yield a single dose and schedule to take forward to the next phase of development. It should instead provide a set of doses and/or schedules to further consider in the next phase of dose finding which should be a randomized dose-ranging Phase II trial. One of the struggles the oncology research community has in moving into a new paradigm, such as that proposed by Ratain, is the terminology of our trials. Historically, Phase I, II, and III each have their own distinct role in the development of anticancer agents. The problem with this is that the three-phase paradigm is not flexible enough to address the modern era of novel therapeutics. As was pointed out by Piantadosi "some widely used terminology regarding trials is unhelpful" and it can be counteracted by alternative terminology which more accurately describes the true intent of a trial [64]. Nowadays, the term "Phase I" tells us very little about the primary goal and scope of an early phase oncology trial. Trials should be designed and developed such that the design (including the sample size) is consistent with the primary objective(s). Forms requiring investigators to label their trials as Phase I, II, or III should be revised, and review committees and IRBs should evaluate trials holistically, with an emphasis on the context of the trial in terms of the type of agent and patient population, the preliminary data, risks and benefits for patients, and given the success of the current trial, what the next phase of development would be for the agent in question.

3.6 SUMMARY

In 2015, the American Society of Clinical Oncology published a policy statement on Phase I trials in cancer research stating that "phase I trials have a much greater potential as a treatment option for many patients with cancer than they did in 1997" [65]. This is due in part to evolution of Phase I trials from small toxicity-based studies in heterogeneous patient populations to large trials, incorporating cohorts which specifically target disease sub-groups with agents with markedly different toxicity profiles then those developed decades ago. As a result, of the move toward targeted agents and immunotherapies, our approach for dose finding should adapt to most efficiently identify optimal doses.

References

[1] Common Terminology Criteria for Adverse Events (CTCAE); 2009.
[2] Storer BE. Design and analysis of phase I clinical trials. Biometrics 1989;45(3):925–37.
[3] Chiuzan C, Garrett-Mayer E, Yeatts SD. A likelihood-based approach for computing the operating characteristics of the 3 + 3 phase I clinical trial design with extensions to other A + B designs. Clin Trials 2015;12(1):24–33.
[4] Paoletti X, Ezzalfani M, Le Tourneau C. Statistical controversies in clinical research: requiem for the 3 + 3 design for phase I trials. Ann Oncol 2015;26:1808–12.
[5] Jaki T, Clive S, Weir CJ. Principles of dose finding studies in cancer: a comparison of trial designs. Cancer Chemother Pharmacol 2013;71(5):1107–14.
[6] Iasonos A, Wilton AS, Riedel ER, Seshan VE, Spriggs DR. A comprehensive comparison of the continual reassessment method to the standard 3 + 3 dose escalation scheme in Phase I dose-finding studies. Clin Trials 2008;5(5):465–77.
[7] Garrett-Mayer E. The continual reassessment method for dose-finding studies: a tutorial. Clin Trials 2006;3(1):57–71.
[8] O'Quigley J, Pepe M, Fisher L. Continual reassessment method: a practical design for phase 1 clinical trials in cancer. Biometrics 1990;46(1):33–48.
[9] Piantadosi S, Fisher JD, Grossman S. Practical implementation of a modified continual reassessment method for dose-finding trials. Cancer Chemother Pharmacol 1998;41(6):429–36.
[10] Goodman SN, Zahurak ML, Piantadosi S. Some practical improvements in the continual reassessment method for phase I studies. Stat Med 1995;14 (11):1149–61.
[11] Faries D. Practical modifications of the continual reassessment method for phase i cancer clinical trials. J Biopharm Stat 1994;4(2):147–64.
[12] Møller S. An extension of the continual reassessment methods using a preliminary up-and-down design in a dose finding study in cancer patients, in order to investigate a greater range of doses. Stat Med 1995;14 (9–10):911–22 discussion 923.
[13] Babb J, Rogatko A, Zacks S. Cancer phase I clinical trials: efficient dose escalation with overdose control. Stat Med 1998;17(10):1103–20.
[14] Rogatko A, Schoeneck D, Jonas W, Tighiouart M, Khuri FR, Porter A. Translation of Innovative designs into phase I trials. J Clin Oncol 2007;25(31):4982–6.
[15] Riviere M-K, Le Tourneau C, Paoletti X, Dubois F, Zohar S. Designs of drug-combination phase I trials in oncology: a systematic review of the literature. Ann Oncol Off J Eur Soc Med Oncol 2015;26(4):669–74.
[16] Thall PF, Millikan RE, Mueller P, Lee SJ. Dose-finding with two agents in Phase I oncology trials. Biometrics 2003;59(3):487–96.
[17] Wages NA, Conaway MR, O'Quigley J. Dose-finding design for multi-drug combinations. Clin Trials 2011;8 (4):380–9.
[18] Tighiouart M, Piantadosi S, Rogatko A. Dose finding with drug combinations in cancer phase I clinical trials using conditional escalation with overdose control. Stat Med 2014;33(22):3815–29.
[19] Wang K, Ivanova A. Two-dimensional dose finding in discrete dose space. Biometrics 2005;61(1):217–22.
[20] Bailey S, Neuenschwander B, Laird G, Branson M. A Bayesian case study in oncology Phase I combination dose-finding using logistic regression with covariates. J Biopharm Stat 2009;19(3):469–84.
[21] Yin G, Yuan Y. A latent contingency table approach to dose finding for combinations of two agents. Biometrics 2009;65(3):866–75.

[22] Yin G, Yuan Y. Bayesian dose finding in oncology for drug combinations by copula regression. J R Stat Soc Ser C Appl Stat 2009;58(2):211–24.

[23] Ivanova A, Wang K. A non-parametric approach to the design and analysis of two-dimensional dose-finding trials. Stat Med 2004;23(12):1861–70.

[24] Ji Y, Liu P, Li Y, Nebiyou Bekele B. A modified toxicity probability interval method for dose-finding trials. Clin Trials 2010;7:653–63.

[25] Yuan Y, Hess KR, Hilsenbeck SG, Gilbert MR. Bayesian optimal interval design: a simple and well-performing design for phase I oncology trials. Clin Cancer Res 2016;22(17):4291–301.

[26] Horton BJ, Wages NA, Conaway MR. Performance of toxicity probability interval based designs in contrast to the continual reassessment method. Stat Med 2017;36(2):291–300.

[27] Cheung YK, Chappell R. Sequential designs for phase I clinical trials with late-onset toxicities. Biometrics 2000;56(4):1177–82.

[28] Ivanova A, Wang Y, Foster MC. The rapid enrollment design for phase I clinical trials. Stat Med 2016;35 (15):2516–24.

[29] Penel N, Adenis A, Clisant S, Bonneterre J. Nature and subjectivity of dose-limiting toxicities in contemporary phase 1 trials: comparison of cytotoxic versus noncytotoxic drugs. Invest New Drugs 2011;29(6):1414–19.

[30] Le Tourneau C, Diéras V, Tresca P, Cacheux W, Paoletti X. Current challenges for the early clinical development of anticancer drugs in the era of molecularly targeted agents. Target Oncol 2010;5(1):65–72.

[31] Van Meter EM, Garrett-Mayer E, Bandyopadhyay D. Proportional odds model for dose-finding clinical trial designs with ordinal toxicity grading. Stat Med 2011;30(17):2070–80.

[32] Bekele BN, Thall PF. Dose-finding based on multiple toxicities in a soft tissue sarcoma trial. J Am Stat Assoc 2004;99(465):26–35.

[33] Chen Z, Krailo MD, Azen SP, Tighiouart M. A novel toxicity scoring system treating toxicity response as a quasi-continuous variable in phase I clinical trials. Contemp Clin Trials 2010;31(5):473–82.

[34] Lee SM, Cheng B, Cheung YK. Continual reassessment method with multiple toxicity constraints. Biostatistics 2011;12(2):386–98.

[35] Yuan Z, Chappell R, Bailey H. The continual reassessment method for multiple toxicity grades: a Bayesian quasi-likelihood approach. Biometrics 2007;63 (1):173–9.

[36] Ezzalfani M, Zohar S, Qin R, Mandrekar SJ, Le Deley M-C. Dose-finding designs using a novel quasi-continuous endpoint for multiple toxicities. Stat Med 2013;32(16):2728–46.

[37] Thall PF, Cook JD. Dose-finding based on efficacy – toxicity trade-offs. Biometrics 2004;60:684–93.

[38] Wages NA, Slingluff CL, Petroni GR. Statistical controversies in clinical research: early-phase adaptive design for combination immunotherapies. Ann Oncol 2017;28:696–701.

[39] Chiuzan C, Garrett-Mayer E, Nishimura M. An adaptive dose-finding design based on both safety and immunologic responses in cancer clinical trials. J Biopharm Stat 2017.

[40] Riviere M-K, Yuan Y, Dubois F, Zohar S. A Bayesian dose finding design for clinical trials combining a cytotoxic agent with a molecularly targeted agent. J R Stat Soc Ser C Appl Stat 2015;64(1):215–29.

[41] Lee J, Thall PF, Ji Y, Müller P. Bayesian dose-finding in two treatment cycles based on the joint utility of efficacy and toxicity. J Am Stat Assoc 2015;110 (510):711–22.

[42] Zhang W, Sargent DJ, Mandrekar S. An adaptive dose-finding design incorporating both toxicity and efficacy. Stat Med 2006;25(14):2365–83.

[43] Braun TM. The bivariate continual reassessment method: extending the CRM to phase I trials of two competing outcomes. Control Clin Trials 2002;23(3):240–56.

[44] Thall PF, Russell KE. A strategy for dose-finding and safety monitoring based on efficacy and adverse outcomes in phase I/II clinical trials. Biometrics 1998;251–64.

[45] Iasonos A, O'Quigley J. Design considerations for dose-expansion cohorts in phase I trials. J Clin Oncol 2013;31(31):4014–21.

[46] One Hundred Twelfth Congress of the United States of America, S.3187 Food and Drug Administration Safety and Innovation Act; 2012. p. 94–96.

[47] Food and Drug Administration. Guidance for industry: expedited programs for serious conditions – drugs and biologics. 2014;910:1–36.

[48] Khoja L, Butler MO, Kang SP, Ebbinghaus S, Joshua AM. Pembrolizumab. J Immunother Cancer 2015;3 (1):36.

[49] Patnaik A, et al. Phase i study of pembrolizumab (MK-3475; Anti-PD-1 monoclonal antibody) in patients with advanced solid tumors. Clin Cancer Res 2015;21(19):4286–93.

[50] Topalian SL, et al. Safety, activity, and immune correlates of anti−PD-1 antibody in cancer. N Engl J Med 2012;366:2443–54.

[51] Brahmer JR, et al. Safety and activity of anti-PD-L1 antibody in patients with advanced cancer. N Engl J Med 2012;366(26):2455–65.

[52] Garon EB, et al. Pembrolizumab for the treatment of non−small-cell lung cancer. N Engl J Med 2015;372 (21):2018–28.

[53] Emanuel EJ, Wender D, Grady C. What makes clinical research ethical? JAMA J Am Med Assoc 2000;283 (20):2701–11.

[54] Theoret MR, et al. Expansion cohorts in first-in-human solid tumor oncology trials. Clin Cancer Res 2015;21 (20):4545–51.

[55] Prowell TM, Theoret MR, Pazdur R. Seamless oncology-drug development. N Engl J Med 2016;374 (21):2001–3.

[56] Lee SM, et al. Case example of dose optimization using data from bortezomib dose-finding clinical trials. J Clin Oncol 2016;34(12):1395–401.

[57] Paoletti X, Doussau A, Ezzalfani M, Rizzo E, Thiébaut R. Dose finding with longitudinal data: simpler models, richer outcomes. Stat Med 2015;34(22):2983–98.

[58] Simon R, Freidlin B, Rubinstein L, Arbuck SG, Collins J, Christian MC. Accelerated titration designs for phase I clinical trials in oncology. J Natl Cancer Inst 1997;89(15):1138–47.

[59] Eisenhauer EA, et al. New response evaluation criteria in solid tumours: revised RECIST guideline (version 1.1). Eur J Cancer 2009;45(2):228–47.

[60] Nishino M, Tirumani SH, Ramaiya NH, Hodi FS. Cancer immunotherapy and immune-related response assessment: the role of radiologists in the new arena of cancer treatment. Eur J Radiol 2015;84(7):1259–68.

[61] Hodi FS, et al. Evaluation of immune-related response criteria and RECIST v1.1 in patients with advanced melanoma treated with pembrolizumab. J Clin Oncol 2016;34(13):1510–17.

[62] Dahlberg SE, Shapiro GI, Clark JW, Johnson BE. Evaluation of statistical designs in phase i expansion cohorts: the Dana-Farber/Harvard cancer center experience. J Natl Cancer Inst 2014;106(7).

[63] Ratain MJ. Targeted therapies: redefining the primary objective of phase I oncology trials. Nat Rev Clin Oncol 2014;11(9):503–4.

[64] Piantadosi S. Clinical trials: a methodologic perspective. New York: Wiley-Interscience; 2005.

[65] Weber JS, et al. American Society of Clinical Oncology policy statement update: the critical role of phase i trials in cancer research and treatment. J Clin Oncol 2015;33(3):278–84.

Evolving Early Phase Trial Designs: A Regulatory Perspective

Marc R. Theoret, Lee Pai-Scherf, Christy Osgood, Abhilasha Nair and Patricia Keegan

U.S. Food and Drug Administration, Silver Spring, MD, United States

4.1 INTRODUCTION

With the enactment of Kefauver Harris-amendments to the Food, Drug, and Cosmetic Act in 1962, when the requirement for "substantial evidence of effectiveness" was added to the existing requirement (1938) for demonstration of the safety of a drug, the traditional clinical trial paradigm was established consisting of a sequential phases of standalone trials spanning the earliest, first-in-human (FIH) clinical trial to the late-phase trial intended to provide the clinical evidence required for marketing approval [1]. These sequential trial phases are codified and described in the Code of Federal Regulations under the Investigational New Drug Application (IND) Regulations as Phase 1, Phase 2, and Phase 3 trials [2]. The International Conference for Harmonization (ICH), an international body to standardize regulatory requirements for drug development globally, provides different nomenclature that defines phases of an investigation based on the underlying objectives (i.e., human pharmacology trials, therapeutic exploratory trials, and therapeutic confirmatory trials), but the principles are the same [3]. In the Office of Hematology and Oncology Products of the Food and Drug Administration, we have seen that FIH trials are increasingly evolving toward a seamless oncology drug development paradigm, with IND sponsors adding cohorts with unique cohort-specific patient eligibility criteria, treatment regimens, and goals (expansion cohorts) to existing protocols through amendments, rather than submission of new later-phase protocols [4,5].

The intersection of better understanding of the biological underpinnings of cancer with identification of suitable molecular targets, as well as greater understanding of the host immune response to cancer, has resulted in evidence of antitumor activity early in the drug development program. FDA has four formal programs to expedite the review and development of drugs and biologics for patients with serious or life-threatening illnesses and unmet

Novel Designs of Early Phase Trials for Cancer Therapeutics
DOI: https://doi.org/10.1016/B978-0-12-812512-0.00004-X

medical needs [6]. Accelerated approval, one of the four FDA expedited programs, provides the regulatory framework for satisfying the statutory standards for effectiveness based on surrogate or intermediate endpoints that are reasonably likely to predict clinical benefit, with the requirement to confirm or further describe benefits in subsequent trials [7,8]. In a single-arm trial, objective response rate as assessed by an independent review committee per standardized tumor-response criteria when coupled with the evaluation of duration of response is a common surrogate endpoint to support accelerated approval for oncology drugs [9]. Development of drugs with a large magnitude of antitumor activity that may be evaluated in single-arm trials—within the context of regulatory flexibility for applying the statutory standards of effectiveness and safety to promising drugs for treatment of patients with serious or life-threatening illnesses—has fostered the seamless oncology expansion cohort drug development paradigm [6,10,11].

4.2 FDA EXPEDITED PROGRAMS FOR EXPEDITING THE DEVELOPMENT AND REVIEW OF DRUGS FOR SERIOUS OR LIFE-THREATENING CONDITIONS

To expedite the development of drugs and biologics to fill an unmet medical need for a serious or life-threatening condition, FDA has developed four programs: fast track, breakthrough therapy, priority review, and accelerated approval (Table 4.1) [6]. These programs are intended to help ensure that therapies for serious conditions are approved and available to patients as soon as it can be concluded that the therapies justify their risks.

All four expedited programs represent efforts to address an unmet medical need in the treatment of a serious condition. An unmet medical need is a condition whose treatment or

diagnosis is not addressed adequately by available therapy. If there is no available therapy, there is clearly an unmet medical need. Alternatively, when available therapy exists, a new treatment could be considered to address an unmet medical need if it meets any of the following criteria:

• has an effect on a serious outcome of the condition that is not known to be influenced by available therapy,
• has an improved effect on a serious outcome of the condition compared with available therapy,
• has an effect on a serious outcome of the condition in patients who are unable to tolerate or failed to respond to available therapy,
• can be used effectively with other critical agents that cannot be combined with available therapy,
• provides efficacy comparable to those of available therapy, while avoiding serious toxicity, or
• provides efficacy and safety comparable to those of available therapy but has a documented improvement in compliance.

For the purposes of these programs, a serious condition is defined as follows [12]:

> A disease or condition associated with morbidity that has substantial impact on day-to-day functioning. Short-lived and self-limiting morbidity will usually not be sufficient, but the morbidity need not be irreversible if it is persistent or recurrent. Whether a disease or condition is serious is a matter of clinical judgment, based on its impact on such factors as survival, day-to-day functioning, or the likelihood that the disease, if left untreated, will progress from a less severe condition to a more serious one.

4.2.1 Fast Track Development Program Designation

Fast track designation is intended to facilitate development and expedite review of drugs

TABLE 4.1   Overview of FDA's Expedited Programs for Serious Conditions [6]

	Type of Data Required	Qualifying Criteria	Benefits
Fast track designation	Preliminary nonclinical, mechanistic, or clinical data	Drug or biologic that is intended to treat a serious condition and nonclinical or clinical data that demonstrate the potential to address an unmet medical need	• Opportunities for frequent interactions with FDA • Rolling review • Possible eligibility for priority review
Breakthrough therapy designation	Preliminary clinical data	Drug or biologic that is intended to treat a serious condition and preliminary clinical evidence indicates that the drug may demonstrate substantial improvement on a clinically significantly endpoint(s) over available therapies	• Opportunities for frequent interactions with FDA • Rolling review • Possible eligibility for priority review • Intensive guidance on efficient drug development program • Organizational commitment involving FDA senior managers
Priority review designation	Data contained in the final NDA submission	An application (original or efficacy supplement) for a drug that treats a serious condition and that if approved would provide a significant improvement in safety or effectiveness	• Period for review of marketing application reduced by 4 months
Accelerated approval	Justification that endpoint is reasonably likely to predict clinical benefit	Drug or biologic that treats a serious condition, generally provides a meaningful advantage over available therapies, and demonstrates an effect on a surrogate endpoint that is reasonably likely to predict clinical benefit or on a clinical endpoint that can be measured earlier than irreversible morbidity or mortality (IMM) that is reasonable likely to predict an effect on "IMM" or other clinical benefit	• Approval based on an effect on a surrogate or intermediate clinical endpoint that is reasonably likely to predict a drug's clinical benefit

to treat serious and life-threatening conditions so that an approved product can reach the market expeditiously. Section 506 of the Food and Drug Administration Modernization Act (FDAMA) of 1997 authorized the fast track provisions. The criteria for a product to qualify for the fast track program is that the product is intended to treat a serious or life-threatening condition and demonstrates the potential to address unmet medical need for the condition. The fast track designation applies to the product and the specific indication for which it is being studied.

A request for fast track designation should include information about the serious condition the drug is intended to treat and the unmet medical need, as well as a plausible basis for the assertion that the drug has potential to address such unmet medical needs. The request must include the specific indication for which it is intended to be studied. The indication includes both the condition for which the drug is intended and the anticipated or established benefit of use. Finally, the request must include a development plan, at a level of detail appropriate for the stage of development, designed to evaluate the potential of the drug to establish the benefit of use described in the indication.

If a drug is granted fast track designation, the drug development program would be eligible for some or all of the following:

- More frequent meetings with FDA to discuss the drug's development plan and ensure collection of appropriate data needed to support drug approval.
- More frequent written communication from FDA about the adequacy of drug development plans such as the design of proposed clinical trials and the use of biomarkers.
- Eligibility for accelerated approval and priority review if relevant criteria are met.
- Rolling review, which allows a pharmaceutical company to submit to FDA complete sections of a Biologic License Application (BLA) or New Drug Application (NDA) for review rather than waiting until every section of the application is completed before the entire application can be reviewed [13].

4.2.2 Breakthrough Therapy Development Program Designation

Breakthrough therapy designation is meant to expedite the development and review of drugs intended to treat a serious condition, based on preliminary clinical evidence that the drug may demonstrate substantial improvement over available therapy. Breakthrough therapy designation was enacted on July 9, 2012, with the ratification of the Food and Drug Administration Safety and Innovation Act (FDASIA). Section 902 of FDASIA provides the two general criteria for a drug to receive

breakthrough therapy designation. First, the drug must be intended alone or in combination with one or more other drugs to treat a serious or life-threatening disease or condition. Second, preliminary clinical evidence must indicate that the drug may demonstrate substantial improvement over existing therapies on one or more clinically significant endpoints. Unlike fast track designation, the second criterion means that data from studies in animals or conducted in vitro showing that a drug has promise are not sufficient to justify this designation; data from clinical trials in humans are needed.

An application for breakthrough therapy designation can be submitted with an original IND or anytime thereafter and is ideally submitted prior to initiation of clinical trial(s) intended to serve as the primary basis for demonstration of efficacy. The application must include preliminary clinical evidence that indicates that the drug may demonstrate substantial improvement over available therapies on one or more clinically significant endpoints.

Substantial improvement is often a matter of judgment and depends on the magnitude of the drug's effect on a clinical significant endpoint, including the duration of the effect and the importance of the observed effect to the treatment of the serious condition or serious aspect of the condition. Approaches to demonstrating substantial improvement may include the following: comparison of the drug to available therapy showing a much greater response; if there is no available therapy, the drug shows a clinically meaningful effect on an important outcome; the drug plus available therapy results in a much greater response compared to available therapy alone; the drug reverses or inhibits disease progression in contrast to available therapy that only provides symptomatic improvement; or the drug has an important safety advantage compared with available therapy and has similar efficacy.

For the purposes of breakthrough therapy designation, clinically significant endpoints refer to an endpoint that measures an effect on morbidity or mortality or on symptoms that represent serious consequences of the disease. Clinically significant endpoints can also refer to an established surrogate endpoint, an effect on a surrogate endpoint considered reasonably likely to predict clinical benefit, an effect on a pharmacodynamic biomarker that does not meet criteria for a surrogate endpoint, but strongly suggests the potential for a clinically meaningful effect on the underlying disease, or a significantly improved safety profile compared to available therapy with evidence of similar efficacy.

Once a drug receives breakthrough therapy designation, the sponsor is able to receive all of the benefits of fast track designation described earlier as well as intensive guidance on an efficient drug development program and organizational commitment involving FDA senior managers. The intensive guidance includes comprehensive high-level discussions of the expedited development program, including planned clinical trials to generate substantial evidence to support accelerated or regular approval, plans for expediting the manufacturing development strategy, and expanded access programs if applicable. The organizational commitment involving senior managers and intensive involvement of experienced reviewers and regulatory health project management staff results in a proactive, collaborative, cross-disciplinary review.

4.2.3 Priority Review Designation of a New Drug Application/Biologics License Application

Under the Prescription Drug User Act (PUDFA) of 1992, specific goals for improving the drug review time were implemented. This included a two-tiered system of review times, standard review and priority review. Compared with standard review timelines, a priority review designation means that the FDA will decrease by 4 months the timeline to take action on an application. FDA decides on the review designation for every application; however, an applicant may expressly request priority review as well. Priority review is granted when a BLA, NDA, or efficacy supplement is filed for a drug or new indication that, if approved, would provide a significant improvement in the safety or effectiveness of the treatment, diagnosis, or prevention of a serious condition. Significant improvement may be demonstrated by providing evidence of increased effectiveness in treatment, prevention, or diagnosis of a condition; elimination or substantial reduction of treatment-limiting drug reactions; documented enhancement of patient compliance that is expected to lead to an improvement in serious outcomes; or evidence of safety and effectiveness in a new subpopulation. Designation of an application for a priority review does not alter the standard for efficacy and safety required for approval or the quality of evidence necessary for approval.

4.2.4 Accelerated Approval and Regular Approval

Marketing approval of drugs and biologics requires substantial evidence of effectiveness from adequate and well-controlled investigations. For a regular approval, the product is expected to demonstrate effectiveness on an endpoint representative of clinical benefit, such as prolongation of life, the improvement in how a patient feels or functions, or an established surrogate for these endpoints. To meet the above criteria for regular approval, it can take many years to complete the clinical investigations. To provide a faster approval mechanism for drugs intended to treat serious conditions that will fulfill an unmet medical need, FDA initiated the accelerated approval regulations in 1992 [7,8]. These regulations allow for drug approval based on substantial evidence of an effect on a surrogate endpoint that is reasonably likely to predict clinical benefit. In 2012, Section 901 of FDASIA amended the FD&C to expand accelerated approval. Specifically, the criteria for accelerated approval are that the drug is intended to treat a serious condition, that it will provide a meaningful therapeutic benefit over existing treatments, and that it demonstrates an effect on an endpoint that is reasonably likely to predict clinical benefit or an intermediate endpoint that is reasonably likely to predict clinical benefit. Surrogate endpoints are indicators of a change in the disease that are believed likely to predict clinical benefit. An intermediate endpoint is a therapeutic effect that can be measured sooner than an effect on irreversible morbidity or mortality and is considered reasonably likely to predict the drug's effect on irreversible morbidity or mortality or other clinical benefit. For example, an intermediate endpoint could be used to support accelerated approval in a situation where a clinical study demonstrates a relatively short-term clinical benefit and assessing the durability of the clinical benefit is essential for regular approval. Examples of clinical endpoints that have been used to support accelerated approval for oncology products include objective response rate with duration of response, disease-free survival, progression-free survival, major or complete cytogenetic response rate, and improved safety endpoints (i.e., improved creatinine clearance or decreased rates of cardiomyopathy) [14].

Drugs granted accelerated approval must meet the same statutory standard for safety and effectiveness as those granted full approval [15,16]. This standard is substantial evidence based on adequate and well-controlled clinical investigations and having sufficient information to determine whether the drug is safe for use under the conditions prescribed, recommended, or suggested in the proposed labeling [17,18].

Following accelerated approval, pharmaceutical companies have been required to conduct postapproval clinical trials to confirm that the drug provides clinical benefit, as predicted by the surrogate or intermediate endpoint. If a company does not confirm clinical benefit by conducting a postapproval clinical trial(s) with due diligence, the regulations allow the drug to be removed from the market. Postapproval trials to confirm clinical benefit need not be conducted in the same population as the trial that was considered for the accelerated approval and may be conducted in patients with less advanced disease [19].

4.3 MULTIARM EXPANSION COHORTS IN EARLY PHASE TRIALS

4.3.1 Traditional Drug Development Paradigm and Seamless Oncology Expansion Cohort Drug Development Paradigm

Traditionally, clinical drug development followed an orderly sequence of clinical trials, termed phases of an investigation, that build upon information gained from the earlier trial to inform the objectives and design of subsequent trials (see Fig. 4.1A). Phase 1 clinical trials, which includes the initial introduction of the new drug into humans (i.e., a first-in-human (FIH) trial), are designed to evaluate the metabolism and pharmacologic actions of an investigational drug in humans, assess the side effects across doses, and, when possible, provide preliminary effectiveness of the new drug [2,20]. In this paradigm, the FIH Phase 1 trial should obtain sufficient information about the pharmacokinetics and pharmacological effects of the drug to permit the design of subsequent well-controlled, scientifically valid

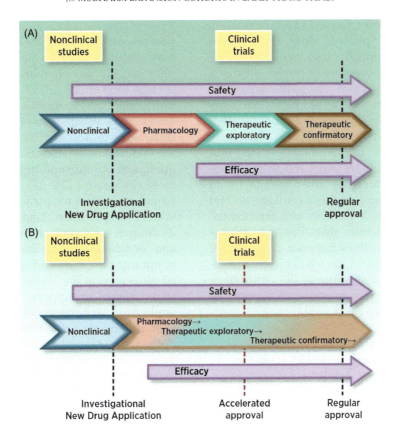

FIGURE 4.1 Evolving drug development paradigm. (A) Traditional drug development paradigm. (B) Seamless oncology-drug development paradigm [4]. Source: *Reprinted with permission from the American Association for Cancer Research [4].*

safety and efficacy trials. As described in the FDA regulations, the total number of subjects included in Phase 1 studies is typically in the range of 20–80 subjects or patients, but this number varies across drug development programs. FDA regulations and guidances do not recommend a specific design for an FIH trial—the design of the clinical protocol as proposed by the sponsor in the IND should ensure that it can meet the stated objectives of the protocol. The clinical trial protocol is but one component of the IND that must be filed to conduct an FIH trial. A description of the other components is beyond the scope of this chapter and is detailed in FDA guidances and regulations [21,22].

Recently, based in part on scientific advances in understanding the biology of cancer and immune biology, rationally designed oncology drugs have demonstrated unprecedented efficacy early in the drug development process [23]. This, along with a regulatory framework supporting expedited development, review, and approval of drugs intended to treat patients with serious and life-threatening diseases in the context of an unmet medical need, as well as a desire from multiple stakeholders to accelerate the drug development and approval process, has led to a reevaluation of the traditional "phased" drug development paradigm for potentially transformative drugs and to sponsors' proposals to pursue seamless oncology trials, which include expansion cohort trials [4,5]. In a seamless oncology expansion cohort paradigm, the drug development objectives typical of each trial phase may be evaluated not in standalone trials, but within separate cohorts proposed in the original design or added as amendments to an existing FIH protocol. In this paradigm, an FIH may enroll over 1000 patients and the nomenclature used to identify this "Phase 1" trial is inadequate, as the lines between distinct trial phases are blurred and the trial objectives evaluated in the FIH may serve as the entire drug development program intended to support an initial approval (see Fig. 4.1B) [4].

4.3.2 Examples of Expansion Cohorts in Seamless Oncology Trials

Designs of FIH trials using expansion cohorts may include one or more objectives in the following types of expansion cohorts:

- Expansion cohort to further explore safety. This type of expansion cohort is designed to further explore the dose that was determined reasonably safe in the traditional dose-escalation phase. Because limited numbers of patients are exposed to the investigational drug at the different dose levels explored in the dose-escalation phase using either 3 + 3 or Bayesian designs, expansion cohorts can further explore the safety of the maximum tolerated dose (MTD) identified in the dose-escalation phase. Expansion cohorts can also provide insight into the long-term tolerability of an investigational drug or explore interventions to minimize specific toxicities such as using supportive care medications for reducing the incidence of febrile neutropenia.

- Expansion cohort to evaluate specific clinical pharmacology endpoints. Expansion cohorts may evaluate specific aspects of the pharmacokinetics of an investigational drug such as food effects, effects of organ impairment on pharmacokinetics, or drug interactions. Whether conducted in standalone protocols or incorporated into the FIH trial as expansion cohorts, FDA guidances provide additional details for these evaluations [24–27].
- Expansion cohort for further dose and schedule exploration. Traditionally, "Phase 2" designs have explored multiple doses and/or schedules of an investigational agent to optimize the dose and schedule to be administered in the "Phase 3" randomized trial designed to support a marketing application. Expansion cohorts with a primary objective of determining the optimal dose(s) and dosing schedule(s), preferably in randomized designs, are being incorporated into the FIH protocols.
- Expansion cohort to further evaluate preliminary efficacy. Increasingly, expansion cohorts are included in the FIH protocol to further explore antitumor activity or obtain preliminary estimates of efficacy, typically in a selected tumor type or biomarker-defined subgroup [28]. In some instances, large disease-specific, single-arm expansion cohorts have supported accelerated approval of drugs with a large magnitude of antitumor activity as evidenced by objective response rates and prolonged duration of responses [29–34]. Considerations for expansion cohorts to further evaluate antitumor activity and obtain preliminary estimates of efficacy are described later in this chapter.
- Expansion cohort for biomarker selection. An expansion cohort may be designed to identify one or more biomarkers that may help enrich future trials for efficacy or to identify specific subpopulations in which

the drug is deemed safer. With the advent of molecularly targeted agents and modern diagnostic assays, such types of expansion cohorts have increased the complexity of expansion cohort trial designs through the requirement for codevelopment of the drug and its potential companion diagnostic assay.

- Expansion cohort to evaluate a new product formulation. Expansion cohorts may be designed to investigate the relative pharmacokinetics, optimal dosage regimen, and safety of multiple formulations of an investigational drug. These cohorts may enroll specific tumor types in which such formulations are intended to be used, such as a liquid formulation for head and neck cancer patients who may have difficulties swallowing a capsule formulation.

- Expansion cohort to explore combination therapies. Expansion cohorts may be designed to explore the combination of the investigational agent with an approved product in an "add on" design. Some expansion cohorts may explore an investigational agent in combination with another investigational agent. In the latter instance, preliminary safety data are ordinarily available for each investigational agent administered as single agents, such that potential overlapping toxicities can be considered in the selection of initial doses of each drug and in developing the safety monitoring plan.

- Expansion cohorts to explore activity in the pediatric population. Expansion cohorts may include one or more cohorts of pediatric patients with various tumor types, especially if there is strong scientific rationale for the role of the cancer pathway that the investigational agent targets in the development of pediatric cancers. Such cohorts may eliminate the need for a separate protocol for exploring the clinical activity in pediatric tumors. Ordinarily,

sufficient pharmacokinetic and safety experience in adults are available to guide dosing and anticipate risks prior to initiation of enrollment in pediatric tumor cohorts.

4.3.3 Regulatory Considerations of Seamless Oncology Expansion Cohort FIH Trials—Opportunities and Challenges

4.3.3.1 *Safety Considerations*

The primary objective of a Phase 1 clinical trial is to assess the safety and tolerability of an investigational product or a combination of products, to determine the MTD and establish a recommended Phase 2 dose (RP2D). Traditionally, the MTD is determined based on data observed in 6–12 patients per dose level enrolled in the dose-escalation phase of the study and the RP2D is selected based on a small expansion cohort of 10–20 subjects treated at the MTD. FIH clinical trials with expansion cohort designs should allow for continuing assessment of the safety profile of an investigational product as more data become available at the MTD, providing opportunities for reestimation and refining of the MTD. When toxicity data from Phase 1 protocols using expansion cohorts were reevaluated, Iasonos et al. demonstrated that there is a high likelihood that a new, higher MTD will be recommended compared with the level reached using the initial dose-escalation data alone [35].

Patients enrolled in expansion cohort studies are exposed to increased risks, in part due to the complexity of the trial design and lack of discrete periods for assessment of safety data across multiple simultaneously enrolling cohorts. These risks must be thoroughly addressed. As indicated in the previous section, expansion cohort protocols undergo frequent modifications either to add a new patient population, a new dose/regimen, or a new drug combination; hence, altering the risks to patients to be enrolled in the existing study. While a clinical study, including the informed consent form, may not be initiated until it has been reviewed and approved by an investigational review boards (IRBs), it remains subject to continuing review by an IRB [36]. Multiple amendments to the protocol over a short interval might preclude real-time assessment and thorough review of all safety information obtained from the ongoing cohorts and timely communication of new safety signals to all investigators and IRBs. This may result in patients being exposed to an investigational product without a thorough risk−benefit assessment to justify the proposed changes.

As experience with these trials has increased, sponsors and investigators conducting multiple expansion cohort trials have implemented, early in the design of the trial, systematic safety monitoring and reporting plans to safeguard patients from harm, including the unnecessary exposure of a large number of patients to a potentially ineffective and toxic agent. For example, the protocol may require a rapid communication plan for all serious safety issues to all investigational sites and regulatory authorities under IND safety reporting regulations [37,38]. Additionally, well-designed expansion cohort FIH protocols have added a prospective plan—e.g., based on total accrual or initiation of a particular expansion cohort—to establish an independent safety committee to review all serious adverse events, meeting periodically to assess the safety data, and charged with making recommendations to the sponsor regarding protocol modifications or other actions to mitigate risks to patients enrolled in the study. Expansion cohort protocols must update the informed consent document periodically with new safety and efficacy information from the ongoing study, as new information may alter a patient's decision to participate in the trial. Lastly, to allow the IRB to serve its function of continuing review and more fully evaluate the risks to patients

enrolled in protocols with one or more expansion cohorts, the investigator should provide cumulative safety information, summary of study progress, and other reports received from the product sponsor, including reports from the Independent Safety Committee at more frequent intervals than annually.

4.3.3.2 *Efficacy Considerations*

As drug development proceeds under IND from the FIH Phase 1 trial to submission of Phase 2 and later trials, the IND regulations place increasing importance not only on assuring the safety of human subjects, which is the main focus of regulatory review of Phase 1 trials, but also on the scientific integrity of the trial in order to ensure it meets its stated objectives. A potential advantage of FIH seamless oncology expansion cohort trials is that, as a hybrid design that includes components of Phase 1 and 2 trials, expansion cohorts may be added—in response to findings in the dose-escalation and expansion component of the trial—to provide a preliminary assessment of efficacy in disease-specific cohorts, potentially defined by tumor type or by a biomarker depending on what is known about the effects of the drug. This type of trial not only exposes patients to higher risks, but may be considered unethical if it is not carefully designed to address specific scientific questions relevant to each specific cohort. Therefore, providing sufficient detail, both in the initial protocol and in protocol amendments, on the goals and conduct of the clinical protocol in a well-defined population, mitigates potential risks to patients and to the drug development program.

While FIH, seamless, expansion cohort trial would contain the elements of a protocol described in the FDA regulations and ICH guidance, amendments to protocols to add expansion cohorts intended to evaluate preliminary efficacy would pay particular attention to inclusion of cohort-specific protocol elements such as scientific rationale for evaluation of efficacy in the specified population, clearly defined objectives, rationally designed eligibility criteria, specific treatment and monitoring plans that encompass disease-specific considerations, and a detailed statistical analysis plan for the cohort [3,21,39]. In these FIH trials, accrual to activity-estimating, disease-specific expansion cohorts for preliminary efficacy, at least initially, will likely be best suited to settings where patients in all expansion cohorts have similar risk tolerance considering natural history, underlying comorbidities, and susceptibility for adverse reactions based on tumor histology, and have similar considerations for the effectiveness of alternative therapy, if any. Within a cohort intended to assess preliminary efficacy, inclusion of detailed eligibility criteria ensures enrollment of a homogeneous population where appropriate (e.g., specifies extent and type of prior therapy, stage of disease, presence or absence of driver mutations) and all criteria necessary to mitigate serious risks to patients, taking into account the known adverse reaction profile of the drug(s). If patient selection is predicated on the identification of a biomarker, sufficient detail on the in vitro diagnostic (IVD) device should be provided to allow an assessment of the reliability of the assay to ensure enrollment of a homogeneous population and mitigate the risk of enrolling patients with false positive or negative results. If an investigational IVD is to be used in a clinical trial, the requirements of the Investigational Device Exemption (IDE) regulation would need to be assessed [40]. These requirements may vary, depending on the level of risk that the device presents to study subjects (i.e., significant risk or nonsignificant risk) as well as other criteria.

Clearly defined objectives and endpoints, including adequate description of the type and timing of the endpoint assessments, for each expansion cohort evaluating preliminary efficacy facilitates the ability of the protocol to achieve its scientific objectives.

Disease-specific expansion cohorts to assess preliminary efficacy of the investigational drug are generally limited in the number of patients, e.g., enrollment of 20–40 patients is typical in a Simon 2-stage single-arm trial model, but the sample size may vary based on design considerations to achieve the objectives, such as the underlying statistical assumptions as well as the requirement for randomization [41]. In a review of expansion cohorts included in "Phase 1" trials over a 25-year period single-institution review, Dahlberg et al. determined that nearly two-thirds of trials failed to provide statistical justification for the number of patients in the expansion cohort [42]. Inclusion of adequate justification in the protocol for each expansion cohort of the maximum sample size and stopping rules for lack of activity/efficacy serves not only to minimize the number of patients exposed to a potentially ineffective drug, but also to limit the accrual of more patients than needed to achieve the cohort's objectives, thereby avoiding inefficiencies and delay in proceeding to the next phase in drug development. Furthermore, exploratory comparisons across cohorts that "over-interpret" the findings observed may inappropriately limit future development, e.g., selection of dosage regimens or biomarker-selected populations based on ad hoc between cohort comparisons. Additionally, the regulatory intent of an expansion cohort to evaluate efficacy within the FIH trial impacts trial conduct considerations, e.g., data capture, site monitoring, independent oversight, and incorporation of independent radiologic review.

If preliminary clinical evidence in the drug development program suggests that a drug may provide substantial improvement over available therapies on a clinically significant endpoint(s) in a patient population with a high unmet medical need, e.g., a breakthrough therapy designated product, modification of the expansion protocol to include an adequately powered disease-specific, single-arm expansion cohort intended to characterize the preliminary efficacy of an investigational drug to support a marketing application (e.g., an accelerated approval based on objective response rate with a prolonged duration of response) may align with the goals and concepts described by FDA's expedited programs. Importantly, the design, conduct, and analysis of an expansion cohort intended to provide substantial evidence for regulatory approval would need to meet the standard of an adequate and well-controlled trial and adequately assess risks to patients [43].

4.4 SUMMARY

Seamless, FIH, dose-escalation and expansion cohort trials represent a hybrid design that seeks to address the objectives of Phase 1 and Phase 2 trial(s) under a single protocol. Expansion cohorts may be proposed in the original protocol, but may also be added following observation of promising antitumor activity early on in the dose-finding portion of the trial to further assess and characterize preliminary efficacy in specific patient populations (e.g., defined by tumor tissue types and/or the presence of a biomarker). The flexibility to modify the protocol through the addition of new cohorts in response to early findings in the trial can, if thoughtfully designed and implemented, provide efficiencies in the drug development program by using the existing trial infrastructure—clinical, operational, and regulatory—to bring highly effective drugs to patients as early as possible without compromising standards for safety and efficacy. In rare instances, the FIH expansion cohort trial has served as the entire clinical drug development program supporting an initial accelerated approval. However, this expedited approach presents increased risks to patients as well as challenges for drug development that must be

thoroughly addressed to ensure the potential efficiencies outweigh the risks of a seamless oncology expansion cohort approach.

References

[1] Junod SW. FDA and clinical drug trials: a short history. In: Davies M, Kerimani F, editors. A quick guide to clinical trials. Washington, DC: Bioplan, Inc; 2008. p. 25−55.
[2] 21 Code of Federal Regulations (CFR) 312.21. <https://www.ecfr.gov/cgi-bin/text-idx?SID = 0bdd88f9c5803af07244a53e51aea78e&mc = true&tpl = /ecfr-browse/Title21/21cfr312_main_02.tpl> [accessed 26.07.17].
[3] International Conference on Harmonization (ICH) of technical requirements for registration of pharmaceuticals for human use, ICH harmonized tripartite guideline, General Considerations for Clinical Trials, E8, <http://www.ich.org/fileadmin/Public_Web_Site/ICH_Products/Guidelines/Efficacy/E8/Step4/E8_Guideline.pdf>; July 17, 1997 [accessed 26.07.17].
[4] Theoret MR, Pai-Scherf LH, Chuk MK, Prowell TM, Balsubramaniam S, Kim T, et al. Expansion cohorts in first-in-human solid tumor oncology trials. Clin Cancer Res 2015;21:4545−51.
[5] Prowell TM, Theoret MR, Pazdur R. Seamless oncology-drug development. N Engl J Med 2016;374:2001−3.
[6] U.S. Food and Drug Administration. Guidance for industry: expedited programs for serious conditions − drugs and biologics, <https://www.fda.gov/ucm/groups/fdagov-public/@fdagov-drugs-gen/documents/document/ucm358301.pdf>; May 2014 [accessed 31.07.17].
[7] 21 CFR 314, subpart H. <https://www.ecfr.gov/cgi-bin/text-idx?SID = 0bdd88f9c5803af07244a53e51aea78e&mc = true&tpl = /ecfrbrowse/Title21/21cfr314_main_02.tpl> [accessed 26.07.17].
[8] 21 CFR 601, subpart E. <https://www.ecfr.gov/cgi-bin/text-idx?SID = 0bdd88f9c5803af07244a53e51aea78e&mc = true&tpl = /ecfrbrowse/Title21/21cfr601_main_02.tpl> [accessed 31.07.17].
[9] U.S. Food and Drug Administration. Guidance for industry: clinical trial endpoints for the approval of cancer drugs and biologics, <https://www.fda.gov/ucm/groups/fdagov-public/@fdagov-drugs-gen/documents/document/ucm071590.pdf>; May 2007 [accessed 26.07.17].
[10] 21 CFR 314.105. <https://www.ecfr.gov/cgi-bin/text-idx?SID = 0bdd88f9c5803af07244a53e51aea78e&mc =

true&tpl = /ecfrbrowse/Title21/21cfr314_main_02. tpl> [accessed 31.07.17].

[11] 21 CFR 312.84. <https://www.ecfr.gov/cgi-bin/text-idx?SID = 0bdd88f9c5803af07244a53e51aea78e&mc = true&tpl = /ecfrbrowse/Title21/21cfr312_main_02. tpl> [accessed 31.07.17].

[12] 21 CFR 312.300(b). <https://www.ecfr.gov/cgi-bin/text-idx?SID = 0bdd88f9c5803af07244a53e51aea78e&mc = true&tpl = /ecfrbrowse/Title21/21cfr312_main_02.tpl> [accessed 31.07.17].

[13] Section 506(d)(1) of the Food, Drug, & Cosmetic Act (FD&C Act).

[14] Johnson JR, Ning Y, Farrell A, Justice R, Keegan P, Pazdur R. Accelerated approval of oncology products: The Food and Drug Administration experience. J Natl Cancer Inst 2011;103:636−44.

[15] Section 505(d) of the FD&C Act.

[16] Section 351(a) of the Public Health Service Act.

[17] Section 505(d)(5) of the FD&C Act.

[18] Section 505(d)(1) of the FD&C Act.

[19] Section 506(c)(2)(A) of the FD&C Act.

[20] Temple R. Current definitions of phases of investigation and the role of the FDA in the conduct of clinical trials. Am Heart J 2000;139:S133−5.

[21] 21 CFR 312.23. <https://www.ecfr.gov/cgi-bin/text-idx?SID = 0bdd88f9c5803af07244a53e51aea78e&mc = true&tpl = /ecfrbrowse/Title21/21cfr312_main_02. tpl> [accessed 31.07.17].

[22] U.S. Food and Drug Administration. Guidance for industry: content and format of investigational new drug applications (INDs) for phase 1 studies of drugs, including well-characterized, therapeutic, biotechnology-derived products, <https://www.fda.gov/ucm/groups/fdagov-public/@fdagov-drugs-gen/documents/document/ucm071597.pdf>; November 1995 [accessed 26.07.17].

[23] Blumenthal GM, Kluetz PG, Schneider J, Goldberg KB, McKee AE, Pazdur R. Oncology drug approvals: evaluating endpoints and evidence in an era of breakthrough therapies. Oncologist 2017;22:762−7.

[24] U.S. Food and Drug Administration. Guidance for industry: food-effect bioavailability and fed bioequivalence studies food effect, <https://www.fda.gov/ucm/groups/fdagov-public/@fdagov-drugs-gen/documents/document/ucm070241.pdf>; December 2002 [accessed 26.07.17].

[25] U.S. Food and Drug Administration. Draft Guidance for industry: pharmacokinetics in patients with impaired renal function—study design, data analysis, and impact on dosing and labeling, <https://www.fda.gov/ucm/groups/fdagov-public/@fdagov-drugs-gen/documents/document/ucm204959.pdf>; March 2010 [accessed 31.07.17].

[26] U.S. Food and Drug Administration. Guidance for industry: pharmacokinetics in patients with impaired hepatic function: study design, data analysis, and impact on dosing and labeling, <https://www.fda.gov/ucm/groups/fdagov-public/@fdagov-drugs-gen/documents/document/ucm072123.pdf>; May 2003 [accessed 26.07.17].

[27] U.S. Food and Drug Administration. Draft Guidance for industry: drug interaction studies—study design, data analysis, implications for dosing, and labeling recommendations, <https://www.fda.gov/ucm/groups/fdagov-public/@fdagov-drugs-gen/documents/document/ucm292362.pdf>; February 2012 [accessed 26.07.17].

[28] Manji A, Brana I, Amir E, Tomlinson G, Tannock IF, Bedard PL, et al. Evolution of clinical trial design in early drug development: systematic review of expansion cohort use in single-agent phase I cancer trials. J Clin Oncol 2013;31:4260−7.

[29] Chuk MK, Chang JT, Theoret MR, Sampene E, He K, Weiss SL, et al. FDA approval summary: accelerated approval of pembrolizumab for second-line treatment of metastatic melanoma. Clin Cancer Res 2017;23:5666−70 Published online February 24, 2017.

[30] Sul J, Blumenthal GM, Jiang X, He K, Keegan P, Pazdur R. FDA approval summary: pembrolizumab for the treatment of patients with metastatic non-small cell lung cancer whose tumors express programmed death-ligand 1. Oncologist 2016;21:643−50.

[31] Kazandjian D, Blumenthal GM, Luo L, He K, Fran I, Lemery S, et al. Benefit-risk summary of crizotinib for the treatment of patients with ROS1 alteration-positive, metastatic non-small cell lung cancer. Oncologist 2017;21:974−80.

[32] Khozin S, Blumenthal GM, Zhang L, Tang S, Brower M, Fox E, et al. FDA approval: ceritinib for the treatment of metastatic anaplastic lymphoma kinase−positive non−small cell lung cancer. Clin Cancer Res 2015;21:2436−9.

[33] Apolo AB, Ellerton JA, Infante JR, Agrawal M, Gordon MS, Aljumaily R, et al. Updated efficacy and safety of avelumab in metastatic urothelial carcinoma (mUC): pooled analysis from 2 cohorts of the phase 1b Javelin solid tumor study. J Clin Oncol 2017;35 (suppl; abstract 4528).

[34] U.S. Food and Drug Administration. Medical and statistical review for durvalumab BLA (BLA 761069), <https://www.accessdata.fda.gov/drugsatfda_docs/nda/2017/761069Orig1s000MedR.pdf> [accessed 31.07.17].

[35] Iasonos A, O'Quigley J. Design considerations for dose-expansion cohorts in phase I trials. J Clin Oncol 2013;31:4014−21.

[36] 21 CFR 56.103. <https://www.ecfr.gov/cgi-bin/text-idx?SID = dc93a58336ab94509ca71938d09d1470&mc = true&tpl = /ecfrbrowse/Title21/21cfr56_main_02.tpl> [accessed 26.07.17].

[37] 21 CFR 312.32. <https://www.ecfr.gov/cgi-bin/text-idx?SID = dc93a58336ab94509ca71938d09d1470&mc = true&tpl = /ecfrbrowse/Title21/21cfr312_main_02.tpl> [accessed 26.07.17].

[38] 21 CFR 312.33. <https://www.ecfr.gov/cgi-bin/text-idx?SID = dc93a58336ab94509ca71938d09d1470&mc = true&tpl = /ecfrbrowse/Title21/21cfr312_main_02.tpl> [accessed 26.07.17].

[39] International Conference on Harmonization (ICH) of technical requirements for registration of pharmaceuticals for human use, ICH harmonized tripartite guideline, Statistical principles for clinical trials, E9, <http://www.ich.org/fileadmin/Public_Web_Site/ ICH_Products/Guidelines/Efficacy/E9/Step4/E9_ Guideline.pdf>; July 17, 1997 [accessed 26.07.17].

[40] 21 CFR 812. <https://www.ecfr.gov/cgi-bin/text-idx?SID = 33b1f63036bcaa7a20bf0767b9922665&mc = true&tpl = /ecfrbrowse/Title21/21cfr812_main_02.tpl> [accessed 26.07.17].

[41] Simon R. Optimal two-stage designs for phase II clinical trials. Control Clin Trials 1989;10:1−10.

[42] Dahlberg S, Shapiro GI, Clark JW, Johnson BE. Evaluation of statistical designs in phase I expansion cohorts: The Dana-Farber/Harvard Cancer Center Experience. J Natl Cancer Inst 2014;106:1−6.

[43] 21 CFR 314.126. <https://www.ecfr.gov/cgi-bin/text-idx?SID = dc93a58336ab94509ca71938d09d1470&mc = true&tpl = /ecfrbrowse/Title21/21cfr314_main_02.tpl> [accessed 26.07.17].

The Challenges of Implementing Multiarmed Early Phase Oncology Clinical Trials

David Hong[1] and Pedro C. Barata[2]

[1]The University of Texas MD Anderson Cancer Center, Houston, TX, United States
[2]Cleveland Clinic Foundation, Cleveland, OH, United States

5.1 INTRODUCTION

Cancer figures among the leading causes of death worldwide. In 2016, more than 1.65 million new cases of cancer were diagnosed in the United States and approximately 0.6 million people died from the disease [1,2]. Nevertheless, among men and women of all major racial/ethnic groups, death rates have been declined over the past decades [3]. Overall, the development of novel anticancer drugs has contributed to the absolute improvement in 5-year overall survival by 19% [4,5]. This development is a consequence of the significant effort being made by the different contributors in this field. Two years ago, there were more than 750 drugs under development for cancer, more than in any other disease area, and more than in any other area of medicine [5,6].

However, this process is time-consuming and highly costly. The drug development timeline for oncology drugs ranges from 2.5 to 8 years and is estimated to take 1.5 years longer than in other diseases [7,8]. Furthermore, the success rate for oncology compounds remains low, with only 18% of Phase 2 studies progressing into Phase 3 trials, and around 50% of confirmatory Phase 3 studies have failed to show a beneficial benefit or been rejected at regulatory submission [9,10]. Overall, the likelihood of approval of an oncology drug is less than 10%, and the cost of a single product to be approved is estimated to be between 1.2 and 1.3 billion [11,12].

In the present chapter, we address how early phase studies have changed and evolved to optimize the process of drug development. We also discuss the challenges/implications that both investigators and institutions have to face as a result of this changing field. Finally, we summarize a number of recommendations both researchers and research centers may adopt to improve the efficiency of Phase 1 trials.

5.2 EVOLUTION OF EARLY PHASE CLINICAL TRIALS

The main goal of early phase clinical trials is to determine the recommended dose to move forward for future clinical studies. Initially, preclinical data are generated in the laboratory, using both cellular models and animals before human studies, to assess the absorption, distribution, metabolization, and excretion of a specific drug and also, to investigate whether a compound has promising anticancer activity [13].

Classical chemotherapy agents are not usually "targeted." They have steep dose–response relationships with higher doses frequently resulting in greater toxicity, and their dose escalation is often limited by organ toxicity. As a consequence, the maximum tolerated dose (MTD) is the most common endpoint for Phase 1 trials, and the quantification of tumor control (response rate, RR) is typically an exploratory endpoint for evaluating efficacy.

In recent years, drug development in oncology has shifted from classical cytotoxic chemotherapy to the novel molecularly targeted agents (MTAs) [14]. Unlike cytotoxic chemotherapy, MTAs inhibit specific proteins (i.e., receptors and enzymes) within intra/extracellular pathways known to be, directly or indirectly, involved in the processes of oncogenesis, cell growth, and metastatic spread [15].

Trials with "one size fits all" approach do not take into consideration the well-established patient-to-patient variation that exists in the molecular drivers of both cancer and drug sensitivity [16]. With advent of MTAs, several aspects of early phase studies have evolved to adapt to the changing nature of cancer therapies and to expedite clinical translation [17].

Their safety profile is often characterized by low-grade, chronic toxicities and "off-target" effects are uncommon and may be caused by nonspecific binding, pathway homology, or previously unknown expression of the target molecule in healthy tissues [14,18]. As a result, and unlike cytotoxic therapies, the use of toxicity as the primary determinant of the recommended Phase 2 dose might not be a predictor of efficacy. Indeed, there are several examples to support the concept that a higher dose does not always yield optimal biological activity [19,20].

In the era of targeted therapy, study objectives of early clinical trials have expanded to give greater focus on evaluation of efficacy and detecting response signals, in addition to safety [18,21]. Furthermore, alternative endpoints such as target modulation of downstream molecular effects may represent relevant surrogates of drug efficacy, helping to select which drugs can move forward. The early integration of predictive biomarkers, such as pharmacokinetics and pharmacodynamics, in the drug discovery process can help to improve our understanding of key pathways in cancer, and may support optimal clinical trial designs yielding better results [16,22]. Predictive biomarkers are crucial to accelerating the drug development process, and some successful examples include ERBB2/trastuzumab, BCR-ABL/imatinib, and EGFR/erlotinib [23–27].

Since MTAs may be active in only a subgroup of patients, the identification of predictive biomarkers is crucial for patient selection and success rates [5,28]. With the increasing use of biomarker-driven patient selection, more patients need to be screened to identify potential candidates for trial inclusion, excluding those who likely will not benefit from that particular study [15,16].

5.2.1 Endpoints

In general, biological agents often have a cytostatic rather than cytotoxic effect, inhibiting tumor growth without direct cytotoxicity [15].

5.2.2 Trial Designs

Rule-based designs, also referred to as "3 + 3" designs, where patients are enrolled into small cohorts at different dose levels, are based on the assumption of a linear dose–response relationship [14]. While they generally perform well for cytotoxic drugs, this model seems to be insufficient for MTAs, given its inability to accurately capture chronic low-grade toxicities, the limited number of doses that can be tested efficiently, or when nonlinear dose–response relationships for efficacy and toxicity are present [5,17]. Thus conventional designs and dose-limiting toxicity (DLT) definitions might be inappropriate for MTAs.

Likewise, the number of patients enrolled on the initial Phase 1 studies constitutes an important factor to predict toxicities and final dose in confirmatory studies. In retrospective analysis of 61 drugs approved by Food and Drug Administration (FDA) for adult cancers between 1990 and 2012, Jardim et al. [29] demonstrated that Phase 1 studies enrolling less than 60 patients were less likely to predict clinical relevant toxicity in later trials. Likewise, Phase 1 trials with MTAs were less predictive of the final approved dose.

Overall, these limitations have led to the development of newer trial designs, which are making their way into current Phase 1 studies. Novel dose-escalation approaches have been proposed to address these issues, including accelerated-titration and adaptive model-trial designs [14,16]. The accelerated-titration model is characterized by a rapid initial dose escalation, where a single patient is enrolled to each dose level until a prespecified level of toxicity (grade ≥ 2) is observed. This method allows more patients to be treated at therapeutic doses, with a faster escalation in the same number of patients [30]. However, it might not be appropriate for agents with a narrow therapeutic index because of the increased risk of DLTs [31].

By contrast, the design of adaptive trials is based on data from previous patients that becomes available during the clinical trial [32–35]. Many model-based designs are based on Bayesian adaptive methods, and were developed in order to determine a more precise MTD using mathematical modeling [16,36]. In general, these designs allow adaptive dose escalation/deescalation, early stopping for efficacy, futility or toxicity, adding or dropping new treatment arms, and sample size reestimation [5,14,37,38]. As a result, adaptive designs have the potential to be more flexible and efficient, treating more patients near optimal doses, and use fewer dose levels [38]. Its use has been recommended by international institutions (European Medicine Agency (EMA) [39], FDA [40]) and free software packages are available to download from several organizations to facilitate its implementation [41,42]. However, they require permanent biostatistical support during the conduct of the study, which has resulted in their use in a minority of clinical studies [43]. Moreover, lack of familiarity with the novel methods proposed and fear that the use of some of the models to decide dose escalations removes control from investigators may also contribute to this suboptimal implementation [36].

Of interest, more recent Bayesian designs, such as the Bayesian optimal interval (BOIN) design, are easy to implement in a way similar to the standard "3 + 3" design, but with a better performance that is comparable to the more complex model-based designs [44]. Advantages include a high probability of identifying the personalized optimal dose, a lower risk of overdosing patients, and the wide availability of user-friendly free software [45].

5.2.3 Multiarmed Trials and the Regulatory "Effect"

In opposition to the traditional approach of testing each agent in a separate study, the use of multiple expansion cohorts for investigational drugs that show preliminary activity allows for the simultaneous testing of different treatments in a cheaper and faster way [46,47]. Current dose- and tumor-expansion cohorts add an additional number of patients who are treated at the established MTD based on the predose-expansion data. These multiple expansion cohorts have emerged to address multiple objectives, including assessing drug efficacy in separate subpopulations of patients with various tumor types. In fact, the proportion of Phase 1 trials with expansion cohorts has been significantly increasing in the last few years, from 12% in 2006 to 38% in 2011, and the median sample size of these studies almost doubled (34 vs 56 patients) in the same period of time [48,49].

The opportunity to expedite breakthrough therapy for approval has impacted the design and conduct of clinical trials, and the regulatory agencies have played an important role in this process [5]. In 2012 in the FDA Safety and Innovation Act, the FDA promoted four different programs ("breakthrough therapy," "fast track," "priority review," and "accelerated approval") to expedite access to these therapies in new indications with high unmet medical need [50–54]. While the first three programs are designations granted by FDA in response to a request by the commercial sponsor of the drug, the "accelerated approval" program represents a pathway intended to provide earlier access of drugs to patients with serious conditions based on positive surrogate or intermediate clinical endpoints that likely predict clinical benefit [47].

Successful examples of these breakthrough therapies include different molecules with unique mechanisms of action, such as the tyrosine kinase inhibitors, gefitinib and geritinib; the selective inhibitor of the cyclin-dependent kinase CDK4/6, palbociclib; and the monoclonal antibodies targeting programmed death-1, pembrolizumab and nivolumab [55–57]. Several studies clearly suggest the success of these programs, including shorter trial periods and regulatory process times, and allow these therapies to reach the market months to years earlier [58–60].

The cases of pembrolizumab and nivolumab are good examples of how FDA expedited programs have contributed to the increased use of expansion cohorts. For example, in a first-in-human study initiated in 2011, Patnaik et al. planned to administer pembrolizumab to approximately 18 patients with advanced melanoma or any type of refractory carcinoma, using a modified "3 + 3" dose-escalation method and enrolled an additional 14 patients with melanoma and renal-cell cancer in two disease-specific expansion cohorts [61]. The protocol expanded to a planned accrual of more than 1000 patients and approximately 3 years later, data from the melanoma cohorts provided substantial evidence of treatment considered reasonable likely to predict clinical benefit in the context of a favorable benefit–risk profile, meeting the criteria of accelerated approval." Pembrolizumab was granted marketing approval under the "accelerated approval" pathway in September 2014 by FDA, with the requirement to conduct further trials for verification and description of its clinical benefit [55].

In a different Phase 1 trial assessing safety, dose–response and clinical activity profile of nivolumab, Topalian et al. enrolled advanced cancer patients in five different escalation cohorts (16 patients per cohort)—non-small cell lung cancer, advanced melanoma, renal-cell cancer, metastatic castration resistant prostate cancer, and colorectal adenocarcinoma—followed by five expansion cohorts of approximately 16 patients each [62]. This Phase 1 trial had a notable success especially in the melanoma, lung, and kidney cancer cohorts, with overall RR between 18% and 27%, and low (14%) incidence of grade 3 or 4 adverse reactions were seen. The data observed in this study preceded different randomized Phase 3 trials for patients with advanced melanoma. nivolumab was granted "accelerated approval" by FDA in December 2014, based on preliminary evidence of clinical benefit including objective responses and durable durations of response in the first 120 patients with metastatic melanoma enrolled in the Phase 3 trial, with a minimum follow up of 6 months. Phase 1 data from non-small cell lung and renal-cell cancer patients also supported the approval of this therapy in each of these settings [63–65].

5.2.4 Logistical Challenges for Institutions and Investigators

The changes in the goals and conduct of Phase 1 trials have resulted in a shift toward multi-institutional studies and centralized management, with a significant impact on the structure of Phase 1 programs [66]. Recently, the enrollment process consists of allocating patients slots to multiple institutions participating in a single Phase 1 study. The desire to accelerate patient recruitment results in the selection of centers based on their ability to enroll, rather than experience and quality of their Phase 1 program. Interestingly, when compared with single institution studies, multi-institutional trials don't decrease the time to study completion, as shown by Dowlati et al., in an extensive review of all published Phase 1 studies between 1998 and 2006 [67]. Generally, the responsibility for allocating patients lies on the sponsor, requiring a significant coordination among participation sites [67]. In addition, slots in each cohort are frequently assigned on a "first-come-first-serve" basis, leading to a limited availability of trial slots per site. As a consequence, institutions need to open a higher number of clinical trials to accommodate the same amount of patients enrolled in studies with experimental therapies [5].

With the emersion of multi-expansion cohorts studies, there may be multiple cohorts enrolling patients with different tumors, requiring the participation of different departments/divisions from each research center. Plus, the introduction of advanced technologies and new techniques in clinical trials has prompted the need for increased training and credentialing of personnel in

participating centers [68]. Thus there is an increased number of requirements that can easily overload the level of logistical resources devoted to these studies, because of the growing demands for real-time monitoring, assessment of toxicities, evaluation of adverse events (AEs), and rapid communication in the form of frequent conference calls between participants [69,70]. The allocation of the necessary resources to fulfill these requirements, including additional staff, constitutes significant challenges to institutions. The potential safety risks inherent to such efforts are considerable, but the gains are not always clear [70].

Additionally, the experience of Phase 1 studies may be influenced by multi-institutional trials and pose potential challenges to younger investigators. Clinicians at one center can only gain limited experience with a novel agent, as disease-specific Phase 1 trials are more likely to be multi-institutional in nature [67]. Activation of a trial may happens at different times by participating institutions, thus, preventing investigators from acquiring experience with investigational drugs. The extent of this impact in the ability of clinicians to recognize diverse AEs is unknown.

Clinical research organizations and not research centers are now frequently leading clinical trials and responsible for overseeing operations, to standardize trial conduct and data collection. Junior faculty/fellows/trainees may be limited to obtain comprehensive training at all aspects of early drug development process, and many more years are required for Phase 1 investigators to become fully competent in designing and conducting early phase trials [5,71].

Finally, with the development of multi-armed studies, the use of traditional Phase 2 studies will tend to diminish. By adding dose-expansion cohorts to Phase 1 studies, investigators obtain signs of efficacy in specific patient population, in the context of a single trial, rather than using multiple classical, Phase 2 trials for these purposes [16,46,72]. Despite the known limitations of single-arm Phase 2 studies, a decrease in number of clinical trials for a specific cancer may, eventually, lead to loss of tumor-specific expertise by investigators [72,73].

5.3 DIRECTIONS FOR FUTURE

With the emergence of MTAs, early phase trials have evolved into complex studies, and trial designs have changed with it. Nonetheless, the development of these drugs remains slow and expensive and the rate of drug approvals is suboptimal. We summarize a number of actions that participants involved in clinical research may adopt to overcome barriers and improve efficiency of late stage trials evolving Phase 1 methodologies.

As pointed out earlier, the clinical use of biomarkers in early drug development is rapidly evolving [74]. The use of predictive biomarkers, scientifically validated in preclinical and clinical studies and corresponding drugs (see Section 5.2.1), is assuming a key role in guiding the individualization/personalization of such therapies to patients, based on specific molecular and genomic characteristics of their tumors [16,74]. The advances in next-generation sequencing and the ability to rapidly scan genomic profile of tumors and identify potential targets have helped to build this concept of "precision medicine." There are now several examples of successful development of therapeutic agents targeting some of these cancer drivers, resulting in enhanced clinical outcomes [23]. Patient preselection, or the ability to recognize those patients who are sensitive to the targeted therapies using these "selection" or "proof-of-principle" biomarkers, is an important step to enhance the efficiency of the development process [74]. Moreover, a larger magnitude of effect can be proven in a smaller sample size, which is expected to accelerate the conduct of these studies.

Secondly, the use of pharmacodynamics biomarkers, together with pharmacokinetics data, should be included in the early drug development process. Their information should be used to confirm that first-in-class drugs inhibit its putative biological target and help identifying the biologically active dose range of these therapies [16].

Once the process of selecting patients has been refined, the dose seeking part of drug development can be combined with antitumor activity in the same setting. To achieve this, the design of clinical trials needs to continue to evolve, anticipating the possibility of rapid acceleration, with the creation of multiple expansion cohorts of patients to screen for anti-tumor activity. Investigators should avoid the traditional "3 + 3" design and use other designs that are known to confer greater patient safety and efficiency [28,75–77]. By using these methods that explore signals of activity, one may potentially accelerate the process by going directly to randomized Phase 1/3 studies with mandatory interim analysis and early stopping rules [16].

Finally, the regulatory process will continue to be optimized to accelerate drug development, including more flexible rules for rapid approval of molecular targeted cancer drugs and aggressive timelines for activation times.

In conclusion, cancer drug development has shift from cytotoxic chemotherapy to MTAs, and Phase 1 trials are evolving to adapt to these new era. Study objectives have expanded to provide much more information about efficacy and detection of response signals, in addition to safety. Some of the important changes include novel designs, such as multiarm early phase studies, that allow rapid expansion and acceleration, and the exploration of predictive biomarkers to optimize patient selection.

As we acknowledge the challenges that institutions and investigators face as a result of the changing landscape of Phase 1 trials, the drug development process needs to continue to ameliorate to efficiently discard un-promising compounds and expedite those agents that improve clinical outcomes and ultimately help our patients.

References

[1] Ryerson AB, Eheman CR, Altekruse SF, Ward JW, Jemal A, Sherman RL, et al. Annual Report to the Nation on the Status of Cancer, 1975–2012, featuring the increasing incidence of liver cancer. Cancer 2016;122:1312–37.

[2] Siegel RL, Miller KD, Jemal A. Cancer statistics, 2016. CA Cancer J Clin 2016;66:7–30.

[3] Edwards BK, Noone AM, Mariotto AB, Simard EP, Boscoe FP, Henley SJ, et al. Annual Report to the Nation on the status of cancer, 1975–2010, featuring prevalence of comorbidity and impact on survival among persons with lung, colorectal, breast, or prostate cancer. Cancer 2014;120:1290–314.

[4] Hiom SC. Diagnosing cancer earlier: reviewing the evidence for improving cancer survival. Br J Cancer 2015;112(Suppl. 1):S1–5.

[5] Wong KM, Capasso A, Eckhardt SG. The changing landscape of phase I trials in oncology. Nat Rev Clin Oncol 2016;13:106–17.

[6] Butler T, Maravent S, Boisselle J, Valdes J, Fellner C. A review of 2014 cancer drug approvals, with a look at 2015 and beyond. Pharm Ther 2015;40:191–205.

[7] DiMasi JA, Hansen RW, Grabowski HG. The price of innovation: new estimates of drug development costs. J Health Econ 2003;22:151–85.

[8] Sleijfer S, Verweij J. The price of success: cost-effectiveness of molecularly targeted agents. Clin Pharmacol Ther 2009;85:136–8.

[9] Arrowsmith J. Trial watch: Phase II failures: 2008–2010. Nat Rev Drug Discov 2011;10:328–9.

[10] Arrowsmith J. Trial watch: Phase III and submission failures: 2007–2010. Nat Rev Drug Discov 2011;10:87.

[11] DiMasi JA, Feldman L, Seckler A, Wilson A. Trends in risks associated with new drug development: success rates for investigational drugs. Clin Pharmacol Ther 2010;87:272–7.

[12] Siddiqui M, Rajkumar SV. The high cost of cancer drugs and what we can do about it. Mayo Clin Proc 2012;87:935–43.

[13] Coupe N, Gupta A, Lord SR. Early phase cancer clinical trials: design, ethics and future directions. Br J Hosp Med (Lond) 2015;76:409–13.

[14] Bradbury P, Hilton J, Seymour L. Early-phase oncology clinical trial design in the era of molecularly targeted therapy: pitfalls and progress. Clin Invest 2011;1:33–44.

[15] Brunetto AT, Kristeleit RS, De bono JS. Early oncology clinical trial design in the era of molecular-targeted agents. Future Oncol 2010;6:1339–52.

[16] Yap TA, Sandhu SK, Workman P, De bono JS. Envisioning the future of early anticancer drug development. Nat Rev Cancer 2010;10:514–23.

[17] Verweij J, De jonge M, Eskens F, Sleijfer S. Moving molecular targeted drug therapy towards personalized medicine: issues related to clinical trial design. Mol Oncol 2012;6:196–203.

[18] Mussai FJ, Yap C, Mitchell C, Kearns P. Challenges of clinical trial design for targeted agents against pediatric leukemias. Front Oncol 2014;4:374.

[19] Jain RK, Lee JJ, Hong D, Markman M, Gong J, Naing A, et al. Phase I oncology studies: evidence that in the era of targeted therapies patients on lower doses do not fare worse. Clin Cancer Res 2010;16:1289–97.

[20] Postel-Vinay S, Arkenau HT, Olmos D, Ang J, Barriuso J, Ashley S, et al. Clinical benefit in Phase-I trials of novel molecularly targeted agents: does dose matter? Br J Cancer 2009;100:1373–8.

[21] Hamberg P, Ratain MJ, Lesaffre E, Verweij J. Dose-escalation models for combination phase I trials in oncology. Eur J Cancer 2010;46:2870–8.

[22] Schwaederle M, Zhao M, Lee JJ, Lazar V, Leyland-Jones B, Schilsky RL, et al. Association of biomarker-based treatment strategies with response rates and progression-free survival in refractory malignant neoplasms: a meta-analysis. JAMA Oncol 2016;2:1452–9.

[23] Fang B, Mehran RJ, Heymach JV, Swisher SG. Predictive biomarkers in precision medicine and drug development against lung cancer. Chin J Cancer 2015;34:295–309.

[24] Fong PC, Boss DS, Yap TA, Tutt A, Wu P, Mergui-Roelvink M, et al. Inhibition of poly(ADP-ribose) polymerase in tumors from BRCA mutation carriers. N Engl J Med 2009;361:123–34.

[25] Piccart M, Lohrisch C, Di leo A, Larsimont D. The predictive value of HER2 in breast cancer. Oncology 2001;61(Suppl. 2):73–82.

[26] Smith AD, Roda D, Yap TA. Strategies for modern biomarker and drug development in oncology. J Hematol Oncol 2014;7:70.

[27] Yeung DT, Hughes TP. Therapeutic targeting of BCR-ABL: prognostic markers of response and resistance mechanism in chronic myeloid leukaemia. Crit Rev Oncol 2012;17:17–30.

[28] Ivy SP, Siu LL, Garrett-Mayer E, Rubinstein L. Approaches to phase 1 clinical trial design focused on safety, efficiency, and selected patient populations: a report from the clinical trial design task force of the

national cancer institute investigational drug steering committee. Clin Cancer Res 2010;16:1726−36.

[29] Jardim DL, Hess KR, Lorusso P, Kurzrock R, Hong DS. Predictive value of phase I trials for safety in later trials and final approved dose: analysis of 61 approved cancer drugs. Clin Cancer Res 2014;20:281−8.

[30] Simon R, Freidlin B, Rubinstein L, Arbuck SG, Collins J, Christian MC. Accelerated titration designs for phase I clinical trials in oncology. J Natl Cancer Inst 1997;89:1138−47.

[31] Heath EI, Lorusso PM, Ivy SP, Rubinstein L, Christian MC, Heilbrun LK. Theoretical and practical application of traditional and accelerated titration Phase I clinical trial designs: the Wayne State University experience. J Biopharm Stat 2009;19:414−24.

[32] Iasonos A, O'Quigley J. Adaptive dose-finding studies: a review of model-guided Phase I clinical trials. J Clin Oncol 2014;32:2505−11.

[33] Lorch U, O'kane M, Taubel J. Three steps to writing adaptive study protocols in the early phase clinical development of new medicines. BMC Med Res Methodol 2014;14:84.

[34] Petroni GR, Wages NA, Paux G, Dubois F. Implementation of adaptive methods in early-phase clinical trials. Stat Med 2017;36:215−24.

[35] Brahmachari B, Bhatt A. Adaptive design − an innovative tool in drug development. Indian J Med Res 2011;133:243−5.

[36] Harrington JA, Wheeler GM, Sweeting MJ, Mander AP, Jodrell DI. Adaptive designs for dual-agent phase I dose-escalation studies. Nat Rev Clin Oncol 2013;10:277−88.

[37] Mahajan R, Gupta K. Adaptive design clinical trials: methodology, challenges and prospect. Indian J Pharmacol 2010;42:201−7.

[38] Zang Y, Lee JJ. Adaptive clinical trial designs in oncology. Chin Clin Oncol 2014;3.

[39] Use, C.F.M.P.F.H. European Medicines Agency Committee for Medicinal Products for Human Use (CHMP) guideline on the evaluation of anticancer medicinal products in man. London: European Medicines Agency; 2006.

[40] FDA, U. Guidance for Industry: Adaptive design clinical trials for drugs and biologics. FDA Draft Guidance; 2010.

[41] Division of Quantitative Sciences − Department of Biostatistics, T. U. O. T. M. A. C. C. Software Download Site [Online]. Available: <https://biostatistics.mdanderson.org/SoftwareDownload/>; 2010 [accessed January 2017].

[42] Berry SM, Carlin BP, Lee JJ, Muller P. Bayesian adaptive methods for clinical trials. Boca Raton, FL: CRC Press; 2010.

[43] Rogatko A, Schoeneck D, Jonas W, Tighiouart M, Khuri FR, Porter A. Translation of innovative designs into Phase I Trials. J Clin Oncol 2007;25:4982−6.

[44] Yuan Y, Hess KR, Hilsenbeck SG, Gilbert MR. Bayesian optimal interval design: a simple and well-performing design for Phase I oncology trials. Clin Cancer Res 2016;22:4291−301.

[45] Guo B, Yuan Y. Bayesian Phase I/II Biomarker-based dose finding for precision medicine with molecularly targeted agents. J Am Stat Assoc 2016;112:508−20.

[46] Iasonos A, O'Quigley J. Early phase clinical trials—are dose expansion cohorts needed? Nat Rev Clin Oncol 2015;12:626−8.

[47] Theoret MR, Pai-Scherf LH, Chuk MK, Prowell TM, Balasubramaniam S, Kim T, et al. Expansion cohorts in first-in-human solid tumor oncology trials. Clin Cancer Res 2015;21:4545−51.

[48] Dahlberg SE, Shapiro GI, Clark JW, Johnson BE. Evaluation of statistical designs in Phase I expansion cohorts: the Dana-Farber/Harvard Cancer Center experience. J Natl Cancer Inst 2014;106 dju163.

[49] Manji A, Brana I, Amir E, Tomlinson G, Tannock IF, Bedard PL, et al. Evolution of clinical trial design in early drug development: systematic review of expansion cohort use in single-agent Phase I cancer trials. J Clin Oncol 2013;31:4260−7.

[50] Brower V. Fast tracking drugs to patients: drug approval agencies are frequently criticised for either being too slow or too fast. EMBO Rep 2002;3:14−16.

[51] FDA, U. Food and Drug Administration Safety and Innovation Act (FDASIA) [Online]. Available: <https://www.fda.gov/RegulatoryInformation/Laws EnforcedbyFDA/SignificantAmendmentstotheFDCAct/FDASIA/default.htm>; 2012 [accessed February 2017].

[52] Johnson JR, Ning YM, Farrell A, Justice R, Keegan P, Pazdur R. Accelerated approval of oncology products: the food and drug administration experience. J Natl Cancer Inst 2011;103:636−44.

[53] Kramer DB, Kesselheim AS. User fees and beyond--the FDA Safety and Innovation Act of 2012. N Engl J Med 2012;367:1277−9.

[54] Sherman RE, Li J, Shapley S, Robb M, Woodcock J. Expediting drug development—the FDA's new "breakthrough therapy" designation. N Engl J Med 2013;369:1877−80.

[55] FDA, U. FDA approves Keytruda for advanced melanoma [Online]. Available: <https://www.cancer.org/latest-news/fda-approves-keytruda-pembrolizumab-for-melanoma.html>; 2014 [accessed February 2017].

[56] Horning SJ, Haber DA, Selig WKD, Ivy SP, Roberts SA, Allen JD, et al. Developing standards for breakthrough therapy designation in oncology. Clin Cancer Res 2013;19:4297−304.

[57] Luo FR, Ding J, Chen HX, Liu H, Fung MC, Koehler M, et al. Breakthrough cancer medicine and its impact on novel drug development in China: report of the US Chinese Anti-Cancer Association (USCACA) and Chinese Society of Clinical Oncology (CSCO) Joint Session at the 17th CSCO Annual Meeting. Chin J Cancer 2014;33:620−4.

[58] Kesselheim AS, Tan YT, Avorn J. The roles of academia, rare diseases, and repurposing in the development of the most transformative drugs. Health Aff (Millwood) 2015;34:286−93.

[59] Kesselheim AS, Wang B, Franklin JM, Darrow JJ. Trends in utilization of FDA expedited drug development and approval programs, 1987−2014: cohort study. BMJ 2015;351:h4633.

[60] Shea M, Ostermann L, Hohman R, Roberts S, Kozak M, Dull R, et al. Regulatory watch: impact of breakthrough therapy designation on cancer drug development. Nat Rev Drug Discov 2016;15:152.

[61] Patnaik A, Kang SP, Rasco D, Papadopoulos KP, Elassaiss-Schaap J, Beeram M, et al. Phase I Study of Pembrolizumab (MK-3475; Anti-PD-1 Monoclonal Antibody) in patients with advanced solid tumors. Clin Cancer Res 2015;21:4286−93.

[62] Topalian SL, Hodi FS, Brahmer JR, Gettinger SN, Smith DC, Mcdermott DF, et al. Safety, activity, and immune correlates of Anti−PD-1 antibody in cancer. N Engl J Med 2012;366:2443−54.

[63] Motzer RJ, Escudier B, Mcdermott DF, George S, Hammers HJ, Srinivas S, et al. Nivolumab versus Everolimus in advanced renal-cell carcinoma. N Engl J Med 2015;373:1803−13.

[64] Borghaei H, Paz-Ares L, Horn L, Spigel DR, Steins M, Ready NE, et al. Nivolumab versus Docetaxel in advanced nonsquamous non−small-cell lung cancer. N Engl J Med 2015;373:1627−39.

[65] Weber JS, D'angelo SP, Minor D, Hodi FS, Gutzmer R, Neyns B, et al. Nivolumab versus chemotherapy in patients with advanced melanoma who progressed after anti-CTLA-4 treatment (CheckMate 037): a randomised, controlled, open-label, phase 3 trial. Lancet Oncol 2015;16:375−84.

[66] Bairu M, Chin R. Global clinical trials playbook: capacity and capability building. San Diego, CA: Academic Press; 2012.

[67] Dowlati A, Manda S, Gibbons J, Remick SC, Patrick L, Fu P. Multi-institutional phase I trials of anticancer agents. J Clin Oncol 2008;26:1926−31.

[68] Ibbott GS, Followill DS, Molineu HA, Lowenstein JR, Alvarez PE, Roll JE. Challenges in credentialing institutions and participants in advanced technology multi-institutional clinical trials. Int J Radiat Oncol Biol Phys 2008;71:S71−5.

[69] Craft BS, Kurzrock R, Lei X, Herbst R, Lippman S, Fu S, et al. The changing face of phase 1 cancer clinical trials: new challenges in study requirements. Cancer 2009;115:1592−7.

[70] Tolcher AW, Takimoto CH, Rowinsky EK. The multifunctional, multi-institutional, and sometimes even global phase I study: a better life for phase I evaluations or just "living large"? J Clin Oncol 2002;20:4276−8.

[71] Nature editorial. Early-career researchers need fewer burdens and more support. Nature 2016;538:427.

[72] Sargent DJ, Taylor JMG. Current issues in oncology drug development, with a focus on Phase II trials. J Biopharm Stat 2009;19:556−62.

[73] Grayling MJ, Mander AP. Do single-arm trials have a role in drug development plans incorporating randomised trials? Pharm Stat 2016;15:143−51.

[74] Sawyers CL. The cancer biomarker problem. Nature 2008;452:548−52.

[75] Ballman KV. Phase I trial improvement: a question of patient selection, trial design, or both? J Clin Oncol 2014;32:489−90.

[76] Tolcher AW. The evolution of phase I trials in cancer medicine: a critical review of the last decade. Chin J Cancer 2011;30:815−20.

[77] Wages NA, Conaway MR, O'quigley J. Dose-finding design for multi-drug combinations. Clin Trials 2011;8:380−9.

Designing Trials for Drug Combinations

Susan P. Ivy[1] and Timothy A. Yap[2]

[1]National Institutes of Health, Bethesda, MD, United States [2]The University of Texas MD Anderson Cancer Center, Houston, TX, United States

6.1 INTRODUCTION

In the current age of precision medicine, since the number of drugs that are highly effective as single agents is limited, the development of combinatorial regimens that will enhance antitumor efficacy with minimal adverse events is a high priority in cancer medicine. Fig. 6.1 uses a consort approach to describe the 745 trials of targeted therapy combination Phase 1 trials listed on ClinicalTrials.gov between 2015 and 2017. The development of effective and rational combinations mandates the use of hypothesis-driven clinical investigations, which leverage clinical synthetic lethality, as well as strategies to circumvent adaptive and intrinsic resistance and evidence-driven disruption of cell cycle and immune checkpoints [1].

Current approaches to the development of combination therapies are by necessity broad and general [1]. For instance, the determination of the most promising agents to combine is daunting in its complexity and may be context and disease dependent. The National Cancer Institute's Cancer Therapy Evaluation Program has been studying investigational drug combinations since 2001 (Fig. 6.2A and B). The systematic evaluation of every possible regimen to assess combinatorial additivity or synergy is not practical clinically in view of the fiscal and operational burdens involved, potentially insufficient numbers of patients, and limited time to design and conduct rational clinical trials. Although taking a blunderbuss approach preclinically in multiple cell lines and xenograft models has led to several interesting leads, often no specific disease indication for combination evaluation is established [2]. This line of approach is not without merit and does not suggest that the preclinical evaluation of combination therapy is unimportant. The concept of clinical synthetic lethality, where two drugs are combined that have minimal activity individually, and that possibly would not proceed in development as single agents, should be considered. When combined, these drugs may have superadditive effects, leading to exceptionally high response rates clinically, improved overall survival in patients, and potentially enhanced treatment effects in diseases where no therapeutic advances have been observed. Such a combination approach

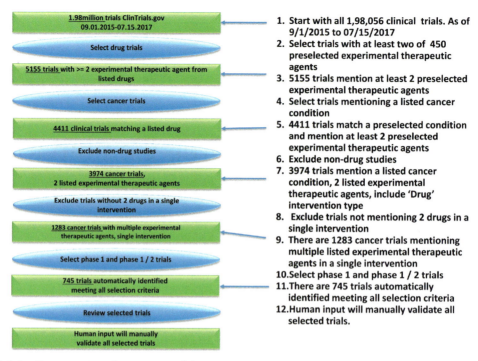

FIGURE 6.1   Consort review of investigational drug combination clinical trials listed in www.clinicaltrials.gov between 2015 and 2017.

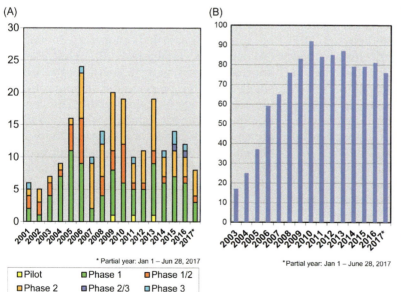

FIGURE 6.2   (A) Investigational combination clinical trials activated for enrollment from the National Cancer Institutes' Cancer Therapy Evaluation Program. This bar graph depicts investigational combination trials of all development phases being activated for patient enrollment annually on the X-axis from 2001 to 2017. The Y-axis indicates the number of trials activated. (B) Investigation combination clinical trials enrolling patients from the National Cancer Institutes' Cancer Therapy Evaluation Program. This bar graph depicts the combination trials actively enrolling patients on treatment by calendar year on the X-axis. The Y-axis indicates the number of trials enrolling patients.

requires robust preclinical evaluation and rapid clinical testing.

6.2 FEATURES OF RATIONAL COMBINATION TRIALS

Conducting investigational combination trials is a great opportunity for clinical research, but there are potential pitfalls [3] (Table 6.1). Although the approaches to combination therapy are diverse, there are common features that are critical to the development of rational combination treatment regimens. First, a hypothesis-driven approach should carefully consider the disease context in which they will be used as combination therapy [3]. Second, a hypothesis-driven approach should leverage standard principles of cancer biology used for the interrogation of conserved pathways and processes that are critical for homeostasis and wellness [3]. Third, the proposed drug combination should use drugs that are molecularly targeted small molecules or biologics that have completed or nearly completed single agent Phase 1 trial testing, and for which a dose and schedule is already known [4]. Fourth, the pathway or process being targeted should have biomarkers that can be used for patient or treatment selection or stratification to assess pharmacokinetic or pharmacodynamic effects. With the advent of precision medicine, we have gained exceptional insights into the cancer genome, transcriptome, transcription interference (loss- or gain-of-function), receptors, and other factors that drive cancers or normal body functions. Fifth, the risk for drug–drug interactions (DDIs) [5] and overlapping toxicity profiles should be determined [6] (Fig. 6.3). Sixth, pharmacokinetics for DDIs or interference and/or normal body functions should be formally evaluated [6]. Seventh, documentation of biochemical or biological effects of the regimen to isolate the individual contributions of each drug in the combination should be planned; there should be a thorough understanding of the pharmacodynamic effects of the combination. Eighth, clinical combination testing of the hypothesis evaluating outcomes and validated biomarker modulation to assess early or intermediate endpoints, such as pharmacodynamic modulation or response to therapy in small or large expansion cohorts should be undertaken [6,7]. Ninth, comparative analysis of trial results should evaluate patient outcomes with in-depth studies of the molecular differences between responders and nonresponders. Exceptional responders should be studied to

TABLE 6.1 Opportunities and Pitfalls of Combination Therapies

Opportunities	Pitfalls
Validate novel biological hypotheses	Unreliable preclinical models
Synergize antitumor effect without synergizing toxicity	Not achieving optimal selection of drugs and targets to study in combination
Increase therapeutic index/window	Not achieving optimal sequence and dose of combination therapy
Synthetic lethality: optimize combination use of single agents with limited single agent activity	Risk overlapping toxicity
Counteract primary and secondary resistance	Lack of standard design for Phase 1/2 combination therapies
Develop novel indications for existing and approved drugs	Competing interests of researchers, corporations, and institutions to combine treatments

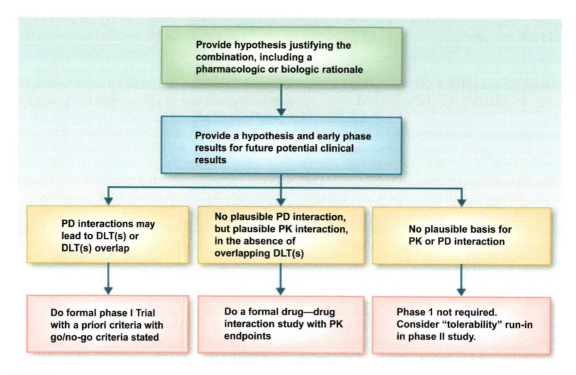

FIGURE 6.3 Pragmatic considerations for early phase clinical trials. When considering combinations, the investigator should have a hypothesis and pharmacological and/or biological rationale. Further to this point, the anticipated clinical results should be stated. The next level of decision making is related to evaluation of overlapping toxicities and anticipated pharmacokinetic/pharmacodynamic (PK/PD) interactions. The fourth and final level for consideration describes the type of clinical investigation to be performed. Source: *Adapted from Paller CJ, Bradbury PA, Ivy SP, Seymour L, Lorusso PM, Baker L, et al. Design of phase I combination trials: recommendations of the Clinical Trial Design Task Force of the NCI Investigational Drug Steering Committee. Clin Cancer Res 2014;20:4210−7.*

gain an understanding of what characteristics made them responsive and what data may be used as future selection markers [8]. Progressors should also be studied to understand the underlying etiology of treatment failure, including but not limited to intrinsic, compensatory, and acquired mechanisms of resistance to therapy [9]. Elucidating the plasticity of malignancies that allows them to adapt and survive has the potential to potentiate the development of optimal and precise combination therapies that are context and disease specific. Tenth, an optimized approach should promote a systematic evaluation of both individual and

population-based cancers [10]. Finally, an optimized approach should result in a systematic evaluation of individual and population-based understanding of cancer in its many forms and stages.

Such a stepwise and system-based approach to general drug development and drug combinations is the foundation for optimized precision medicine. Workman first described this compelling need to understand pharmacology and pharmacodynamics in drug development [11]. This hypothesis-driven, evidence-based approach developed into the pharmacological audit trail, the latest reiteration of which incorporated basic molecular testing and monitoring [12]. Expanding on this concept, the addition of more detailed and comprehensive molecular characterization of patient specimens during the conduct of early phase clinical trials adds another layer of elements to what could now be called the molecular and pharmacological audit trail (MoPhAT) (Fig. 6.4). Expansion of the concepts and approaches provided above will be discussed in this chapter on designing trials of combination therapies.

As with all hypothesis-driven research, the investigator should begin with the end in mind. Define what tumor or tumors would be expected to respond to the planned combination therapy. Is there sufficient evidence of activity in these tumors with either drug to expect modest single agent activity? Do the tumors studied share a genetic, metabolic, or other aberration that is associated with their genotype or phenotype? For example, tumors such as cholangiocarcinoma and glioblastoma multiforme harbor isocitrate dehydrogenase (IDH) 1 and 2 mutations produce an oncometabolite that suppresses homologous recombination, thus creating a "BRCAness" phenotype and potentially sensitizing them to poly (ADP-ribose) polymerase (PARP) inhibitors [13]. Neither of these tumors is treated in a similar fashion. Alternatively, can targeting two independent processes, such as the cell cycle and DNA replication and repair, be an effective approach? The cell cycle checkpoint kinase 1/2 (CHK1/2) inhibitor LY2606368 and the PARP inhibitor olaparib were hypothesized to act synergistically as the CHK1/2 inhibitor prevents RAD51 foci formation, fostering sensitivity to PARP inhibition and further limiting DNA damage repair. This combination was demonstrated to have synergistic activity in high-grade serous ovarian cancer cell lines. Although the combination of cell cycle inhibitors with PARP inhibitors awaits further clinical testing, what is clear is that the preclinical data supporting the hypothesis are strong. If DNA replication and repair is blocked at various stages along the cell cycle and if the cell cycle is inhibited, mitosis is stalled, which leaves highly proliferative cells vulnerable since cellular regulators and checkpoints are disrupted [14]. The combination of two drugs, cediranib and olaparib, both reasonably active but not sufficient for further single agent development in ovarian cancer, targeted the tissue microenvironment, hypoxia, angiogenesis, and DNA repair. When combined, these drugs had superadditive clinical effects [15]. In these examples, the common theme is that the hypothesis for the combination drives both the preclinical and clinical development of the combination, which is often undertaken in a context/disease-dependent fashion.

6.3 BIOMARKERS

Biomarkers play a critical role in the development of combination therapies as they are used to isolate the effects of individual agents in the regimen. The use of biomarkers in combinatorial clinical trials is essential to the activity or efficacy of the combination outcome by allowing for the discrimination of individual drug effects. Biomarkers may be stratified in several categories: descriptive (diagnostic and pharmacodynamics), predictive, prognostic, and surrogate (Fig. 6.5A). A prognostic biomarker is clinically meaningful, measurable, and provides individual patient information independent of the treatment or treatment regimen that a patient has received. A predictive biomarker is also clinically meaningful and measurable but provides individual patient information that is directly associated to the response to treatment intervention or toxicity. Descriptive biomarkers may provide information on factors that describe the pharmacodynamic effects of treatment or define diagnostic elements. Surrogate biomarkers are used as a substitute for a clinically meaningful endpoint [16]. The biomarkers

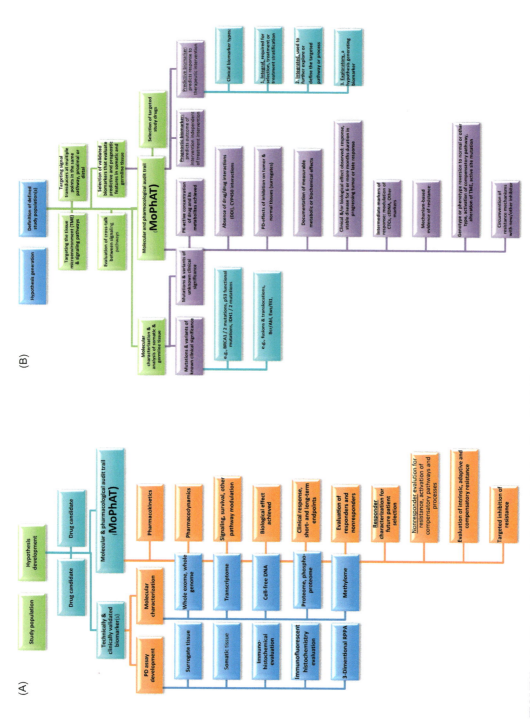

FIGURE 6.4 The molecular and pharmacological audit trail (MoPhAT). (A) The flow diagram provides the steps necessary for the sequential development of molecular targeted combination therapies. (B) The panel addresses the questions and processes for evaluation of combination therapy following the MoPhAT audit trail for combination drug development.

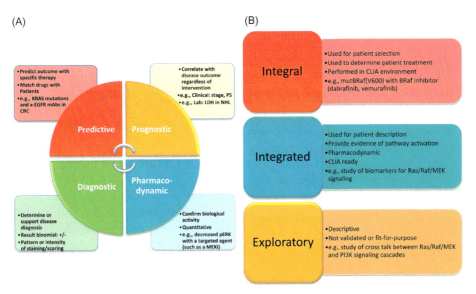

FIGURE 6.5 (A) The contribution of biomarkers in early and late phase trials. The roles of descriptive and pharmacodynamic markers are described. Prognostic biomarkers are treatment independent and predictive biomarkers are treatment dependent. (B) Outline of the definitions and utility of integral, integrated, and exploratory biomarkers. A description of each type of biomarker and how, when, and where it is used is provided.

with the highest level of interest are those that predict response to treatment.

When clinically evaluating biomarkers, they may be categorized as integral, integrated, or exploratory (Fig. 6.5B). The integral marker is used for patient selection, treatment assignment, or stratification. Inherent to the study, integral biomarkers must be performed at the time of study entry, or prior to therapy. Furthermore, integral biomarkers must be analytically and technically validated, performed in a CLIA laboratory environment, and may require an investigational device exemption when used in later phases of trial settings. All integral biomarkers require mandatory acquisition of tissue for participation in a clinical trial.

Integrated biomarkers are used to identify assays or tests that further define the molecular or pharmacodynamic features of a patient's tumor during exposure to treatment. In general, the integrated marker is also being evaluated for future use and whether it may

prove predictive. The marker may be used to define on target effects that may predict response to therapy and be used for patient selection in the future. As with integral biomarkers, a prespecified statistical plan for the evaluation and analysis of integrated biomarkers is essential. Integrated biomarkers may be defined as mandatory if an invasive procedure with increased risk is required for collection of the specimen.

The exploratory biomarker does not have mandatory tissue collection requirements, but rather is used to generate new data and is meant to be hypothesis-generating. The exploratory marker does not require the level of analytical and technical validation necessary for assay development of an integral or integrated biomarker. The data generated from exploratory biomarkers are not critical and fundamental to the combination trial completion and analysis.

All biomarkers must be prioritized within the context of the combination clinical trial.

The lack of prioritization is a fundamental flaw in many clinical trials and often leads to the inability to evaluate the biomarkers in the context of outcome results. Each biomarker must be clearly identified, characterized, and analyzed using a defined statistical analysis plan. Another serious shortfall of biomarker analysis is the lack of complete or any characterization and analysis. The most egregious error an investigator can make is to collect tissue and never analyze the specimen. Another issue is that poor biomarker planning without prioritization may result in the most critical assays of the study not being performed, leading to an uninterpretable study. Biomarkers provide a wealth of information on precious clinical specimens and should not be wasted due to poor planning, characterization, and analysis. All biomarkers planned for clinical studies must have strong scientific and laboratory underpinnings and directly add value to the investigation.

6.4 FIT-FOR-PURPOSE ASSAYS AND ANALYSES

All biomarker assays and analyses should be fit-for-purpose (Fig. 6.6A) [17]. Assays that are analytically and technically valid share the

(A)

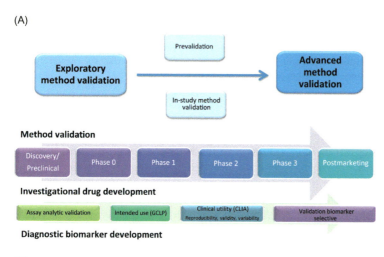

(B)

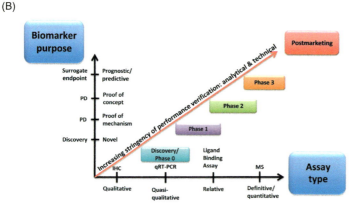

FIGURE 6.6 (A) Fit-for-purpose drug and biomarker development. The flow diagrams illustrate concurrent assay and methodology validation throughout phases of drug development for a diagnostic biomarker. (B) Fit-for-purpose biomarker and drug development related to biomarker purpose and assay type. The biomarker purpose changes over time progressing from novel to proof of mechanism and purpose to an analytically and technically validated predictive or prognostic biomarker performed in the context of a clinical trial and in a CLIA environment. The stringency of the assay moves from qualitative to definitive and quantitative. The requirements for a fit-for-purpose marker increase in stringency the later the phase of clinical development.

following common features: (1) they are reliable and reproducible with limited inter- and intravariation of results; (2) these assays are accurate, precise, and measurable; (3) they are sensitive and specific, and the analyte is studied in duplicate or triplicate at a minimum; and (4) they are robust, not prone to operator error, and are defined by locked standard operating procedures. Another feature of a robust assay is that all the preanalytical variables have been evaluated and preferably tested to assure limited operator and institutional variability in specimen collection, handling, and storage conditions. Finally, the stringency of testing and validation of biomarkers increases as the phase of study changes and matures. The analytical and technical validation of the biomarker assay is highest when it is used as an integral biomarker for patient or treatment selection (Fig. 6.6B).

Assay development is a highly collaborative process as the test moves from discovery to clinical utility. For example, clinical validation requires the skills of laboratory scientists, bioinformaticians, and clinicians, while analytical validation requires computational scientists and statisticians. The result is a clinically useful assay or test.

A final note of caution is not to confuse diagnostic assays with pharmacodynamic assays that require a dynamic range for performance. For example, a diagnostic assay is commonly used for tumor marker identification with immunohistochemistry performed at saturating concentrations of antibody in a CLIA-certified laboratory. However, the same assay is not fit-for-purpose when being used quantitatively to measure the modulatory effects of a drug on the same diagnostic specimen, even though used in a CLIA environment. The pharmacodynamic assay is evaluating the same epitope with the same antibody, but not at saturating concentrations, as a measurable dynamic range of modulatory activity is being evaluated.

6.5 MANAGEMENT OF ADVERSE EVENTS WITH COMBINATION TREATMENT

6.5.1 Overlapping Toxicity Management in Combination Trials

A major challenge that remains in the development of combinatorial approaches is the management of overlapping toxicities. Key issues include the use of rational dosing and scheduling, causality attribution of adverse events, and addressing chronic low-grade toxicities, which may not have been picked up during the single agent or combination therapy dose-limiting toxicity period. To enable these issues to be addressed effectively, it is important for each component drug to already have completed monotherapy Phase 1 trial testing with the maximum tolerated dose or recommended Phase 2 dose established, and to have data available from pharmacokinetic, pharmacodynamic (biologically effective dose), and other biomarker studies. For example, by knowing the maximum tolerated and biologically effective dose ranges of both drugs, we can rationally select a limited number of focused dose levels for the combination regimen to rapidly reach the recommended monotherapy Phase 2 doses of both drugs if feasible [3]. In addition, such key monotherapy data will also aid in the design of both the dose and schedule of the combination trial and the incorporation of hypothesis-testing combination assessments.

6.5.2 Drug–Drug Interactions and Toxicity

Understanding DDIs is a critical part of the drug development process as polypharmacy has become commonplace in many therapeutic areas, including the cancer patient population. Many small molecule targeted agents are cytochrome P450 (CYP) inducers, inhibitors, or substrates; thus, investigating CYP-mediated

DDI profiles for therapies used in the oncology setting is of critical importance when treating cancer patients who have complex medical conditions [18,19]. The concomitant medications administered with CYP interactive agents can potentially alter the effective concentrations of the cancer therapy and may even increase concentrations to toxic levels. Evaluating DDI preclinically and being attuned to clinical risks is important, as the outcomes and endpoints of an early phase trial will be affected (Fig. 6.3).

6.5.3 Acute and Chronic Adverse Events in Combination Clinical Trials

The combination of molecularly targeted agents will commonly involve overlapping toxicities, especially gastrointestinal ones through the combination of orally administered agents, and nonspecific adverse events, such as fatigue. Chronic toxicities, including mild grade 2 toxicities, which limit the long-term administration of a combination regimen, should also be considered when establishing the recommended Phase 2 combination dose. This is especially important since there is now evidence that Phase 1 studies underestimate toxicities when recommending doses of small-molecule targeted agents, albeit based on modest numbers of patients. In a retrospective study, it was estimated that approximately 45% of patients in large Phase 3 trials required dose modifications from doses/schedules established in Phase 1 trials due to drug-related toxicities observed [20]. Such issues will certainly come to the fore with the emergence of novel combination regimens involving such targeted agents.

6.6 CLINICAL COMBINATION TRIAL CONSIDERATIONS

While strategies to deal with such overlapping toxicities need to be individualized depending on the agents involved, potential solutions may involve the use of high-dose, pulsatile schedules of one or both drugs, in contrast to continuous low doses to improve tolerability and potentially widen the therapeutic window of combinatorial regimens (Fig. 6.7A). The pulsatile dosing of drugs will also permit more target and pathway blockade compared with continuous dosing, and may potentially minimize tumor cell adaptation and eventual secondary drug resistance. To guide dose and scheduling in clinical trials, it will be important to preclinically define the extent and duration of target and signaling pathway inhibition required for an optimal antitumor benefit and an acceptable therapeutic window.

Another key challenge in the development of combination regimens is determining if the combination is biologically and clinically "active" (i.e., Do two drugs have synergistic activity?). While the well-established method of proving this is through suitably powered, randomized Phase 3 clinical trials, it is important to minimize the risk of failure of such combination studies in early phase clinical trials. One could provide valuable proof-of-concept for a combination by assessing a "reversal-of-resistance" approach in Phase 1/2 trials by adding the combination at disease progression to the single agent (Fig. 6.7B). Early determination of the superiority of the combination is important in view of the large number of potential drug combinations that can be evaluated.

Although the primary approaches to combination therapy involve concurrent drug administration, in some instances, these prove to be too toxic. This may be due to overlapping toxicity profiles for the two drugs, CYP interactions, DDI, or pharmacokinetic/pharmacodynamic interference. Regardless of the cause, two other approaches to trial design should be considered. The first and most practical is an alternating approach where each drug is given for one or multiple cycles and then followed by the other

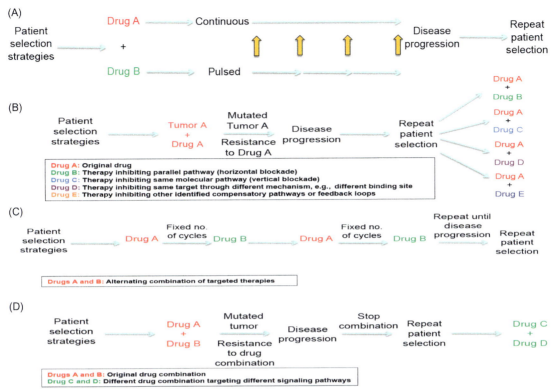

FIGURE 6.7   (A) Pulsed dosing approach: After patient selection strategies, two appropriate therapies are commenced, with one drug administered on a continuous dosing schedule and the partner drug augmenting the combination administered on a pulsed schedule. Such a strategy may reduce the potential for the development of antitumor drug resistance. This strategy should be continued until disease progression, when repeat patient selection is undertaken. (B) Reversal of resistance approach: By using gene sequencing strategies, it may be possible to select appropriate patient populations to target with a potent and specific targeted therapy. When drug resistance to tumor A develops, with resulting disease progression, patient selection strategies should be repeated and an appropriate drug (Drugs B–E) added to Drug A to reverse such acquired drug resistance. (C) Alternating approach: By using gene sequencing strategies, it may be possible to select appropriate patient populations to target with a potent and specific targeted therapy. When drug resistance to Tumor A develops, with resulting disease progression, patient selection strategies should be repeated and an appropriate drug (Drugs B–E) added to Drug A to reverse such acquired drug resistance. (D) Sequential approach: With this approach, the combined targeting of appropriate signaling pathways with Drug A and Drug B should be undertaken after appropriate patient selection strategies. Once disease progression ensues because of drug resistance, the original combination should be stopped. Patient selection strategies should be repeated and a new combination of drugs started.

drug or drugs. This alternating sequence is repeated until progression of disease or loss of clinical benefit (Fig. 6.7C). The second is perhaps the most traditional approach in which combination regimens are given sequentially, thus minimizing overlapping toxicity, and perhaps, DDI (Fig. 6.7D). Each of these approaches

presents opportunities and challenges that will provide options for clinicians planning to perform combination clinical trials with investigational drugs using an evidence-based and hypothesis-driven approach (Table 6.2).

It is noteworthy that there has been an increase in the number of seamless Phase 1/2

TABLE 6.2   Approaches to Combination Therapies

Approaches	Pitfalls
Pulsed	Arguably more likely to impact survival if tolerability is an issue
Reversal of resistance	Proof of concept when one drug has antitumor activity
Alternating	Rational for study of agents that cannot be combined
Sequential	Traditional approach generally used in medical oncology

trials, which will likely lead to fewer single-arm Phase 2 trials in the future. Such Phase 1/2 trials have the advantages of speed and the potential fiscal benefits of avoiding the setup of completely new Phase 2 trials, which are often not powered to address key combination therapy questions [12]. These seamless Phase 1/2 studies should be designed to justify randomized Phase 2/3 trials, which can then be suitably powered to enable the regulatory approval of such combination regimens, or be discontinued for futility through predefined interim analyses. In the likely rare situation where the combination regimen demonstrates significant antitumor efficacy and safety in a well-defined tumor or molecular context within the Phase 1/2 trial, accelerated regulatory approval should be obtained directly as guided by the FDA.

The current conventional Phase 1 trial design for novel therapies usually involves dose and/or schedule escalation/deescalation in distinct patient cohorts. The use of intrapatient dose escalation schemas in combination studies have recently been proposed [3]. With such a strategy, intrapatient dose escalation is undertaken in individual patients receiving different schedules of the combination. Dose schedules found to be toxic or that have poor pharmacokinetic–pharmacodynamic profiles are discontinued, whereas promising schedules are taken forward through expanded cohorts of patients, preferably involving those with specific molecularly defined tumor types. Bayesian adaptive design models incorporating

the analysis of data from multiple doses and schedules may also be considered with such a design. Such an approach has the potential to optimize drug exposures in individual patients, compare multiple combination schedules, and reduce the need for a large Phase 1 trial.

There are also important biological and ethical reasons for pursuing an intrapatient dose escalation study for combinatorial regimens. For example, since interpatient pharmacokinetic variability and interpatient tumor heterogeneity remains an issue with many oral antitumor agents, optimizing drug exposures at an individual level to minimize the number of patients receiving inactive drug doses may prove effective. One could assess drug trough levels for pharmacokinetic studies, perform pharmacodynamic detailed profiling of target and/or pathway blockade using serial normal or tumor tissue sampling, or perform functional molecular imaging to determine target modulation at different patient disease sites. A more clinical approach might be monitoring patients clinically while undertaking intrapatient dose escalation until a well-recognized predefined toxicity measure is detected, such as skin rash with epidermal growth factor receptor or Mitogen-activated protein kinase (MAPK)/Extracellular Signal-regulated kinase (ERK) = (MEK) inhibitors. In using such approaches, it will be important to establish the maximum tolerated dose and biologically active dose ranges in single agent trials to ensure that both safety and drug disposition data will be available for both drugs.

6.7 TRIAL OPTIMIZATION FOR COMBINATION THERAPIES

Although approaches to combination clinical trials may be varied, several challenges and issues are relatively common, including biological challenges, pharmacological issues, toxicity issues, trial design approaches and issues, intellectual property issues, and ethical issues related to patients. While considering these challenges, the investigator may also avail themselves of the opportunities presented to directly address problems common to combination therapy development with defined approaches to optimize combination studies [3].

One of the primary biological challenges is the approach to the optimal selection of drugs and their targets. All drugs in the same class may each act in a context-dependent fashion, thus suggesting that each may be used in unique clinical settings. To effectively address this challenge, hypothesis-driven biological and preclinical evidence should be developed. The other challenge is the lack of a wide repertoire of investigational drugs and potential targets. The predictive value of preclinical models for combination therapies as with single-agent preclinical evaluation is also relatively poor. At present, newer types of models, such as transgenics and patient-derived xenografts, hold enormous potential, as do high-throughput screening platforms for combination analysis. Furthermore, patients may have highly variable pharmacokinetics, and thus dose optimization can become an issue. A high degree of tumor heterogeneity with documented inter- and intrapatient variability highlights the need for upfront patient selection and intrapatient dose escalation. The use of surrogate biomarkers in normal tissue may not reflect the same outcomes in tumor. Each of these challenges should be directly addressed, and whenever possible, resolved prior to trial initiation.

The pharmacological issues that arise often relate to the inhibition of target or complete pathway blockade, as well as duration and degree of signaling suppression. An approach is to determine the pharmacokinetic/pharmacodynamic exposures and target them using high-throughput preclinical models. Furthermore, the determination of antitumor activity of an active drug or drug substance using crossover designs at the time of progression can assist in the clinical evaluation of the study agent. Another critical step is the clinical assessment of the target and pathway blockade by obtaining tumor tissue to determine pharmacokinetic/pharmacodynamic profiles and using multiplexed kinase assays to evaluate both tumor and normal tissue. Optimizing the dose, schedule, and sequence of combination drug administration allows for determination of the optimal dose, schedule, and sequence of the study agents. A variety of schedules can be explored in parallel. The use of intrapatient dose escalation can minimize the number of patients required to complete a clinical combination study efficiently. A final pitfall is the incomplete or inaccurate understanding of the underlying mechanism of action for each drug in the combination. The performance of meticulous preclinical studies that are biologically driven and that study both single agents and the combination can be of value.

Overlapping toxicity issues are often due to a very narrow therapeutic index for one or both study drugs, and either drug may have cumulative toxicity due to pharmacokinetic clearance. An approach to this problem is to use intermittent or pulsatile dosing to allow plasma concentrations of the drug to decrease. The other pharmacokinetic problem is drug interactions. It may be possible to circumvent this problem by performing extensive pharmacokinetic studies in predictive animal models to prepare for or to ameliorate this problem prior to clinical testing.

Clinical trial design strategies are important as trials fail when they are poorly designed and the outcomes and endpoints become uninterpretable. Very large early phase trials or studies that fail to complete in a timely fashion waste time, effort, and most importantly, patients. Several types of designs that are more adaptive in nature may provide opportunities to efficiently study combination treatment regimens, such as studies using intrapatient dose escalation, accelerated titration limiting the number of patients treated at nontherapeutic dose levels, evaluation of multiple schedules at the same time, and seamless Phase 1/2 trial designs. To avoid inadequate and futile trial designs, it may be beneficial to seek additional guidance from regulatory officials and input from early phase clinical trial experts.

Intellectual property issues have been one of the major challenges to performing investigational/investigational drug combinations. The legal ramifications for two separate sponsors to collaborate remain a hurdle, although this problem is diminishing. A more effective strategy to bridge this problem is through a neutral third party or honest broker, such as government or academia. The structuring of agreements between two parties using nonexclusive, royalty free licenses has also been effective. Defining the regulatory and agreement environment on agreed common principles, when needed, enhances development of either single or combination regimens.

Finally, there are ethical challenges for combination therapy studies in which the individual contributions of both drugs must be teased out. Such studies often require serial tumor biopsies that are invasive in nature. The simplest scenario that presents as an alternative is harvesting circulating tumor cells or cell free DNA. Exposing patients to subtherapeutic doses of drug tests ethical boundaries, but using novel trial designs, such as the accelerated titration design or intrapatient dose escalation, ameliorate this problem to an extent. Switching from concurrent drug administration to pulsatile or alternating dosing regimens will often diminish the cumulative dosing or toxicity effects. Defining the maximum tolerated dose and toxicity profile in single-agent studies initially is often more efficient. Despite all the challenges outlined above, the opportunities afforded to patients to improve outcomes by exploring novel combination treatment regimens generally outweigh the risks associated with minimally invasive procedures.

6.8 SUMMARY AND CONCLUSIONS

Detailed pragmatic considerations for the design of early phase clinical trials, as well as the MoPhAT, which is a framework that includes all the steps necessary for the successful development of molecular targeted combination regimens, have been proposed. Key definitions of the different biomarkers used and how they should be developed, validated, and incorporated in combination clinical trials have been outlined. Finally, several novel trial designs to consider when developing early phase trials involving rational combinations of antitumor agents have been discussed. Overall, clinical trial designs for combination regimens should ideally include toxicity monitoring strategies during dose escalation, mechanism-of-action combinatorial pharmacodynamic studies, detailed pharmacokinetic profiling (including DDI pharmacokinetic studies), and exploratory studies to assess putative predictive biomarkers of response and resistance of the combination. Such biomarker-based studies will enable the clinical testing of rational combinatorial regimens of investigational agents using an evidence-based and hypothesis-driven approach. Such efforts will allow us to fully exploit both our improved understanding of cancer biology and the latest technological advances, leading to accelerated drug development and improved outcomes for patients.

References

[1] Kummar S, Chen HX, Wright J, Holbeck S, Millin MD, Tomaszewski J, et al. Utilizing targeted cancer therapeutic agents in combination: novel approaches and urgent requirements. Nat Rev Drug Discov 2010;9:843−56.

[2] Holbeck SL, Camalier R, Crowell JA, Govindharajulu JP, Hollingshead M, Anderson LW, et al. The National Cancer Institute ALMANAC: a comprehensive screening resource for the detection of anticancer drug pairs with enhanced therapeutic activity. Cancer Res 2017;77:3564−76.

[3] Yap TA, Omlin A, De bono JS. Development of therapeutic combinations targeting major cancer signaling pathways. J Clin Oncol 2013;31:1592−605.

[4] Banerji U, Workman P. Critical parameters in targeted drug development: the pharmacological audit trail. Semin Oncol 2016;43:436−45.

[5] Fulda TR, Valuck RJ, Vander zanden J, Parker S, Byrns PJ, Panel TUPDURA. Disagreement among drug compendia on inclusion and ratings of drug-drug interactions. Curr Ther Res 2000;61:540−8.

[6] Paller CJ, Bradbury PA, Ivy SP, Seymour L, Lorusso PM, Baker L, et al. Design of phase I combination trials: recommendations of the Clinical Trial Design Task Force of the NCI Investigational Drug Steering Committee. Clin Cancer Res 2014;20:4210−17.

[7] Tan DS, Thomas GV, Garrett MD, Banerji U, De bono JS, Kaye SB, et al. Biomarker-driven early clinical trials in oncology: a paradigm shift in drug development. Cancer J 2009;15:406−20.

[8] Abrams J, Conley B, Mooney M, Zwiebel J, Chen A, Welch JJ, et al. National Cancer Institute's Precision Medicine Initiatives for the new National Clinical Trials Network. Am Soc Clin Oncol Educ Book 2014;71−6.

[9] Henning W, Sturzbecher HW. Homologous recombination and cell cycle checkpoints: Rad51 in tumour progression and therapy resistance. Toxicology 2003;193:91−109.

[10] Hood L, Heath JR, Phelps ME, Lin B. Systems biology and new technologies enable predictive and preventative medicine. Science 2004;306:640−3.

[11] Workman P. How much gets there and what does it do?: The need for better pharmacokinetic and pharmacodynamic endpoints in contemporary drug discovery and development. Curr Pharm Des 2003;9:891−902.

[12] Yap TA, Sandhu SK, Workman P, De bono JS. Envisioning the future of early anticancer drug development. Nat Rev Cancer 2010;10:514−23.

[13] Sulkowski PL, Corso CD, Robinson ND, Scanlon SE, Purshouse KR, Bai H, et al. 2-Hydroxyglutarate produced by neomorphic IDH mutations suppresses homologous recombination and induces PARP inhibitor sensitivity. Sci Transl Med 2017;9:eaal2463.

[14] Lin AB, Mcneely SC, Beckmann RP. Achieving precision death with cell-cycle inhibitors that target DNA replication and repair. Clin Cancer Res 2017;23:3232−40.

[15] Liu JF, Barry WT, Birrer M, Lee JM, Buckanovich RJ, Fleming GF, et al. Combination cediranib and olaparib versus olaparib alone for women with recurrent platinum-sensitive ovarian cancer: a randomised phase 2 study. Lancet Oncol 2014;15:1207−14.

[16] Dancey JE, Dobbin KK, Groshen S, Jessup JM, Hruszkewycz AH, Koehler M, et al. Guidelines for the development and incorporation of biomarker studies in early clinical trials of novel agents. Clin Cancer Res 2010;16:1745−55.

[17] Cummings J, Raynaud F, Jones L, Sugar R, Dive C. Fit-for-purpose biomarker method validation for application in clinical trials of anticancer drugs. Br J Cancer 2010;103:1313−17.

[18] Huang SM, Temple R, Throckmorton DC, Lesko LJ. Drug interaction studies: study design, data analysis, and implications for dosing and labeling. Clin Pharmacol Ther 2007;81:298−304.

[19] Waters NJ. Evaluation of drug-drug interactions for oncology therapies: in vitro-in vivo extrapolation model-based risk assessment. Br J Clin Pharmacol 2015;79:946−58.

[20] Roda D, Jimenez B, Banerji U. Are doses and schedules of small-molecule targeted anticancer drugs recommended by Phase I studies realistic? Clin Cancer Res 2016;22:2127−32.

Further Reading

Food and Drug Administration. Guidance for Industry: Co-development of two or more new investigational drugs for use in combination, <https://www.fda.gov/downloads/drugs/guidances/ucm236669.pdf> [accessed 27.07.17].

Dose Selection of Targeted Oncology Drugs in Early Development: Time for Change?

Bahru A. Habtemariam[1], Lian Ma[2], Brian Booth[2], Olanrewaju O. Okusanya[2] and Nitin Mehrotra[3]

[1]Alnylam Pharmaceuticals, Cambridge, MA, United States [2]U.S. Food and Drug Administration, Silver Spring, MD, United States [3]Merck and Co, Kenilworth, NJ, United States

Disclaimer: The views expressed are those of the authors' and do not reflect official policy of the FDA. No official endorsement by the FDA is intended or should be inferred.

7.1 INTRODUCTION

Adequate dose selection for targeted oncology drugs can result in better efficacy and minimize the risk for toxicities that lead to high rates of treatment discontinuation and dose reduction. Less than optimal dose selection in many cases is due to tolerability-driven dose selection that was developed for cytotoxic chemotherapy drugs as far back as the early 1940s. This chapter addresses the following topics: (1) discusses the importance of optimal dose selection from the perspectives of different stakeholders, (2) highlights current dose selection approaches for targeted oncology drugs, and (3) provides proposed approaches for optimal dose selection. A few case studies are provided at the end of the chapter to highlight the different issues discussed in the main text.

7.2 IMPORTANCE OF OPTIMAL DOSE SELECTION

7.2.1 Patient Perspective

Paracelsus, in the 15th century, has been attributed with the saying, "All things are poison, and nothing is without poison, the dosage alone makes it so a thing is not a poison." This adage is supported by our knowledge that drugs have a therapeutic window, which is bound by ineffectiveness at one end and unacceptable toxicity at the other. At very high doses, the drug exposure will be above the therapeutic window and the harm from drug toxicity could outweigh any therapeutic benefit. On the other hand, doses that are too low will not be effective. Therefore, appropriate dose selection to balance efficacy and safety is of great importance. In the past, most cancers were terminal diseases. To prolong survival, it was necessary to administer the highest dose that a patient could reasonably tolerate to maximize efficacy. This was the beginning of the maximum-tolerable-dose (MTD) paradigm in oncology drug development. However, recent breakthroughs in cancer treatment make many cancers more like chronic diseases, with patients surviving longer, and remaining on treatment for longer periods than in the past. Given the longer duration of therapy, dose selection that optimizes efficacy and minimizes toxicity allows the patient to take the drug for a longer period of time which may be conducive to greater tumor growth suppression and the inhibition of metastasis. However, if the selected dose provided for a systemic drug exposure that is too toxic, adverse events could endanger the patient's life or significantly reduce the patient's quality of life. Secondly, the patient could discontinue treatment due to the adverse event(s), and fail to receive the full benefit of the drug, which may result in disease progression and reduced survival. In addition, if a patient is significantly harmed by drug-induced adverse events, the patient may not be strong enough to tolerate the current treatment or other subsequent anticancer treatments, thereby depriving the patient of a therapeutic benefit from alternate treatments [1]. In summary, appropriate dose selection is vital because dose optimality is directly linked to favorable therapeutic outcome.

7.2.2 Drug Development Perspective

Appropriate dose selection during early phase clinical trials is critical and could determine the overall fate of a drug development program [2]. Optimal dose evaluation and selection early in development could help establish the therapeutic window of the drug. This can be useful in avoiding unnecessary confusion and delay in the approval and marketing of the drug, and allow quicker access of effective treatment to patients. In some instances, optimal dose selection in early development can help show the unique safety or activity profile of the drug that could in turn lead to a more informative target product profile for the drug to aid in development. Dose selection, early in development, is important because once the dose decision is made and the registration trial is initiated, it is very difficult and expensive to modify the design or start again with a different dose. This is, in part, because registration trials are typically blinded and the results remain unknown until the trial is completed. Even though preliminary results are sometimes available from interim analysis, starting a new dose finding trial could significantly delay the development program.

When registration trials are conducted with doses that do not optimally balance benefit/risk, the outcome of the trial may be marginal or equivocal or simply unfavorable. In superiority trials, a drug that fails to beat the comparator may not receive regulatory approval. Such uncertainty in dose selection could have disastrous consequence for drug developers and unnecessarily use up valuable trial resources. For example, the marketing application for rociletinib, a selective inhibitor of mutant epidermal growth factor receptor (EGFR) for the treatment of nonsmall cell lung cancer (NSCLC), was withdrawn due to nonoptimal dose selection. The lack of an optimal dose for rociletinib for the proposed indication was highlighted at the Oncologic Drug Advisory Committee (ODAC) meeting. Following a negative opinion on the benefit–risk profile of rociletinib by the ODAC, the company decided to terminate the development of rociletinib and withdrew the marketing authorization application for rociletinib from the European Medicines Agency (more details provided in the Section 7.8) [3,4].

Nonoptimal dose selection that led to Phase 3 results with an unacceptable benefit/risk profile in the studied population was also observed in the development of panobinostat for the treatment of patients with multiple myeloma who have received at least one prior therapy. Panobinostat showed marginal tumor control properties where progression free survival was prolonged by two months compared to the control arm [5]. Higher rates of grade 3 or worse adverse events occurred in the panobinostat arm compared to the control arm, including thrombocytopenia (56.7% vs 24.7%), neutropenia (23.8% vs 8.1%), diarrhea (25.4% vs 7.8%), and fatigue (59.6% vs 24.6%) [5]. In addition, increased incidence of death (7% vs 3.5%) was observed due to myelosuppression, hemorrhage, infection, gastrointestinal (GI) toxicity, and cardiac toxicity in the panobinostat arm compared to the control arm [5]. In light of these findings, the majority of the ODAC members recommended "not to approve" panobinostat [6]. However, after the ODAC deliberations, additional analysis showed improved benefit/risk balance in patients who received at least two prior treatments. The FDA subsequently approved panobinostat for a narrower population than initially proposed by the company [6,7].

Poor dose selection also resulted in temporary suspension of the sales of ponatinib due to the risk of life-threatening toxicities including "heart attack, stroke, loss of blood flow to the extremities resulting in tissue death, and severe narrowing of blood vessels in the extremities, heart, and brain requiring urgent surgical procedures to restore blood flow" [8]. These vascular adverse events occurred in 48% of patients enrolled in Phase 1 clinical trials and 24% of patients enrolled in Phase 2 clinical trials. Ponatinib marketing approval was later

reinstated after the company agreed to the following conditions [8,9]: (1) Revise the indication to restrict its use in a limited patient population and to indicate that the starting dose of ponatinib is unknown, (2) Develop a risk evaluation and mitigation strategy plan, and (3) Conduct five additional clinical studies, including pharmacovigilance, safety, and dose finding studies.

Given the impact of poor dose selection on the drug development pathway, it is clear that dose selection has far reaching implications and could influence regulatory outcome and ultimate success in the market place.

7.3 BRIEF HISTORY OF ONCOLOGY DRUG DEVELOPMENT

Oncology drug development was born out of the toxicological research of chemical warfare agents during World War II [10]. In order to develop potential treatment for chemical warfare agents, scientists were studying the mechanistic basis of nitrogen and sulfur mustard-induced toxicities to cells and human tissues [10]. Such research revealed that nitrogen and sulfur mustards caused widespread systemic toxicities by disrupting cellular metabolism and proliferation activities; and the severity of the toxicities was directly related to the dose [10]. At the same time, the researchers noted that the toxic effects of the mustards were more pronounced in cells and tissues with high rates of proliferation, which made them suitable candidates for the treatment of patients with cancer. In addition to nitrogen and sulfur mustards, other drugs evaluated in the mid-20th century included antifolates, platinum-based drugs, and vinca alkaloids [11,12]. Generally, these drugs were cytotoxic and worked by interfering with DNA synthesis or cell division. Because these early oncology drugs affected cells with rapid growth and proliferation, they have poor selectivity between normal healthy cells that turn over rapidly, and cancerous cells which share some of these same metabolic and proliferative characteristics. For example, GI, hair, and bone marrow cells often showed the deleterious effects of these drugs because of their rapid turnover. Such cytotoxic drugs lacked distinct dose—response curves for efficacy and toxicity, rather, the dose—toxicity and dose—efficacy curves for such drugs increased "monotonically" with the dose [13]. The Phase 1 oncology trials of cytotoxic drugs generally used toxicity matrix as a dose selection method. The goal of the trial was to identify the highest dose that patients could tolerate with manageable toxicities, in an effort to maximize the therapeutic potential. This dose was defined as the MTD. The MTD was generally evaluated in subsequent phases of trial to establish efficacy, with provision for dose reduction for toxicities.

7.4 PROMISE OF TARGETED ONCOLOGY DRUGS

Many oncology drugs discovered and developed in the past two decades are more selective for cancer cells compared to older chemotherapy drugs. Instead of indiscriminately affecting basic biological process such as DNA replication and cell division, targeted oncology drugs are intended to act on distinct biological pathways that promote the proliferation and/or migration of cancerous cells. The approval of imatinib in 2001 ushered in the era of targeted oncology drugs. The drug targeted an abnormal tyrosine kinase created by chromosomal abnormality present in cancerous cells. In addition to prolonging survival compared to the standard of care, the rates of neutropenia and thrombocytopenia were reduced by 50% and 70% in the imatinib-treated patients compared to patients who were treated with Inteferon plus Ara-C, illustrating the reduced toxicities of targeted oncology drugs [14]. With the advent of imatinib on the market, many

new targeted therapies, including biologics have been approved and many more are being evaluated as potential oncology therapies.

7.5 PITFALLS OF CURRENT DOSE SELECTION PRACTICES

In order to fully attain the promise of targeted oncology drugs, improvement is needed in the dose selection approach for targeted oncology drugs. One major obstacle that prevents optimal dose selection for targeted oncology drugs has been the use of toxicity-based dose selection. Despite the difference in the mode of action of targeted oncology drugs relative to traditional chemotherapy drugs, drug developers continue to select doses based on the MTD paradigm, where escalating doses are administered to patients until dose limiting toxicities are observed [15,16]. As such, the dose selection is based on a one-dimensional view of the data, i.e., safety without understanding or considering the efficacy and the overall therapeutic window of the drug. Such view of data for dose selection ignores many other important signals that should be considered in the dose selection process. For a targeted oncology drug, dose selection based solely on the MTD paradigm has the following problems:

- The selected dose could be unnecessarily high, providing systemic exposures that result in high rates of adverse events (Fig. 7.1A).
- The selected dose could have minimal or no additional efficacy, therefore advancing ineffective drug for further development (Fig. 7.1B). This occurs because studies are not designed to assess activity.

The typical justification that is often provided for taking the MTD approach is that one would not want to compromise on efficacy and therefore "the more, the better." While this approach may be appropriate for cytotoxic drugs that do not act through a particular

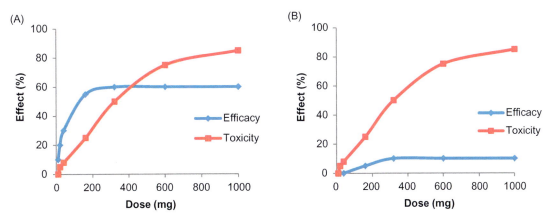

FIGURE 7.1 Dose−response relationship for efficacy and toxicity. The dose−response relationships for efficacy and safety of two hypothetical drugs are depicted (A and B). In (A), the 600 mg dose is selected for further testing based on the MTD approach, despite the fact that maximal effect is achieved at doses between 200 and 400 mg, while the toxicity increases substantially between 200 to 600 mg. In (B), a 600 mg dose is selected for further testing based on the MTD approach despite a very low response rate, increasing toxicity with dose and the lack of additional efficacy beyond 300 mg.

target, it is not a rational approach for dose selection of targeted oncology agents where one can balance safety in the context of the therapeutic window of the drug. In fact, one may argue whether determining MTD should be a goal of Phase 1 trial for targeted oncology agents.

In many cases, drugs approved for oncology indications require dose reductions to address intolerable adverse reactions (ARs) that sometimes develop later during therapy. This phenomenon leads to questions about whether a lower dose may mitigate these ARs without loss of efficacy. The FDA has issued several postapproval postmarketing requirements or commitments between 2011 and 2016 to address these questions. These drugs span several oncology indications and have different mechanisms of action. Several examples are included in Table 7.1.

In summary, a shift in both conceptual framework and methodology should be considered in the development of targeted oncology agents. In other words, the way we think about oncology drugs, how we design the trials, how we set the study objectives and select endpoints, the types of data we collect,

and the types of analyses we conduct should be carefully reevaluated for targeted oncology drug dose selection.

7.6 PROPOSED ONCOLOGY DOSE SELECTION APPROACH

Our experience regarding the evidence that is generated in Phase 1 dose-escalation or dose-selection trials in oncology is summarized in Table 7.2 [30]. The information is categorized by six different attributes and was gathered during the course of drug development to support dose selection. Also shown are three hypothetical scenarios to indicate the current state in oncology dose selection and the potential future state to which we should aspire to. Based on our experience, the evidence generated in Phase 1 dose-escalation or dose-selection trials is somewhere between scenario 1 and 2, while arguably, the goal to strive for scenario 3.

In scenario 1, MTD is the primary goal and exposure−response (ER) analysis is conducted and used to provide support of the selected dose. In scenario 2, apart from identifying the

TABLE 7.1   Summary of Drugs for Which Postmarketing Studies Were Needed to Optimize Dose

Drug	Indication	Reason for PostMarketing Requirement (PMR)/PostMarketing Commitment (PMC)
Vandetanib [17,18]	Symptomatic or progressive medullary thyroid cancer	Dose too high. Significant QT prolongation at the therapeutic dose
Crizotinib [19,20]	Locally advanced or metastatic nonsmall cell lung cancer (NSCLC)	Proposed dose did not achieve maximal efficacy for all patients. Lower ORR and shorter PFS in the lowest quartile of exposure (data not mature), with low incidence of AEs and flat ER for safety
Omacetaxine [21,22]	Chronic or accelerated phase chronic myeloid leukemia	BSA based dosing may not be optimal. Drug response rate and drug concentrations were lower in light weight patients
Cabozantinib [23,24]	Metastatic medullary thyroid carcinoma	Dose maybe too high. Significant tolerability issues at the approved dose. Dose reduction occurred in 60% of patients. Adverse reactions led to treatment discontinuation in 10% of patients
Ponatinib [9,25]	Chronic phase, accelerated phase, or blast phase chronic myeloid leukemia (CML)	Optimal starting dose for initiating therapy is not known. Dose modifications (dose delays or dose reductions) due to adverse reactions occurred in 74% of the patients
Radium-223 dichloride [26,27]	Castration-resistant prostate cancer with symptomatic bone metastases	Dose maybe low. Data indicated that higher dose may produce better efficacy, especially in lower body weight patients ($\leq$73 kg)
Lenvatinib [7,28]	Differentiated thyroid cancer and renal cell cancer	Dose too high. Tolerability issues at the approved dose. Adverse reactions led to dose reductions in 68% of patients and discontinuation in 18% of patients
Panobinostat [7,29]	Multiple myeloma	Significant tolerability issues at the approved dose. Discontinuation due to adverse reactions occurred in 36% of patients. Deaths due to adverse events occurred in 7% of patients in the Panobinostat arm versus 3.5% on the control arm

TABLE 7.2   Regulatory Experience on Evidence Generation and Basis of Dose Selection in Phase 1 Oncology Trials

Attributes	Scenario 1 Safety-Based	Scenario 2 Safety-Based and Some PK	Scenario 3 Safety and Efficacy-Based With Dose Individualization
MTD determination	✓	✓	✓
Modeling and simulation to design trials			✓
Assessing efficacy of lower doses/alternate regimens			✓
Exposure–response (efficacy and safety) based dose justification: IND stage		✓	✓
Dose individualization in registration trials			✓
Exposure–response (efficacy and safety) based dose justification: NDA/BLA	✓	✓	✓

MTD and the submission of ER analysis during the New Drug Application/Biologic License Application (NDA/BLA) submission, dose justification based on ER is evaluated during drug development and discussed with the agency during drug development. In other words, while ER-based dose selection is often submitted as part of regulatory BLA/NDA submission, the justification of dose selection using dose—response, ER, or other quantitative analysis is less common during drug development.

Scenario 3 is the recommended scenario in oncology dose selection. In scenario 3, we propose that doses lower than MTD are evaluated in dose ranging trials to optimize the benefit:risk ratio. In addition, whenever possible, all available data including pharmacokinetic (PK), pharmacodynamic (PD), safety, and efficacy are used for integrated data analyses, modeling, and to simulate different doses and regimens to assess the probability of success of a particular dose or dosing regimen in the registration trial. In addition, we propose that dosing should be individualized in the registration trial if the effect of the certain intrinsic/extrinsic factor on drug exposure is significant and is known *a priori*. This will help gather efficacy and safety information at individualized doses for specific populations rather than employing one-size-fits-all dosing strategy.

There are trends indicating that quantitative benefit/risk analyses are being conducted during drug development to justify dose selection and other drug development decisions. The strategy posed in scenario 3 helps in rationalizing the evidence-based dose selection for registration trials. It is also important to evaluate more than one dose or dosing regimen to adequately characterize the dose/ER relationship in pivotal trials. It has been observed that conducting ER analysis based on just one dose level may lead to an inaccurate conclusion regarding the shape of ER relationships.

Dose selection should be based on the totality of evidence and analysis using all available data that at minimum includes PK, PD, safety, and efficacy at the end of Phase 1 or Phase 2 stages. The rank order of each factor (PK, PD, safety, and efficacy) should be carefully considered when making dosing decisions. While PK, PD, and safety maybe the primary factors in selecting dosing regimen for early phase trials, dosing regimen for pivotal trials should be primarily based on efficacy and safety data. The dose selected for pivotal trial should show preliminary evidence of balanced efficacy and safety.

7.6.1 Preclinical Data

Although preclinical to clinical translation and extrapolation is very difficult in oncology, preclinical data can provide important pieces of information that may be useful in early clinical dose selection. *In vitro* and animal data regarding target engagement, potency, and PK—PD information can be informative in the selection of the range of doses that will be evaluated in Phase 1 dose selection studies. Therefore information from preclinical data should be carried forward to inform the dose selection decision during early clinical development. While the decision regarding starting dose can be based on calculations of no observed adverse effect levels and corresponding human equivalent dose with the appropriate safety factor as described in the FDA's guidance for industry [31], the appropriateness of this starting dose along with subsequent doses to be explored should be informed with these data.

7.6.2 Early Clinical Data

Early dose finding studies should be designed to evaluate several dose levels that span the entire spectrum of the dose—response curve. In order to select doses that balance safety and efficacy, dose-escalation trials should be designed to generate robust and informative activity (efficacy), safety, and PK data. The range of doses to be evaluated should be selected based on the available preclinical data including the target-engagement profile of the drug, preclinical anticancer properties of the drug, and the expected toxicities from animal toxicological evaluations. These doses should also leverage clinical data obtained in other indications, if available. The crucial point here is the need to identify and evaluate a wide range of doses that will provide preliminary evidence of balanced efficacy and safety information that can be used to identify potential doses for further testing in pivotal trial using a variety of different approaches. For example, although the methodological discussion is beyond the scope of this chapter, the MCP-Mod (Multiple Comparison Procedure—Modeling) method has been evaluated by the FDA and EMA and both Agencies have concluded that it is an adequate and appropriate method for the assessment of dose—response [32,33].

The development of carfilzomib reflects the need for the evaluation of a wide range of doses (more details provided in Section 7.8) in Phase 1 dose-escalation trials. The dose of 27 mg/m^2 twice a week was selected based on a response rate of 50% in a cohort of 6 patients with hematologic malignancies after evaluating doses of 1.2–27 mg/m^2 given twice weekly in patients with multiple myeloma [34]. However, the pivotal trial showed a response rate of 23% in patients with multiple myeloma ($N = 266$). In contrast, a follow-on dose finding trial that evaluated doses of 36–70 mg/m^2 showed a response rate of 60% at 56 mg/m^2 twice a week without additional safety findings [35]. It is important to note that leveraging data from the initial Phase 1 trial and the follow-on dose finding provided a more complete picture of the dose—response characteristics of carfilzomib.

The need to leverage information from early clinical and preclinical studies was also observed in the development of idelalisib, a PI3Kδ kinase

inhibitor approved by the FDA for the treatment of indolent non-Hodgkin's lymphoma and relapsed chronic lymphocytic leukemia (CLL). The company evaluated a wide range of dosing regimens in the Phase 1 dose-escalation trial (150–300 mg once daily; 50–350 mg twice a day). In addition, *in vitro* biomarker data and PK simulations at a number of dosing regimens were generated. The availability of these data enabled the use of dose/ER analyses for efficacy and safety to select the 150 mg twice a day dose for the pivotal trials (more details provided in Section 7.8).

Dose—response and ER analyses for efficacy and safety endpoints are at the core of rational dose selection. The dose selection effort is a very critical step in drug development and should involve comprehensive and thorough analysis of all critical data. Minimally, such data should include PK, PD, efficacy, and safety. These data may be leveraged to facilitate dose selection using an integrated data analysis approach (Fig. 7.2). An integrated analysis could include the following: (1) a combined dose—response analysis for safety and activity (efficacy) as shown in Fig. 7.2 or (2) a combined

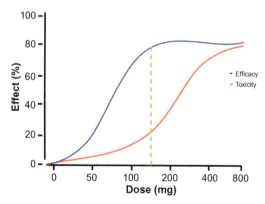

FIGURE 7.2   Dose—response for efficacy and safety for a hypothetical drug. In this scenario, 150 mg dose is selected for further testing based on preliminary determination of risk—benefit using early phase efficacy and safety data.

exposure (AUC, trough concentration) response analysis for safety and efficacy. To the extent possible, innovative data visualization efforts should be used to make the data clear, intuitive, and easy to understand.

7.6.3 Clinical Data From Late Phase or Registration Trials

Dose optimization would be improved immensely if two or more doses were evaluated in late phase studies. This approach would necessitate the inclusion of more patients than that evaluated in the early phase studies in each cohort with a decision made by balancing the observed efficacy and safety. However, the inclusion of additional doses in these studies will provide more information that can be used to optimize or support the selected dose prior to registration. In addition, the data gathered from these trials is also used to assess the effect of various intrinsic and extrinsic factors on the PK of the drug, which may indicate the need for dose adjustment.

7.6.4 Postmarketing Data

Dose optimization does not stop at the approval stage but can be conducted post-approval as well. Although this path of dose selection/optimization is not ideal, it is sometimes unavoidable if the registration trials of the proposed dose result in greater adverse reactions (AR)s than anticipated from earlier trials. There are several examples listed in Table 7.1 where a postmarketing trial was required/recommended to the company for dose optimization.

7.6.5 PK/PD Considerations

In dose-finding studies, the PK/PD sampling schedule should be carefully designed to capture the time course of the PK and PD data.

These data are important in designing appropriate dosing regimens. For example, if the drug has a long half-life (e.g., 12–15 hours), collecting PK samples for just 24 hours would not be sufficiently informative. Instead, PK samples may need to be collected for up to 72 hours. Similarly, for a drug whose PD effect is observed over a long duration, PD assessments should include steady-state in order to fully characterize the magnitude PD effect. If there is good understanding of the PD biomarker of the targeted oncology agent, that information should be utilized toward dose optimization.

PK and PD variability should also be considered when deciding what doses to evaluate in dose-finding trials. If the PK variability is large, one should have a large separation between the doses to gather informative dose–response data. For example, if the between subject PK variability (%CV) for a drug is $>100\%$, evaluating two doses which are only 1.5-fold of each other (e.g., 50 and 75 mg) will not be sufficiently informative for an adequate characterization of dose–response and subsequent dose selection. A more efficient trial may be designed by removing one of the dose cohorts if the efficacy/safety information about that dose cohort can be interpolated using ER analysis. For example, if the plan is to evaluate 50, 75, and 100 mg for a drug with high between subject PK variability (%CV $> 100\%$), one option is to consider removing the 75 mg dose cohort, collecting PK in all patients for 50 and 100 mg cohorts, and utilizing ER analysis to interpolate the predicted efficacy/safety of 75 mg dose.

7.7 OTHER CONSIDERATION FOR THERAPEUTIC OPTIMIZATION

It is important to note that the selection of the optimal dose may require other considerations given that patient's response to treatment

TABLE 7.3   Examples That Highlight Therapeutic Optimizations Based on Intrinsic and Extrinsic Factors

Key Factors	Examples
Physiological factors (body size vs fixed dosing)	*Omacetaxine*: Clearance was not related with BSA. Based on BSA-adjusted dosing, the response rates were lower in lower body weight patients. A PMR issued to study the PK, safety, and preliminary efficacy of a fixed dose regimen in patients with chronic phase (CP) or accelerated phase (AP) chronic myeloid leukemia (CML) who has failed two or more TKI therapies
Pharmacogenetic factors	*Irinotecan*: mutations in UGT1A1 increased the risk for neutropenia
Food effect	*Ceritinib*: 98% of patients experienced GI adverse reactions. Ceritinib is dosed on an empty stomach, but taking the medication with food may alleviate GI toxicities and improve patients' compliance. A PMR issued to conduct clinical trial to evaluate the gastrointestinal tolerability, efficacy, and PK of 450 mg ceritinib taken with a meal as compared with that of 750 mg ceritinib taken in the fasted state in metastatic ALK-positive NSCLC patients

is influenced by intrinsic and extrinsic factors that are unique to each patient (Table 7.3).

The most common clinical pharmacology evaluations in oncology drug development to facilitate dose selection include the following:

- Determination of size-based (mg/kg or mg/m^2) versus fixed dosing;
- Food effect evaluation (e.g., dosing fasted patients);
- Drug–drug interaction (DDI) evaluation;
- Organ impairment evaluation (e.g., reduced dose based on extent of organ dysfunction).

7.7.1 Determination of Size-Based Versus Fixed Dosing

Based on historical practices, early stage oncology trials tend to use body size (weight or body surface area (BSA)) based dosing. However, once the PK of the drug has been characterized, a determination can be made as to whether a fixed-dose or dosing by body size (dosing based on BSA, BMI, or weight) is appropriate. If PK analyses show body size does not influence the PK of the drug and/or if the drug has fairly wide

therapeutic window, then fixed dosing should be considered for subsequent studies. This approach aided in the selection of a fixed dose during the development of ixazomib [36].

While we should aspire to determine the most optimal dosing regimen in the early stage of drug development, dose optimization is a continuous and iterative process that could span from early to late phase development. For example, recommended adult dosing for pembrolizumab was changed from 2 mg/kg to 200 mg every three weeks for all five approved indications, based on previously established population PK model and therapeutic window information derived from dose/ER results in patients with advanced melanoma or NSCLC. The fixed dosing regimen of 200 mg every three weeks was tested and confirmed in five trials across four indications [37]. Similarly, the previously approved recommended body weight-based dosage regimen of 3 mg/kg intravenously every two weeks for nivolumab was modified to a fixed dose of 240 mg intravenously (IV) every two weeks for three indications (renal cell carcinoma, metastatic melanoma, and NSCLC). The approval of these fixed dosing regimens was based on population

PK analyses, modeling and simulation, and robust dose/ER analyses that demonstrated the comparability of the PK, safety, and efficacy of the fixed dosing regimen with the previously approved weight-based regimen [38].

7.7.2 Food Effect

Food has been known to alter the systemic exposure of some orally administered drugs, thereby influencing the safety and efficacy profile of the drugs. The effect of food on the PK of the drug should be evaluated during early development and may be incorporated in the First-in-Human (FIH) trial. Once the effect of food is known, an informed decision regarding the dosing in future trials can be made. Such an approach has several benefits, including:

- Improving drug exposure;
- Removing restrictions with regards to food, when food has no effect;
- Improved patient convenience and compliance;
- Potentially improved GI tolerability.

During the development of venetoclax, the effect of food was evaluated in the dose-escalation part of the FIH trial. It was determined that the administration of venetoclax with either high-fat or low-fat foods increased venetoclax exposure by three- to four-fold relative to when venetoclax was administered fasted [39]. Based on this result, in all subsequent studies, venetoclax was administered with food.

7.7.3 Drug—Drug Interaction

Often, two or more drugs in combination are used in the treatment of cancer. In other cases, patients could be treated with other drugs to manage drug-related adverse events or other comorbidities. Even more importantly, drug-drug interactions (DDI) could influence dose selection in the following ways:

- DDI could increase the concentration of the drug even at low dose levels and lead to adverse events. This could result in underestimation of the MTD dose and even termination of the program due to unexpected adverse events.
- A DDI effect that increase the rate of drug clearance and reduces drug concentrations could result in the overestimation of the recommended Phase 2 dose.

Therefore in order to avoid erroneous dose selection and optimize treatment for patients who need treatment with other drugs, DDI assessments should start with *in vitro* screening studies prior to Phase 1 trials (Fig. 7.3) These studies include *in vitro* studies to identify whether the drug is metabolized by any of the known liver enzymes and whether the drug induces or inhibits the metabolism or transport of other drugs. The need for clinical DDI studies can be assessed by the guidance on DDI of the FDA [40]. It is important to note that DDI can lead to considerable magnitude of exposure change that could influence the safety and efficacy of the drug. For example, venetoclax was found to be metabolized by liver enzyme CYP3A4. A subsequent clinical study showed a 6.4-fold increase in the AUC of venetoclax when it was given with the strong CYP3A4 inhibitor [39], which would increase the risk for toxicity. On the other hand, administration of venetoclax with the strong CYP3A4 inducer decreased the AUC of venetoclax by 71% which may provide suboptimal exposure. Therefore understanding the influence of DDI enables optimal dose selection for the general population and individualization of dosages that ensure safety and efficacy for every patient.

7.7.4 Organ Impairment

In many cases, patients with cancer may have additional significant decreases in the function of their liver or kidneys. This can occur as part of the natural history of the disease, for example, renal impairment in patients with multiple myeloma or as a natural decline in renal function due to age or other comorbid diseases like diabetes. Renal or hepatic impairment may increase systemic drug exposure relative to that observed in patients with normal organ function. The higher drug concentrations in patients with organ impairment could lead to higher rates of toxicities. The decision to enroll patients with renal or hepatic impairment in dose-finding trials should be based on understanding the metabolic and excretion properties of the drug using data from preclinical studies and previous clinical studies. Beaver and colleagues have provided detailed guidance on the enrollment of organ impairment patients in oncology clinical trials [41].

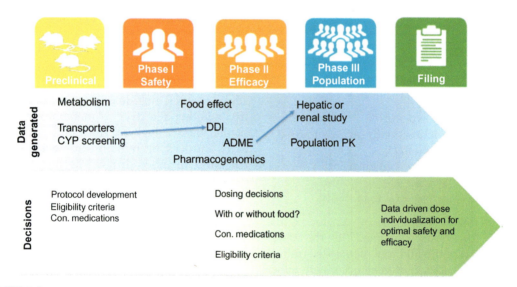

FIGURE 7.3   Development continuum and data needs for therapeutic individualizations.

7.8 CASE STUDIES

CASE STUDY 1: IBRUTINIB [42]

This case study will highlight the following topics:

- The evaluation of doses that cover the full spectrum of the dose—response curve;
- The importance of evaluating PK, PD, efficacy, and safety data for dose selection.

Ibrutinib is an irreversible inhibitor of Bruton's tyrosine kinase (BTK) that binds to a cysteine residue (Cys-481) in the BTK active site. Ibrutinib is approved for treatment of mantle cell lymphoma (MCL) and CLL among other indications [43].

During the development of ibrutinib, a Phase 1, dose-escalation trial was conducted to

(cont'd)

determine MTD, PK, and PD of ibrutinib in patients with recurrent B-cell lymphoma ($N = 66$). The trial did not follow traditional $3 + 3$ trial design, and cohorts with 6−10 subjects per dose level were evaluated until the MTD was reached. Patients were given daily ibrutinib doses of 1.25−12.5 mg/kg. Dose−response relationships for BTK occupancy and clinical response showed that maximum BTK occupancy and maximum response (ORR) were achieved at doses of ∼2.5 mg/kg (∼175 mg for average weight of 70 kg) (Fig. 7.4). Although major Grade 3 + AEs were observed, the MTD was not reached. No dose-dependent safety signals were observed. Weight did not influence the clearance of ibrutinib [44].

Dosing Selection Decisions:

- Safety and efficacy data showed that ibrutinib appears to have a wide therapeutic window, which supported the selection and further evaluation of doses in the plateau part of the dose−response curve.

- The PD data provided additional evidence by showing sufficient receptor occupancy at the selected doses.
- PK data showed that weight does not influence the PK of ibrutinib, as a result, dosing transitioned from weight-based to fixed dosing.

Outcome:

After the completion of the Phase 1 trial, the 420 mg dose was evaluated for the CLL indication and the 560 mg dose was evaluated for the MCL indication in Phase 2 studies. In the Phase 2 trials, robust response rates (Table 7.4) relative to previously approved therapies for CLL and MCL were observed. No exposure−response relationships were observed for Grade 3+ adverse events for doses of up to 840 mg.

Lessons Learned:

- The Phase 1 study provided robust dose−response data suggesting that ibrutinib has a fairly wide therapeutic window.

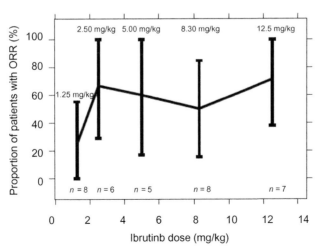

FIGURE 7.4 Ibrutinib dose−response relationship for efficacy.

(cont'd)

- Unlike most Phase 1 oncology studies, the dose-escalation study for ibrutinib did not follow the traditional 3 + 3 study design. As a result, sufficient data were available such

that the Phase 2 doses can be selected based on efficacy.
- PD assessment provided additional evidence of efficacy and avoided the need for toxicity-based dose selection.

TABLE 7.4 Summary of Ibrutinib Efficacy Findings [43,45]

Efficacy Endpoint per IRC[a]	MCL (N = 111) Ibrutinib 560 mg Daily	CLL (N = 48) Ibrutinib 420 mg Daily
ORR	76 (68.5%)	28 (58.3%)
95% CI	(59.0, 77.0)	(43.2, 72.4)
CR	23 (20.7%)	None achieved

[a] Independent review committee.

CASE STUDY 2: IDELALISIB [46]

This case study will highlight the following topic:

- Importance of preclinical PD assessment and determination of target concentration to aid dose selection.
- Idelalisib is a PI3Kδ kinase inhibitor, approved for the treatment of refractory indolent non-Hodgkin lymphoma (iNHL) and relapsed CLL. A Phase 1 dose-escalation study evaluated idelalisib doses of 50, 100, 150, 200, and 350 mg twice daily (BID) and 150 and 300 mg once daily (QD) in patients with NHL and CLL. Safety, PK, and tumor growth (sum of products of greatest perpendicular diameters of index lesions) data were collected. Univariate exposure–response analysis evaluating the relationship between the best reduction in tumor growth and steady-state trough concentrations showed that doses greater than 150 mg BID did not offer any additional antitumor activity and doses below 150 mg BID may lead to lower effect on tumor

reduction and thus reducing efficacy (Figs. 7.5 and 7.6). Accounting for the PK variability, simulations using data from patients with iNHL and CLL demonstrated that most patients (97%) administered doses of 150 mg BID would have exposures sufficient to inhibit the target (125 ng/mL) (Fig. 7.7).

Dosing Selection Decisions:

- Dose selection incorporated clinical tumor growth inhibition data, *in vitro* target inhibition data, and clinical PK data.

Outcome:

Both the PK simulations and the exposure–response analysis led to the selection of 150 mg BID for the iNHL and the CLL population and eventual recommendation of this dose for treatment.

Lessons Learned:

- Phase 1 trial with wide range of doses and extensive PK, PD, and exposure–response analyses enabled optimal dose selection for the registration trials.

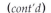

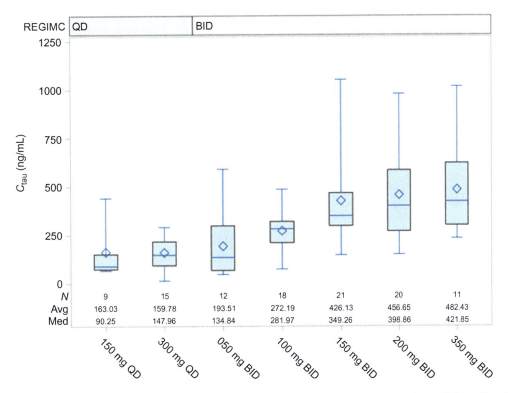

FIGURE 7.5 Boxplots of the predicted steady state trough concentration (C_{tau}) (population PK predicted) in patients with iNHL and CLL after the administration of a range of doses of idelalisib.

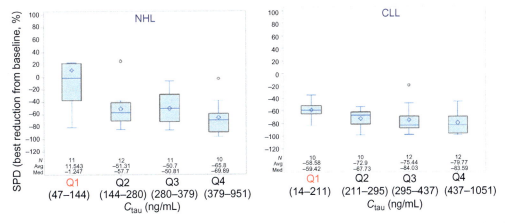

FIGURE 7.6 Pooled exposure−response relationship for efficacy in patients with indolent non-Hodgkin lymphoma (NHL; left) and chronic lymphocytic leukemia (CLL; right) following treatment with 50, 100, 150, 200, and 350 mg BID and 150 and 300 mg QD doses.

(cont'd)

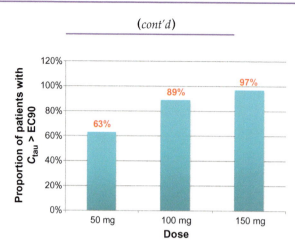

FIGURE 7.7   Proportion of simulated patients with iNHL and CLL given a range of doses (50–150 mg twice daily) predicted to have steady state trough concentrations (C_{tau}) > EC_{90} (125 ng/mL).

CASE STUDY 3: ROCILETINIB [47]

This case study will highlight the following topics:

- The evaluation of a wide range of doses that cover the full spectrum of the dose–response curve;
- The importance of evaluating PK as it relates to safety;
- Traditional tolerability assessment, using data from Cycle 1, may not reflect toxicity following chronic treatment.

Rociletinib is a small molecule epidermal growth factor receptor-small inhibitor (EGFR-TK). Rociletinib demonstrates nonlinear pharmacokinetics and systemic exposures does not increase at doses greater than 500 mg twice daily. The company sought accelerated approval for the treatment of patients with NSCLC with the EGFR T790M mutations who were previously treated with an EGFR-targeted therapy, based on the results of two nonrandomized studies.

An open label, Phase 1/2 study in patients with NSCLC who have progressed after prior treatment with an EGFR-tyrosine kinase inhibitor evaluated the safety, PK, and antitumor activity of rociletinib. The Phase 1 component of the study evaluated rociletinib doses ranging from 150 mg once daily to 1000 mg twice daily. Based on Cycle 1 assessment, the MTD was not reached. The Phase 2 component of the study evaluated rociletinib doses of 500, 750, and 1000 mg BID in patients who have progressed on initial EGFR inhibitor therapy. The overall results showed a high incidence of ARs at the 750 and 1000 mg BID doses, with comparable overall response rates (ORR) among 500, 625, and 750 mg BID dose cohorts.

Exposure–response analyses indicated a relatively flat relationship between ORR and exposure (AUC at steady state) suggesting that no substantial improvement in efficacy was observed with doses above 500 mg BID

(cont'd)

(Fig. 7.8). As such, no additional efficacy could be derived by increasing dose.

The company proposed a 500 mg BID dosing regimen for the initial NDA submission to seek accelerated approval of rociletinib. The ORR for the 500 mg BID cohort was 23% (95% CI: 14, 34). However, during the review process, the company amended their NDA to change the proposed dose to 625 mg BID, in response to a numerically higher ORR of 32% (95% CI: 25, 40) observed in 170 patients who received that dose.

It is important to note that while a MTD was not observed for rociletinib, the drug has two toxic metabolites, M502 and M460, with high accumulation ratios of 20- and 58-fold, respectively. Exposure-safety analyses showed that QTc prolongation increases with increased exposure of these metabolites (Fig. 7.9), suggesting that high drug exposure may be a safety concern.

Dose Selection Decision:

- Doses evaluated have overlapping exposure and do not provide full picture of the dose–response and exposure–response profile of the drug.
- PK and toxicity properties of the metabolites were not carefully considered.

Outcome:

After weighing the benefit–risk profile of rociletinib, the FDA's ODAC voted against the accelerated approval of rociletinib for patients with metastatic EGFR T790M-mutated NSCLC who have previously received an EGFR-targeted therapy. The ODAC recommended that the results of the confirmatory clinical trial (TIGER-3) be submitted before FDA made a regulatory decision on the application. However, the company decided to terminate the development of rociletinib and withdraw its NDA [3].

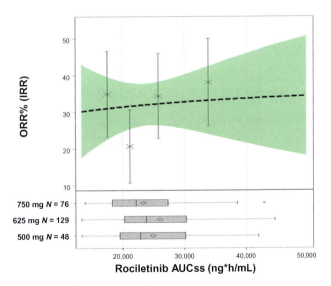

FIGURE 7.8   Rociletinib exposure–efficacy relationship.

(cont'd)

Lessons Learned:

- For targeted drugs, short-term tolerability findings do not reflect toxicity following chronic treatment.

- All available data, including, safety, efficacy, and PK should be carefully evaluated in selecting doses and in deciding further development of the drug.

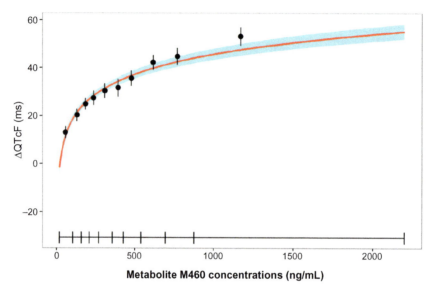

FIGURE 7.9   M460 exposure—safety relationship: QTc prolongation.

CASE STUDY 4: CARFILZOMIB [48]

This case study will highlight the following topics:

- The evaluation of doses that cover the full spectrum of the dose–response curve;
- The importance of evaluating preliminary safety and efficacy outcomes in dose selection decision.

Carfilzomib is a second-generation proteasome inhibitor. It is approved for the treatment of patients with refractory and relapsed multiple myeloma [34].

During the development of carfilzomib, a dosing regimen of 20 mg/m^2 at Cycle 1 and 27 mg/m^2 for Cycles 2 and beyond (given as a 2–10-minute intravenous infusion on Days 1, 2, 8, 9, 15, and 16 of a 28-day treatment cycle) was selected based on results of a Phase 1/2 dose-escalation study. The Phase 1 part of study evaluated carfilzomib doses of 1.2, 2.4, 4, 6, 8.4, 11, 15, 20, and 20 mg/m^2 in Cycle 1 and 27 mg/m^2 in subsequent cycles (20/27 mg/m^2 dose) given on Days 1, 2, 8, 9, 15, and 16 of a 28-day treatment cycle. Carfilzomib showed modest clinical

(cont'd)

responses at doses greater than 15 mg/m^2 (Fig. 7.10) with no major safety signals. Based on these data, the 20/27 mg/m^2 dose was selected for pivotal trial based on clinical response.

Further evaluation of the carfilzomib 20/27 mg/m^2 dose in 266 patients provided an ORR of 23% with no major safety issues observed. Based on these studies, carfilzomib was approved in the United States for patients with relapsed and refractory multiple myeloma using the 20/27 mg/m^2 dose.

Dose Selection Decision:

Response rate was modest with dose selected. Higher doses should have been explored because no maximal response was observed and no dose-related toxicities were observed.

Outcome:

The company conducted an additional dose-finding trial where doses of 36−70 mg/m^2 were explored. Data from this study were pooled with data from the initial dose-finding study. Efficacy outcomes from patients given carfilzomib suggested improved ORR at higher doses, as such, the revised recommended Phase 2 dose was determined to be 20 mg/m^2 in Cycle 1 followed by 56 mg/m^2 in subsequent cycles (20/56 mg/m^2) which had an ORR of 60%. In addition, all adverse events of interest were manageable. Subsequently, the labeling was updated to include the 20/56 mg/m^2 dose as an option.

Lessons Learned:

In early dose-finding studies, a wide range of doses should be explored to fully characterize the dose−response profile of the drug.

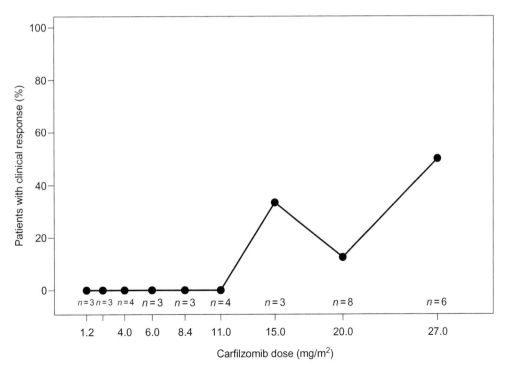

FIGURE 7.10   Dose response versus clinical response in Phase 1 dose escalation study.

7.9 CONCLUSION

Targeted oncology drugs represent a major advance in the treatment of cancer. These drugs are typically more specific for cancer cells, thus enabling patients to better tolerate treatment compared to traditional cytotoxic drugs. This is important given that many patients remain on these agents for long periods of time to suppress tumor growth and to improve survival. However, to fully exploit the full potential of targeted oncology drugs in the fight against cancer, a conceptual and operational change is needed in the dose selection of targeted oncology drugs.

Given the relative specificity of targeted oncology drugs, we need to approach dose-escalation trials for these drugs differently. The goal of such trials should not solely be the determination of the MTD, but rather, to also find the optimal dose(s) with favorable preliminary evidence of balanced efficacy and safety. To achieve this goal, dose-escalation trials should include a wide range of doses that are designed to assess activity as well as safety. The range of doses to be evaluated maybe up to 1 order of magnitude, but should leverage information obtained from preclinical and nonclinical data for the drug. Further, if maximal response or the DLT is not determined in the planned dosing range trial, additional dose levels should be assessed until the collected data provide a full picture of the dose–response curve.

Data from dose-escalation trials should help answer the following key questions:

- What dose/exposure is required to completely saturate the target and achieve maximal anticancer activity?
- What dose(s) should be taken forward for pivotal study evaluation based on integrated analysis of dose, PK, PD, activity, and safety data?

- Does PK and PD, if relevant, suggest that fixed dosing has more consistent exposure than BSA or weight-based dosing?

Other important factors that should be considered include the impact of food on orally administered drugs, and whether the metabolism of the drug will be impacted by chronically administered concomitant medications, and the prevalence of organ impairment in the treatment population. Using this information in its entirety, the best dose(s) can be selected for the next critical phase of development.

References

[1] Minasian L, et al. Optimizing dosing of oncology drugs. Clin Pharmacol Ther 2014;96(5):572–9.
[2] Printz C. Failure rate: why many cancer drugs don't receive FDA approval, and what can be done about it. Cancer 2015;121(10):1529–30.
[3] Breanna Burkart AS. Clovis oncology announces Q1 2016 operating results and corporate update. Available from: <http://www.businesswire.com/news/home/20160505006474/en/Clovis-Oncology-Announces-Q1-2016-Operating-Results>; 2016 [cited 22.05.17].
[4] Broderick JM. Clovis ends development of rociletinib in lung cancer. Available from: <http://www.onclive.com/web-exclusives/clovis-ends-development-of-rociletinib-in-lung-cancer>; 2016 [cited 22.05.17].
[5] FDA Briefing Document: Oncologic Drugs Advisory Committee Meeting. NDA 205353 panobinostat (Farydak); 2014. p. 28.
[6] Summary Minutes of the Oncologic Drugs Advisory Committee Meeting November 6, 2014. Available from: <https://wayback.archive-it.org/7993/20170403224015/https://www.fda.gov/downloads/AdvisoryCommittees/CommitteesMeetingMaterials/Drugs/OncologicDrugsAdvisoryCommittee/UCM430826.pdf>; 2014.
[7] Approval Letter for NDA 206947. Available from: <https://www.accessdata.fda.gov/drugsatfda_docs/appletter/2015/206947Orig1s000ltr.pdf>; 2015.
[8] FDA Drug Safety Communication: FDA asks manufacturer of the leukemia drug Iclusig (ponatinib) to suspend marketing and sales. Available from: <http://wayback.archive-it.org/7993/20161022203734/http://www.fda.gov/Drugs/DrugSafety/ucm373040.htm>; 2013.

[9] Approval Letter for NDA 203469/S-007 & S-008. Available from: <https://www.accessdata.fda.gov/drugsatfda_docs/appletter/2013/203469Orig1s007,s008ltr.pdf>; 2013.

[10] Gilman A, Philips FS. The biological actions and therapeutic applications of the B-chloroethyl amines and sulfides. Science 1946;103(2675):409−36.

[11] Chabner BA, Roberts Jr. TG. Timeline: Chemotherapy and the war on cancer. Nat Rev Cancer 2005;5(1):65−72.

[12] DeVita Jr. VT, Chu E. A history of cancer chemotherapy. Cancer Res 2008;68(21):8643−53.

[13] Le Tourneau C, Lee JJ, Siu LL. Dose escalation methods in phase I cancer clinical trials. J Natl Cancer Inst 2009;101(10):708−20.

[14] Package insert for imatinib mesylate. Available from: <https://www.accessdata.fda.gov/drugsatfda_docs/label/2017/021588s049lbl.pdf>; 2017.

[15] Nie L, et al. Rendering the 3 + 3 design to rest: more efficient approaches to oncology dose-finding trials in the era of targeted therapy. Clin Cancer Res 2016;22(11):2623−9.

[16] Bullock JM, Rahman A, Liu Q. Lessons learned: Dose selection of small molecule-targeted oncology drugs. Clin Cancer Res 2016;22(11):2630−8.

[17] Approval letter for NDA 022405. Available from: <https://www.accessdata.fda.gov/drugsatfda_docs/appletter/2011/022405s000ltr.pdf>; 2011.

[18] Clinical Pharmacology and biopharmaceutics review for NDA022405Orig1s000. Available from: <https://www.accessdata.fda.gov/drugsatfda_docs/nda/2011/022405Orig1s000ClinPharmR.pdf>; 2011.

[19] Clinical pharmacology and biopharmaceutics review for 202570Orig1s000. Available from: <https://www.accessdata.fda.gov/drugsatfda_docs/nda/2011/202570Orig1s000ClinPharmR.pdf>; 2011.

[20] Approval letter for NDA 202570. Available from: <https://www.accessdata.fda.gov/drugsatfda_docs/appletter/2011/202570s000ltr.pdf>; 2011.

[21] Approval letter for NDA 203585. Available from: <https://www.accessdata.fda.gov/drugsatfda_docs/appletter/2012/203585Orig1s000ltr.pdf>; 2012.

[22] Clinical pharmacology and biopharmaceutics review for NDA 203585Orig1s000. Available from: <https://www.accessdata.fda.gov/drugsatfda_docs/nda/2012/203585Orig1s000ClinPharmR.pdf>; 2012.

[23] Approval letter for NDA 203756. Available from: <https://www.accessdata.fda.gov/drugsatfda_docs/appletter/2012/203756Orig1s000ltr.pdf>; 2012.

[24] Clinical pharmacology and biopharmaceutics review for 203756Orig1s000. Available from: <https://www.accessdata.fda.gov/drugsatfda_docs/nda/2012/203756Orig1s000ClinPharmR.pdf>; 2012.

[25] Clinical pharmacology and biopharmaceutics review for NDA 203469/S-007 & S-008. Available from: <https://www.accessdata.fda.gov/drugsatfda_docs/nda/2013/203469Orig1s007,s008.pdf>; 2013.

[26] Approval letter for NDA 203971. Available from: <https://www.accessdata.fda.gov/drugsatfda_docs/appletter/2013/203971Orig1s000ltr.pdf>; 2013.

[27] Clinical pharmacology and biopharmaceutics review for NDA 203971Orig1s000. Available from: <https://www.accessdata.fda.gov/drugsatfda_docs/nda/2013/203971Orig1s000ClinPharmR.pdf>; 2013.

[28] Clinical pharmacology and biopharmaceutics review for 206947Orig1s000. Available from: <https://www.accessdata.fda.gov/drugsatfda_docs/nda/2015/206947Orig1s000ClinPharmR.pdf>; 2015.

[29] Clinical pharmacology and biopharmaceutics review for 205353Orig1s000. Available from: <https://www.accessdata.fda.gov/drugsatfda_docs/nda/2015/205353Orig1s000ClinPharmR.pdf>; 2015.

[30] FDA/AACR workshop titled "Dose-finding of small molecule oncology drugs". Available from: <http://www.aacr.org/AdvocacyPolicy/GovernmentAffairs/Pages/dose-finding-of-small-molecule-oncology-drugs.aspx#.WUtVCesrLDC>; 2015.

[31] Guidance for Industry: Estimating the maximum safe starting dose in initial clinical trials for therapeutics in adult healthy volunteers. U.S. Department of Health and Human Services, Food and Drug Administration; 2005.

[32] FDA letter on MCP-Mod. Available from: <https://www.fda.gov/downloads/Drugs/DevelopmentApprovalProcess/UCM508700.pdf>.

[33] EMA letter on MCP-Mod "Qualification Opinion of MCP-Mod as an efficient statistical methodology for model-based design and analysis of Phase II dose finding studies under model uncertainty". Available from: <http://www.ema.europa.eu/docs/en_GB/document_library/Regulatory_and_procedural_guideline/2014/02/WC500161027.pdf>; 2016.

[34] PRESCRIBING INFORMATION: KYPROLIS® (carfilzomib) for injection, for intravenous use. Available from: <http://pi.amgen.com/~/media/amgen/repositorysites/pi-amgen-com/kyprolis/kyprolis_pi.ashx>; 2012.

[35] Papadopoulos KP, Lee P, Singhal S, Holahan JR, Vesole DH, Rosen S, et al. A phase 1b/2 study of prolonged infusion carfilzomib in patients with relapsed and/or refractory multiple myeloma: updated efficacy and tolerability from the completed 20/56 mg/m2 expansion cohort of PX-171-007. American Society of Hematology Annual Meeting. San Diego, California; 2011.

[36] Clinical pharmacology and biopharmaceutics review for NDA208462Orig1s000. Available from: <https://www.accessdata.fda.gov/drugsatfda_docs/nda/2015/208462Orig1s000ClinPharmR.pdf>; 2015.

[37] Package insert for pembrolizumab. Available from: <https://www.accessdata.fda.gov/drugsatfda_docs/label/2017/125514s014lbl.pdf>; 2017.

[38] Modification of the dosage regimen for nivolumab. Available from: <https://www.fda.gov/Drugs/InformationOnDrugs/ApprovedDrugs/ucm520871.htm>; 2016.

[39] Clinical pharmacology and biopharmaceutics review for NDA208573Orig1s000. Available from: <https://www.accessdata.fda.gov/drugsatfda_docs/nda/2016/208573Orig1s000ClinPharmR.pdf>; 2016.

[40] Draft Guidance for Industry "Drug interaction studies − study design, data analysis, implications for dosing, and labeling recommendations". U.S. Department of Health and Human Services, Food and Drug Administration; 2012.

[41] Beaver JA, Ison G, Pazdur R. Reevaluating eligibility criteria − balancing patient protection and participation in oncology trials. N Engl J Med 2017;376(16):1504−5.

[42] Clinical pharmacology and biopharmaceutics review for NDA2055523Orig1s000. Available from: <https://www.accessdata.fda.gov/drugsatfda_docs/nda/2013/205552Orig1s000ClinPharmR.pdf>; 2013.

[43] Package insert for ibrutinib. Available from: <https://www.accessdata.fda.gov/drugsatfda_docs/label/2013/205552s000lbl.pdf>; 2013.

[44] Marostica E, et al. Population pharmacokinetic model of ibrutinib, a Bruton tyrosine kinase inhibitor, in patients with B cell malignancies. Cancer Chemother Pharmacol 2015;75(1):111−21.

[45] Statistical review for NDA205552; 2013.

[46] Clinical pharmacology and biopharmaceutics review for NDA206545Orig1s000. Available from: <https://www.accessdata.fda.gov/drugsatfda_docs/nda/2014/206545Orig1s000ClinPharmR.pdf>; 2014.

[47] Briefing information for the April 12, 2016 meeting of the Oncologic Drugs Advisory Committee (ODAC). Available from: <https://www.fda.gov/AdvisoryCommittees/CommitteesMeetingMaterials/Drugs/OncologicDrugsAdvisoryCommittee/ucm494781.htm>; 2016.

[48] Clinical pharmacology and biopharmaceutics review for NDA202714Orig1s000. Available from: <https://www.accessdata.fda.gov/drugsatfda_docs/nda/2012/202714Orig1s000ClinPharmR.pdf>; 2012.

Integrating Biomarkers in Early-Phase Trials

Ralph E. Parchment[1], Katherine V. Ferry-Galow[1] and James H. Doroshow[2]

[1]Leidos Biomedical Research, Inc., Frederick National Laboratory for Cancer Research, Frederick, MD, United States [2]National Cancer Institute, Bethesda, MD, United States

8.1 INTRODUCTION

Molecularly targeted cancer therapies offer opportunities not only for the precise partnering of therapeutic agents with particular oncogenic drivers of disease but also for evaluating and tailoring therapeutic regimens based on measurements of target suppression and downstream molecular events. The latter is achieved through the use of molecular pharmacodynamic (PD) biomarkers: quantifiable biological molecules that are altered in response to a therapeutic agent and are therefore essential for establishing mechanism of action (MoA) for reversible, targeted inhibitors. Molecular biomarkers can be broken down into several categories (Table 8.1); PD biomarkers are valuable research tools during drug development and in optimizing dosage regimens but are not used in directing individual patient treatment plans, while "actionable" biomarkers, which can include diagnostic,

prognostic, and predictive biomarkers, effect clinical decision-making and are therefore valuable for improving individual patient outcomes. Thus PD biomarkers have traditionally been less profitable than actionable biomarkers that become commercial diagnostics, but that may be changing with the recent signing into law of the 21st Century Cures Act [1], which emphasizes the use of biomarkers and other surrogate endpoints as sufficient evidence for accelerated drug approval and, as a result, may enhance the financial incentives for PD biomarker development.

Clinical use of PD biomarkers often begins with the fundamental task of establishing proof of mechanism (PoM) in human tumor biopsy samples in Phase 0 or Phase I studies, which can be followed in later stage trials by proof of concept (PoC), wherein a relationship between biomarker modulation and efficacy is demonstrated. Information from PoM and PoC studies can then be applied in several ways,

TABLE 8.1   Biomarker Definitions

Biomarker	Purpose
Pharmacodynamic	Indicates a drug-induced pharmacological effect associated with the therapeutic effect of the drug
Surrogate	Serves as a substitute for a clinical endpoint
Companion diagnostic	Is required for the safe or effective use of a specific targeted agent
Actionable	Impacts clinical decision-making for individual patients; assay must meet Clinical Laboratory Improvement Amendments regulations
Prognostic	Provides information about a patient's intervention-independent disease outcome
Predictive	Indicates probability that a patient may benefit (or experience adverse events) from a specific intervention
Integral	Required for a clinical trial and measured in real-time during trial
Integrated	Examined during a clinical trial to optimize or validate assays for use in future trials; used to test a trial hypothesis
Exploratory/ancillary	Developed during a clinical trial to better understand the therapeutic agent, but not critical for successful completion of the trial

Adapted from Dancey JE, Dobbin KK, Groshen S, et al. Guidelines for the development and incorporation of biomarker studies in early clinical trials of novel agents. Clin Cancer Res 2010;16(6):1745−55.

including: (1) optimization of targeted agent scheduling based on molecular response rather than toxicity or pharmacokinetics (PKs); (2) developing novel, mechanistically based combination therapies targeting the multiple signaling defects that drive many malignancies; and (3) use of diagnostic or actionable biomarkers for patient or treatment selection [2]. Here, we discuss the myriad considerations for developing biomarker assays to establish PoM, explain the aforementioned applications of PD biomarker assays, and provide a framework for incorporating PD biomarker assessments into early-phase clinical trial design.

8.2 ESTABLISHING PROOF OF MECHANISM IN EARLY-PHASE TRIALS

In molecular pharmacodynamics, clinical PoM refers to evidence that the investigational agent engages and functionally alters its intended molecular target in the diseased tissue in a manner already confirmed by preclinical studies. Biomarkers that provide evidence of this target engagement and modulation are referred to as primary PD biomarkers, but PoM studies can also examine the downstream molecular and cellular/physiological consequences of target engagement through the use of secondary and even tertiary PD biomarkers, respectively [2]. For example, in the case of the small-molecule Wee1 kinase inhibitor AZD1775 (MK-1775), clinical PoM was established in a first-in-human (FIH) Phase I trial through use of a primary PD biomarker, phosphorylation of the substrate Cdk1/2 tyrosine residue 15, which was hypothesized and then shown to decrease in patient tumor biopsy samples following AZD1775 treatment, and the secondary PD biomarker γH2AX, which increased as a consequence of downstream DNA damage response activation [3]. A tertiary biomarker could have been the apoptotic marker cleaved caspase 3, which would indicate

AZD1775-mediated tumor cell death. Such thorough demonstration of PoM in early-phase clinical trials is important not only for research purposes but also for improving success rates of later-phase trials, as described below.

8.2.1 Rationale for Integrating Proof of Mechanism in First-in-Human Trials: Improving the Impact of First-in-Human Trials in Cancer Drug Development

Approximately half of all Phase II trials are unsuccessful due to lack of efficacy [4]. A causal analysis of Pfizer Phase II efficacy failures [5] found that the majority of these occurred in cases where drug MoA was not verified in the clinic. With the goal of improving Phase II success rates, the authors put forth three "pillars of survival" to be demonstrated for each candidate agent: (1) required agent exposure at the site of action, (2) kinetically adequate target binding, and (3) sufficient modulation of relevant downstream effector molecules at the site of action. In other words, while pharmacokinetic parameters such as tumor drug concentration are important, they address only the first pillar, and molecular PD biomarker measurements are equally critical. Thus use of PD biomarkers to assess PoM in FIH trials may reduce the number of costly, late-stage drug development failures.

8.2.2 Improving Drug Development by Using Phase 0 Studies

For some agents, Phase 0 (or exploratory investigational new drug) trials may be an efficient method for preventing later stage drug development failures. The FDA's "Exploratory IND Studies" guidance outlines pre-Phase I clinical trial designs for performing pharmacological assessments to accelerate drug development [6]. Such Phase 0 trials entail administration of nontoxic, subtherapeutic doses in a small

number of patients (6–15) over an abbreviated period of time (a few weeks) to acquire critical pharmacological data prior to Phase I studies [7]. Thus Phase 0 trials may be ideal platforms for FIH testing of clinical PoM in a manner far less resource-intensive than a Phase I trial. Phase 0 trials also represent early opportunities for using PD biomarkers to select a dosing schedule that maintains adequate control of target activity (see Section 8.4.1); e.g., PD biomarker results from a Phase 0 trial of poly (ADP-ribose) polymerase (PARP) inhibitor ABT-888 revealed the short duration of PARP inhibition, leading to a BID dosing schedule that was used in several subsequent Phase I and II trials [2,8].

However, it is important to note that not all biomarkers are suitable for Phase 0 trials, depending on the variability of the biomarker signal and the degree to which the signal is modified in response to drug (see Section 8.3) [7]. Furthermore, because Phase 0 trials are not intended to achieve efficacy, many tertiary biomarker responses will not be observed, and these studies are not suitable for demonstrating PoC [2]. Nonetheless, for many targeted agents, Phase 0 trials may represent a relatively low-cost option for FIH assessment of pharmacological responses and, therefore, may improve the efficiency of the clinical drug development process for such agents.

8.3 PHARMACODYNAMIC BIOMARKER SELECTION AND ASSAY DEVELOPMENT: ESTABLISHING FITNESS-FOR-PURPOSE IN A PRECLINICAL SETTING

Determining the appropriate PD biomarkers is critical for establishing PoM, with important selection criteria including not only drug MoA but also the: (1) biological variability, (2) degree of drug-induced biomarker modulation,

(3) therapeutic index of the agent, and (4) temporal dynamics of biomarker response, as related to timing of the biopsy procedure in the clinic [7]. These criteria are empirically derived, rendering biomarker selection heavily reliant on development of robust, clinically suitable, fit-for-purpose (FFP) PD biomarker assays, which begins in a preclinical setting. To facilitate a smooth bench-to-bedside transition, preclinical FFP experiments should replicate the clinical setting as closely as possible; e.g., the NCI PARP assay was validated in a "preclinical Phase 0" approach [9] that modeled the subsequent clinical Phase 0 ABT-888 trial [8].

Most PD biomarker assays can be classified into two broad categories: microscopy-based and tissue extract-based assays. Both categories feature distinct advantages and disadvantages; while a tissue extract-based approach, such as a sandwich enzyme-linked immunosorbent assay (ELISA), allows for high-specificity due to the use of two independent antibodies per analyte, this approach cannot distinguish between signal arising from tumor versus nontumor tissue and can therefore be clouded by sample-to-sample variations in biopsy tumor content (see Section 8.3.4) [2]. In contrast, immunofluorescence microscopy assays (IFAs) using fixed tissue sections allow for differentiation of tumor versus nontumor biomarker signal through the use of H & E staining and/or tumor markers such as MUC1 and CEA [10,11]. However, use of a single detection antibody does not confer high-specificity, which is particularly crucial when examining changes in posttranslational modification sites among highly homologous signaling proteins [12]. Simultaneous implementation of both types of assays is ideal; FIH investigation of a new biomarker may evolve from an initial ELISA demonstrating a general PD response, to a follow-up IFA to demonstrate that the PD response is tumor cell-specific [2]. Regardless of the assay, the range and timing of biomarker response must be established, as discussed below.

8.3.1 Pharmacodynamic Biomarker Levels: Baseline Variability and Drug-Induced Modulation

In establishing whether a PD biomarker is appropriate for an early-phase trial, the degrees of variation in both baseline and posttreatment biomarker levels are key considerations that are dependent on the biomarker itself (biological variability, lability, amplitude of response to drug, etc.) and the sensitivity and precision of the biomarker assay. These factors combine to determine the smallest drug-induced PD effect that can reach statistical significance. The intensity of a baseline biomarker signal often varies widely due to several factors, including inter- and intratumor heterogeneity, tumor biopsy quality and sampling variability, and diurnal variation, among others (see Section 8.3.4). Acceptable ranges of baseline variability depend on the degree of drug-induced biomarker signal changes; the biomarker and assay must allow for distinguishing pre- and posttreatment biomarker levels in patient samples. Furthermore, posttreatment biomarker changes must be detectable at nontoxic doses, rendering therapeutic index a key consideration. Finally, the type of trial conducted must be considered; e.g., a biomarker may be appropriate for both Phase I and Phase 0 studies when the ranges of baseline and posttreatment biomarker levels (at nontoxic doses) do not overlap (Fig. 8.1, left) [7]. However, a biomarker would be inappropriate for a Phase 0 study if a significant difference between baseline and posttreatment biomarker levels is observed only at toxic doses (Fig. 8.1, right); in this case, the biomarker might still be applicable in Phase I or Phase II studies in which it can be assessed at the maximum tolerated dose (MTD).

8.3.2 Pharmacodynamic Biomarker Dynamics

The dynamic nature of PD biomarkers is critical to the mechanistic insight that they

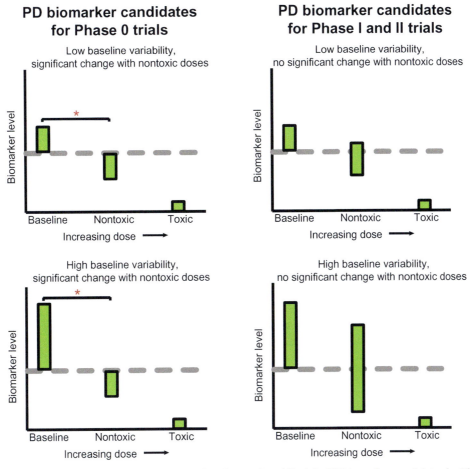

FIGURE 8.1   Evaluating PD biomarker suitability for Phase 0, I, and II trials. PD biomarker candidates for Phase 0 trials are those for which biomarker levels at a nontoxic dose are significantly different from baseline, regardless of whether baseline variability is high or low (left). PD biomarkers for which levels at a nontoxic dose are not significantly different from baseline (right) are not good candidates for Phase 0 studies but may still be suitable for Phase I or Phase II trials, which escalate the dose to levels with acceptable adverse events (toxicity). Source: *Adapted from Doroshow JH, Parchment RE. Oncologic phase 0 trials incorporating clinical pharmacodynamics: from concept to patient. Clin Cancer Res 2008;14 (12):3658–63.*

provide, but it also presents two practical challenges: (1) determining the optimal time frame for biomarker measurements and (2) preserving the biomarker during biopsy sample collection and handling. While pharmacokinetics can provide some insight through measurements of drug concentration over time, sufficient drug concentration, even in tumor, is not always

coupled with molecular target modulation (see Section 8.4.1). Hence, another key aspect of establishing PD biomarker FFP in a preclinical setting is performing time course experiments to profile the temporal pattern of PD biomarker modulation after drug administration [9,13–15]. This knowledge is then used to estimate the clinical sampling time point(s) that will yield the highest likelihood of measuring the largest modulation in biomarker levels [2].

8.3.3 Multiplex Pharmacodynamic Biomarker Analysis

Given that variability in biomarker modulation kinetics increases the potential for missing a biomarker response when biopsying a particular patient at a single time point, use of multiplex PD assays to simultaneously measure levels of two or more biomarkers (within a signaling pathway or across several pathways) is highly valuable ([16]; e.g., see Refs. [15,17]). By selecting a range of markers that are expected, based on preclinical data, to achieve maximum signal modulation (compared to baseline) at different time points, the likelihood of capturing a biomarker response may be increased (Fig. 8.2). Another benefit of multiplex PD biomarker analysis is the ability to simultaneously examine multiple levels (primary, secondary, and tertiary) of PD response to fully characterize drug MoA. Furthermore, because multiplex IFA analysis allows for examination of biomarker colocalization at the single-cell level, information regarding intratumoral heterogeneity of molecular response can be obtained. In addition to the examination of different molecules, multiplex analysis can also be used to examine multiple posttranslational modifications on a single key signaling molecule, such as the various phosphotyrosine residues that result from activation of the MET receptor tyrosine kinase [14].

8.3.4 Establishing Clinical Readiness of a Pharmacodynamic Biomarker Assay

Following preclinical PD biomarker assay development, demonstrating the clinical readiness of the assay is an imperative next step. The criteria for clinical readiness vary depending on whether the biomarker will have an integral, integrated, or exploratory role in the trial (see Table 8.1 and Section 8.5). Regardless,

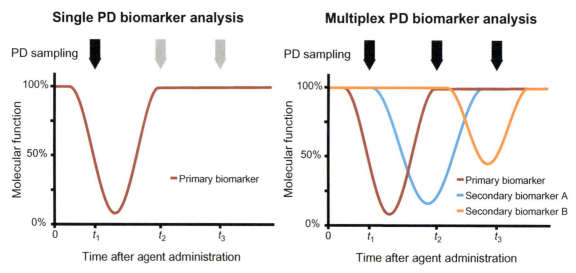

FIGURE 8.2 Multiplex analysis improves likelihood of detecting a PD biomarker response. When a single PD biomarker is assayed (left), the window for detecting a PD response is small (here, sampling at t_1 but not t_2 or t_3 yields a detectable PD biomarker signal). Use of a multiplex PD biomarker assay (right) expands this PD response detection window (sampling at t_1, t_2, or t_3 yields a detectable PD biomarker signal).

the components defining clinical readiness can be divided into three broad categories: (1) preclinical biomarker modeling and assay validation, (2) patient tissue collection and handling, and (3) clinical testing and biomarker quantitation (Table 8.2) [18,19]. The first category comprises properties that are important for any assay, such as accuracy, precision, specificity, and robustness, as well as preclinical quantitation of the assay endpoint using a clinically relevant calibration curve to improve the likelihood of a suitable dynamic range in the clinic [19]. One of the most significant problems encountered during assay development, lot-to-lot reagent quality and consistency, can be addressed at this level through rigorous validation and monitoring of antibodies, buffers, and other reagents by establishing clear assay and reagent performance specifications and using in vitro-derived analyte calibration standards as well as animal model and even clinical test samples remaining from previous studies (though, for the latter, patient consent must be appropriately documented) [17,20].

The second set of clinical readiness considerations pertains to how PD biomarker levels are affected by: (1) the type of tissue collected (tumor biopsies vs surrogate tissues) and (2) preanalytic variables such as the conditions of specimen collection and storage. Sample collection can cause cellular stress and tissue injury that may result from hypothermia, electrolyte disturbance, acidosis, hypoxia, and hypoglycemia, and subsequent tissue handling can result in cold ischemia, UV light exposure, and hyperoxia [12], though the impact of these stressors on PD biomarker levels will depend upon both the tissue type and the stability of the biomarker itself. For example, while a PD biomarker such as gene methylation is evaluable in cell-free plasma or other surrogate tissues and is likely highly stable [21], examination of a more labile PD biomarker such as protein phosphorylation in tumor biopsy samples often necessitates specific time and temperature parameters for specimen processing [14,22,23].

The final stage of establishing PD biomarker assay clinical readiness is the actual clinical testing of assay performance, which involves determining factors such as the clinical dynamic range and lower and upper limits of quantification, the baseline variability in biomarker levels and the contribution of biopsy sample heterogeneity, the effects of prior sampling on subsequent specimen collection (for biopsies), and the timing of sample collection (discussed earlier) [19]. As noted earlier in the case of the ABT-888 Phase 0 study, this final stage can be made less arduous when it is preceded by preclinical studies that replicate closely the clinical scenario [8,9].

A determination of acceptable levels of tumor biopsy sample quality and heterogeneity, both within and across specimens, is also critical

TABLE 8.2 Considerations for Establishing PD Biomarker Clinical Readiness

Preclinical Modeling and Assay Validation	Patient Tissue Collection and Handling	Clinical Testing and Biomarker Quantitation
Assay accuracy and precision	Type of tissue	Dynamic range, LLOQ, ULOQ
Assay specificity	Specimen collection	Baseline variability
Assay robustness	Specimen storage conditions	Biopsy sample quality/heterogeneity
Endpoint quantitation	Specimen processing	Effects of prior sampling
Lot-to-lot reagent quality	Analyte preservation	Timing of specimen collection

LLOQ, lower limit of quantification; *ULOQ*, upper limit of quantification.

TABLE 8.3　NCI PD Assay Biopsy Suitability Scoring System

Biopsy Tumor Content	Suitability for Slide-Based Assay	Suitability for Extract-Based Assay
>50%	Optimal	Optimal
25%–50%	Adequate	Marginal
5%–25%	Marginal	Inadequate
<5%	Inadequate	Inadequate

Tumor content is scored by a pathologist [20]. Required tumor content is higher for assays using tumor extracts because they do not allow for differentiation between biomarker signal in malignant versus nonmalignant tissue.

when considering the clinical readiness of a PD biomarker assay, as such assays require high-quality biopsy samples that feature greater tumor content and better tissue preservation than is necessary for the diagnostic biopsies with which most radiologists and pathologists are familiar. Standards for biopsy quality can be examined in metaanalyses of samples collected across different studies and addressed at the institutional level through implementation of SOPs for biopsy collection and sample processing, lessening the burden of this component during the development of individual PD biomarker assays. To this end, NCI has recently developed a scoring system protocol in which biopsy tumor content and sample handling artifacts are evaluated by a pathologist examining H & E-stained specimen sections [20]; this allows for regular feedback to the clinical team, with the goal of identifying aspects of lesion selection, image guidance, and collection that influence biopsy adequacy. Although biopsy inadequacy has been attributed to several factors, including high mucin content, necrosis, fibrosis, and inadequate biopsy size, the most common failure mode identified in NCI's metaanalysis of a large number of postdiagnostic biopsies collected for PD assays was that the lesion was missed entirely, yielding instead a core of normal tissue. While initial evaluations using this system at the NCI Developmental Therapeutics Clinic found that the majority of paired patient biopsy samples were of insufficient quality for PD biomarker assessment, changes to tissue quality requirements and biopsy sample processing, increasing the number of biopsy passes, and improved communication (Section 8.5.3) have led to improvement in the biopsy success rate, from approximately 50% to 60% (our unpublished results).

One important assay-specific biopsy QC criterion that has been established is overall tumor content; whereas slide-based assays can be performed on biopsy samples with tumor content as low as 5%–25%, the adequacy requirements are more stringent for extract-based assays (Table 8.3). Although H & E evaluation cannot be used to prescreen biopsies slated for whole-tissue extraction assays, NCI's use of the biopsy quality scoring system prior to slide-based assays suggests that as many as 45% of postdiagnostic biopsies collected using current methods contain <25% tumor and are therefore inadequate for extract-based assays (unpublished data).

Though the above criteria for establishing the clinical readiness of a PD biomarker assay are numerous, rigorously addressing all of these points increases the likelihood that the biomarker analysis will result in meaningful data that can inform future trials.

8.3.5 Surrogate Tissues for Pharmacodynamic Biomarker Analysis

While human tumor biopsy samples represent the traditional and most direct tissue for evaluating molecular PD biomarker responses to cancer therapy, the risks associated with biopsies, along with the inherently limited number and frequency of possible biopsies, have warranted the development of PD biomarker assays that instead utilize surrogate tissues, including peripheral blood mononuclear cells (PBMCs), skin, hair follicles, and plasma (for cell-free DNA analysis) [18,21]. Though use of surrogate tissues can ameliorate patient safety concerns and allow for more thorough sampling, it creates additional complications for data interpretation. Due to their nonmalignant nature, surrogate tissues do not contain the genetic and molecular abnormalities characteristic of tumor and therefore may manifest a molecular response to therapy that differs from that of malignant tissue. Thus rather than assuming that a surrogate tissue is an adequate proxy for molecular changes in tumor, an investigator must first demonstrate the occurrence of the molecular response in tumor, followed by demonstration of a statistical correlation between responses in tumor and in surrogate tissue, as was done in the case of PARP inhibition in PBMCs in the ABT-888 Phase 0 trial [8]. Importantly, not all targeted agents are suitable for evaluation in surrogate tissues; e.g., a drug that targets a tumor-specific enzyme-activating mutation may yield a PD biomarker response in tumor but not in normal tissue [12].

In the case of epithelial cancers, another potential surrogate is circulating tumor cells (CTCs). CTC enumeration has been used prognostically, but these cells are also beginning to be used for PD biomarker analysis. CTC isolation from blood has traditionally used antibodies to the epithelial marker EpCAM and defined carcinoma cells by the cytokeratin$^+$/DAPI$^+$/CD45$^-$ phenotype, though these markers together are sufficient only for defining epithelial cells [24]. Such markers must therefore be combined with additional, tumor-specific markers to distinguish the PD response

in tumor cells from that in normal epithelial cells, which are shed into the blood during therapy. Other approaches to isolating and identifying CTCs include negative selection through depletion of normal blood cells, microchip technology, dielectrophoretic field-flow fractionation, and filtration methods, but a universal tumor-specific CTC marker has yet to be identified. Another difficulty in developing CTCs for PD biomarker assessment is that CTC testing in mouse models is challenging. Finally, use of CTCs is complicated by highly variable CTC counts in a single blood sample and the low proportion of early-phase trial patients (20%−40%) that have any detectable CTCs, as determined using conventional isolation techniques [24]. Despite these limitations, use of CTCs for monitoring PD effects has been explored in several trials, including measurement of DNA damage biomarker γH2AX in CTCs from patients undergoing treatment with PARP inhibitors [25−28]. However, further studies demonstrating that PD biomarker changes in CTCs correlate with those occurring in tumor biopsy samples will be needed to establish CTCs as a true surrogate tissue.

8.4 BEYOND PROOF OF MECHANISM: OTHER BIOMARKER APPLICATIONS IN EARLY-PHASE TRIALS

Establishing POM for a given molecularly targeted agent is only one of several clinical uses of mechanistic PD biomarkers. For early-phase trials in particular, PD biomarker data may be complementary, or even superior, to the traditional use of PK information in guiding the optimization of dosage regimens (i.e., doses and schedules) for targeted agents. In addition, PD biomarkers are critical to understanding the molecular basis of drug resistance and how this problem may be combated through combination therapies. Finally, though this chapter has focused on PD biomarkers, the use of actionable and companion diagnostic biomarkers can also be beneficial to early-phase trials.

8.4.1 Pharmacodynamic-Guided Biologically Effective Dosage Regimens as an Alternative to Toxicity- and Pharmacokinetic-Based Guidance

If the goal of molecularly targeted anticancer therapies is to kill malignant cells via molecular target inhibition, a logical parameter for determining the dose and schedule of such agents is the extent and duration of molecular target suppression. Unfortunately, this parameter is often not considered, and instead, dosage regimens are typically selected based on tolerability (a criterion originally developed for systemic chemotherapies) rather than on target control. Given that patients in many trials experience clinical benefit from targeted agent therapy even at doses well below the MTD [29], dosage regimens based on tolerability may not offer improvements in efficacy compared to those that are designed to maintain adequate target suppression. In addition, unnecessarily high doses can lead to toxicity issues and low patient adherence [30]. Thus molecular PD biomarkers are poised to aid in dosage regimen optimization, allowing for determination of the "molecular biologically effective dose" [30] and schedule—the lowest dose that achieves the desired level of target suppression, and the dosing schedule that sustains this level of target suppression during dosing intervals. PD-guided biologically effective dosage regimens (PD-BEDR) may yield greater efficacy and reduced cost and toxicity compared to traditional, MTD-based regimens.

In terms of dosage regimen selection, PD biomarker measurements of target activity represent a more direct and potentially more useful parameter than traditional PK values such as blood or even tumor concentrations of unbound drug. Though PK and PD parameters are often correlated, this is not always the case; e.g., in preclinical experiments with the MET tyrosine kinase inhibitor XL184, target activity recovered after dosing even as tumor drug concentrations remained unchanged [31]. Such cases emphasize the need for monitoring PD biomarker responses over numerous time points to create a "PD effect × time" ($E \times t$) profile analogous to "drug concentration × time" ($C \times t$) profiles in PK analysis. Clinical development of the BCR-Abl inhibitors imatinib and dasatinib further illustrates this problematic reliance on PK guidance; after initial PK- and MTD-based dosage regimens resulted in toxicity issues, several studies eventually revealed that lower doses and/or altered schedules can reduce toxicity without compromising efficacy [32–34]—an outcome that may have been achieved years earlier through PD-BEDR. Of course, plasma PK data are more easily obtained than PD measurements (due to the relative ease and ethics of multiple blood sample collections compared to multiple tumor biopsies), but PK values can be used as surrogates for target inhibition only after conducting a correlative analysis of the PK–PD relationship. Thus PD biomarker levels represent a direct measurement of target inhibition that may complement or even, in some cases, supplant PK data in the optimization of dosage regimens to achieve maximal efficacy with minimal toxicity.

Like establishing PoM, the process of developing a PD-BEDR begins in a preclinical setting, with the selection of adequate primary and/or secondary biomarkers of target activity and clinically suitable biomarker assays. After a PD biomarker response is observed, the next critical aspect of defining a preclinical PD-BEDR is to establish the level of molecular target control (i.e., the target activity threshold) that is required for achieving maximum efficacy (ideally, tumor regression). This can be

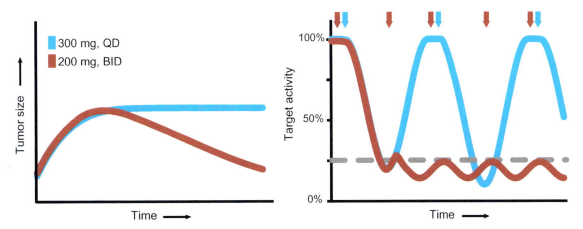

FIGURE 8.3   PD biomarker-guided biologically effective dosage regimens (PD-BEDR). An MTD-based dosage regimen (*blue*) may result in suboptimal tumor regression (left) due to only transient inhibition of the molecular target activity (right), which rebounds above the acceptable activity threshold (*dotted line*) during dosing intervals. In contrast, a dosage regimen that is optimized, through PD biomarker assays, to continuously maintain target activity below this threshold (*red*) may yield tumor regression. Source: *Adapted from Parchment RE, Doroshow JH. Pharmacodynamic endpoints as clinical trial objectives to answer important questions in oncology drug development. Semin Oncol 2016;43(4):514−25.*

done by measuring target activity levels and the rate of target recovery following administration of a single dose at a number of different dose levels, and then designing a dose-schedule (dosage regimen) that will continuously maintain target activity levels at or below the threshold value (i.e., the minimum level of continuous target control that yields the desired tumor response) (Fig. 8.3) [2].

8.4.2 Pharmacodynamic Biomarkers for Developing Novel Combination Therapies

The PD biomarker-based dosage regimen optimization described earlier can also be a powerful approach for developing combination therapies. Whereas efficacy-based assessment of single-agent therapies may erroneously classify some drugs as "inactive" because they do not achieve tumor regression in multifactorial disease, PD-based analysis allows for distinguishing truly molecularly inactive agents (those that do not inhibit their intended target)

from those that are highly active in molecular target inhibition but do not confer substantial antitumor activity due to the presence of compensatory driver mutations that allow the tumor to circumvent the molecular consequences of individual target inhibition [2]. By defining whether or not an agent is active in suppressing its intended target, PD biomarker assessments may uncover novel, previously overlooked agents for clinical use as a component of a combination therapy. The often substantial intra- and interpatient tumor mutational heterogeneity, wherein any given patient with advanced cancer is likely to have tumors containing various multiple driver mutations (as well as many passenger mutations, which do not influence malignancy), underscores the need for such an approach; e.g., a study of late-stage pancreatic adenocarcinomas found that each harbored an average of 63 somatic driver mutations (point mutations and other genetic alterations), mapping to 12 different signaling pathways [35]. Use of PD biomarker analysis to evaluate targeted agents based on target suppression, rather than single-agent efficacy, could allow for a greater diversity of personalized combinations that target the key driver mutations in a particular patient.

8.4.3 Pharmacodynamic Biomarkers as a Prelude to Actionable Biomarkers and Companion Diagnostics

Though this chapter has focused on the research use of molecular biomarkers that are altered in response to the intended mechanism of targeted therapies, some PD biomarkers may be of further use as actionable biomarkers for diagnostic, prognostic, or predictive purposes, with the goal of determining the best course of treatment for individual patients. Indeed, the assays and corresponding instrumentation are similar, if not identical, for both actionable and research-focused PD biomarkers. Thus the transitioning of a PD biomarker to "actionable" confers potential advantages not only for improving patient outcomes but also for mitigating the considerable costs associated with PD biomarker assay development. The latter is important because investments in assay development are not typically recouped through use of the assay for research purposes but may be offset by commercialization of a companion diagnostic biomarker assay that is required to be used together with a particular therapeutic agent [2]. By definition, PD biomarkers must be measured in both baseline and postdose samples; for actionable biomarkers, however, the baseline measurement alone is often the relevant value for determining whether or not a particular molecule represents a reasonable target in a patient. For example, patients with undetectable baseline levels of tyrosine 15-phosphorylated cyclin-dependent kinase 1 (pY15-Cdk1) may not be good candidates for treatment with AZD1775 (MK-1775), an inhibitor of the Wee1 kinase that catalyzes Y15-Cdk1 phosphorylation, because the target

is already suppressed prior to AZD1775 therapy [3]. An important caveat of actionable biomarkers is that even when a patient sample contains suitably high (or low) baseline biomarker levels to suggest that a specific therapy is warranted, this does not indicate whether the biomarker is truly a driver of disease in that patient or what other driver abnormalities may need to be addressed [2]. For combination therapies, a predictive diagnostic biomarker assay may be performed during dosing with the first agent to determine what agent(s) to administer in combination with the first; e.g., an assay that measures specific phosphoisoforms of MET kinase [14] could be used to determine whether patients undergoing therapy with erlotinib, an EGFR inhibitor, have erlotinib resistance-associated elevations in MET kinase activity and may therefore benefit from addition of a MET kinase inhibitor [36].

One critical distinction between the use of a biomarker assay for PD studies versus diagnostic or predictive purposes is that the latter is regulated by the Clinical Laboratory Improvement Amendments (CLIA) program and/or the FDA because the resulting measurements are used to direct patient treatment plans. Assays for actionable biomarkers should be performed in accordance with the appropriate FDA guidance documents, such as the Laboratory Developed Test guidance, and the laboratory in which the assay is conducted must be CLIA approved. If an assay for a diagnostic biomarker is integral to safe and effective use of an agent, it must be approved by the FDA as a companion diagnostic for use with the agent [37]. In such cases, the agent and companion diagnostic are often codeveloped and approved simultaneously, requiring close cooperation between the sponsor of the drug and the entity developing the companion diagnostic. Though the FDA strongly recommends that companion diagnostics are validated and demonstrated to be FFP and clinically suitable before the clinical trial begins, this sometimes occurs only later, when necessitated by efficacy or safety issues. Despite these complexities, a number of FDA-approved companion diagnostics exist, and this process represents a logical extension of PD biomarker assays into commercially valuable space, which could offset the large costs associated with PD biomarker research and development.

8.5 DESIGNING CLINICAL TRIALS TO INCORPORATE PHARMACODYNAMIC BIOMARKER STUDIES

An overarching consideration for the design of clinical trials involving biomarkers is whether the biomarker will be integral, integrated, or exploratory; e.g., integral biomarkers, when used to direct clinical decision-making for an individual patient, must be assessed in accordance with CLIA regulations (Table 8.1). In contrast, the use of integrated biomarkers, which often involves clinical validation of the biomarker assay for utilization in subsequent trials, is not CLIA regulated but must be described in detail (including statistical design, specimen collection, and data analysis) in the clinical protocol. Regulatory requirements for exploratory biomarkers, which are not fundamental to the trial, are considerably less stringent (Table 8.1). Because early-phase trials often involve the use of exploratory biomarkers to investigate MoA in a relatively small number of patients using biomarker assays that may not be extensively characterized, the biomarker-related hypotheses tested and subsequent conclusions may be limited [19]. However, the less stringent regulatory requirements for exploratory PD biomarker assays do *not* translate into less rigorous assay validation, clinical readiness, and fitness-for-purpose requirements because clinically meaningful results are much more likely when trials use assays that meet these standards, adopted from clinical lab medicine and pathology; this is an important principle that was overlooked in a previous metaanalysis of the value of PD biomarker studies in Phase I trials [38].

8.5.1 Pharmacodynamic Biomarker Insights From Early-Phase Trials

When incorporating biomarkers in the clinical evaluation of a targeted agent, one must design the trial or series of trials based on which pharmacodynamic insights can be gained during each stage of clinical testing (Fig. 8.4). Phase 0 trials are an excellent platform for establishing biomarker assay clinical readiness, molecular target engagement and secondary PD effects (PoM), and a preliminary understanding of the time course of PD biomarker response(s) to nontoxic, nonefficacious

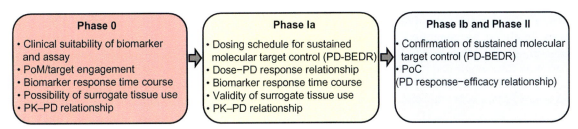

FIGURE 8.4 Workflow for integrating pharmacodynamic biomarker assessments into early-phase clinical trials. The critical PD components that can be determined in each trial phase (Phase 0, Phase Ia (dose escalation), Phase Ib (MTD expansion), and Phase II) are shown.

doses of an agent. This biomarker response time course can then be more thoroughly explored in a subsequent Phase Ia (dose escalation) study, wherein multiple time points may be examined by either randomly assigning individual patients or an entire dose level cohort of patients to each time point [2]. When use of a surrogate tissue for biomarker analyses is desired, Phase 0 and Phase Ia trials are also early opportunities for demonstrating surrogate tissue validity by comparing PD biomarker responses in surrogate tissue versus tumor. Ideally, in Phase 0 or Phase Ia studies, samples for PK analysis should be collected simultaneously with PD biomarker samples so that the relationship between biomarker changes and plasma and/or tumor drug levels can be explored, providing evidence that changes in PD biomarker levels occur as drug levels rise and fall. The Phase Ia setting may also allow for a preliminary understanding of the dose—PD response relationship, provided that dose-concentration (PK) and concentration-response (PD) relationships are not unusual. In addition, by providing information about the temporal dynamics of the PD biomarker response, a Phase Ia study allows for initial selection of a dosage regimen that can achieve sustained molecular target control (PD-BEDR; see Section 8.4.1). Though PD biomarker analyses are sometimes delayed until the Phase Ib (MTD expansion) stage, incorporation of such analyses in Phase 0 or Phase Ia is advantageous because it allows for assay evaluation and clinical optimization early in clinical development so that useful data are more likely to be generated in Phase Ib and later-phase trials; early PD-BEDR determination may also maximize the chances of observing clinical responses while minimizing toxicities in Phase Ib [12].

Finally, Phase Ib MTD expansion studies and Phase II trials represent opportunities for dosage regimen optimization (PD-BEDR) and preliminary examination of associations between biomarker response and efficacy (PoC), though the latter can be difficult due to the small numbers of patients relative to a Phase III study [19]. There are trade-offs for the use of a Phase Ib versus Phase II trial to establish PoC; while a Phase Ib trial, with mandatory biopsies, likely yields a greater number of patient specimens, the histologically heterogeneous and generally drug-resistant advanced disease stage may render PoC analysis difficult. On the other hand, optional biopsies in a Phase II trial may yield fewer tumor samples for research, but a more defined patient population can improve response rates [12].

8.5.2 Writing Clinical Protocols That Include Pharmacodynamic Biomarker Analyses

A prerequisite to clinical PD biomarker studies is incorporating the proper rationale and experimental design details into the clinical protocol. In a 2010 document [19], the NCI Investigational Drug Steering Committee (IDSC) Biomarker Task Force presented recommendations for investigators submitting proposals for clinical trials that incorporate PD biomarker studies (Fig. 8.5). The first of these is the statement of a biomarker-related hypothesis and corresponding justification, including the a priori rationale (based on the putative drug MoA), empirical information (preclinical and possibly clinical data), and an explanation of how and why the biomarker assay will be used in the trial, including whether the biomarker will be integral, integrated, or exploratory. Investigators should also include information demonstrating assay validity and clinical readiness, assay and biomarker fitness-for-purpose in the context of the study, and the experience of the investigators with performing the assay.

Beyond these assay-related details, one must also include a statement regarding statistical

- Provide a hypothesis and rationale for biomarker utility and a description of the impact on therapeutic agent development based on the following considerations:
  - biological and/or mechanistic rationale with data to support relationship between biomarker and agent effects
  - intended use within the proposed study
  - preclinical in vitro,in vivo, and clinical results if available.
- Describe the assay method's validity and appropriateness for the study.
- Describe the investigator's experience and competence with the proposed assays.
- Provide the data supporting the degree of biomarker "fit for purpose" and clinical qualification.
- Justify the number of patients and specimens
  - to demonstrate feasibility
  - to demonstrate that studies are likely to produce interpretable and meaningful results.
- Give thoughtful consideration to the risk to the patient of obtaining samples, specimens, or data for biomarker studies in the context of data on biomarker validity and degree of clinical qualification.

FIGURE 8.5   NCI Investigational Drug Steering Committee Biomarker Task Force recommendations for investigators proposing biomarker studies in new clinical trials. Source: *From Dancey JE, Dobbin KK, Groshen S, et al. Guidelines for the development and incorporation of biomarker studies in early clinical trials of novel agents. Clin Cancer Res 2010;16(6):1745—55.*

considerations: a justification of the number of patients and specimens required to draw meaningful conclusions about the biomarker-related hypothesis [19]. The required sample sizes will depend on numerous factors, including the nature of the biomarker-related study objective (e.g., whether the aim is to demonstrate feasibility of the biomarker assay application or to produce clinically meaningful results), the role of the biomarker (integral, integrated, or exploratory), the type of trial (Phase 0, I, or II), the degree of biomarker modulation required to reach statistical significance (estimated from previous data), and the anticipated sample quality and heterogeneity (e.g., biopsy tumor content). For example, a Phase 0 trial with the aim of demonstrating the feasibility of measuring changes in an exploratory primary biomarker would require far fewer patients than a Phase II trial in which the aim is to use that same biomarker in an integrated fashion for PoC. Generally, assuming a normal distribution of biomarker levels in the patient population, the larger and more histologically well-defined Phase II patient population allows for greater confidence in biomarker-related

conclusions [19]. In some cases, PoC and other conclusions may not be confidently established until a much larger Phase III trial.

Finally, the impact of the proposed biomarker studies on the patient risk—benefit assessment must be addressed. Prior demonstration of biomarker assay validity, clinical readiness, and FFP is ethically imperative given the risk to patients conferred by tissue sample collection, particularly for biopsies [12]. This risk must be adequately balanced with the potential benefits arising from the biomarker study and must also be communicated in both the clinical protocol and patient consent forms [19].

8.5.3 An Interdisciplinary Team Approach to Biomarker Studies

A critical (and often overlooked) aspect of incorporating biomarker analyses into clinical trials is the multidisciplinary team of clinicians and scientists required and the importance of establishing communication and training infrastructures to ensure optimal PD biomarker results (Fig. 8.6) [12].

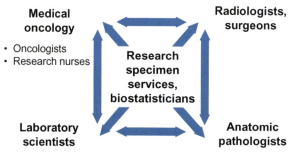

FIGURE 8.6   Multidisciplinary communication is necessary for clinical PD biomarker studies.

8.5.4 Defining "Clinical Correlation" in Proof of Concept Pharmacodynamic Biomarker Studies

When seeking to demonstrate an association between PD biomarker response and clinical outcome for solid tumors, reliance on traditional RECIST (Response Evaluation Criteria in Solid Tumors) guidelines may be problematic. Given the high levels of intrapatient tumor heterogeneity, attempts to correlate a molecular response that occurs in a small portion of a single lesion (i.e., the site of biopsy) with the RECIST-defined clinical response, as compiled from analysis of a number of lesions, may miss biologically meaningful relationships. Thus we recommend that clinical protocols stipulate a distinct radiological assessment and scoring of the biopsied lesion(s) exclusively, which can be used for tumor PD biomarker PoC studies.

8.6 THE FUTURE OF PHARMACODYNAMIC BIOMARKERS IN EARLY-PHASE TRIALS

Despite the value of PD biomarker assays in improving the drug development process and

clinical outcomes, key challenges and opportunities for innovation remain; some of these are inherent to current technologies, while others stem from new directions in the development of molecularly targeted cancer therapeutics. In particular, the increasing number of oncology trials involving immune-modulating targeted agents necessitates improved methodologies for examining the associated complex, multicellular MoAs; this emerging field of immuno-pharmacodynamics requires microscopy to visualize the spatial relationships among different cell types, juxtaposed with the biomarker responses occurring in each [39]. Likewise, the design of single agents that target multiple molecules (i.e., "multitarget drugs") requires expanding the capacity of multiplex imaging tools to examine several biomarkers for each of the desired targets [2]. Several of the critical challenges pertaining to these and other uses of PD biomarker assays are outlined below.

8.6.1 Improved Biopsy Instrumentation

Because many biomarker analyses are performed using tumor tissue, and given the difficulties with obtaining high tumor content tissue samples (Section 8.3.4), improvements in biopsy collection technology translate to improvements in the quality of clinical PD biomarker analyses. To this end, numerous image-guided biopsy efforts are underway, in which sensors embedded in the biopsy needle allow for real-time visualization of the tissue encountered by the needle, allowing radiologists to better target the lesion [40,41]. One can also imagine devices that would enable continuous sampling of a lesion and, hence, construction of a comprehensive "$E \times t$" (PD effect × time) profile (Section 8.4.1). Though the benefits of continuous PD sampling are numerous, and an "$E \times t$" profile highly useful, this will require substantial technological innovation, such as development of fixed-location, "central access" biopsy needles that allow for repeated sampling at a single lesion site.

8.6.2 Identification of Biomarkers for Tumor Content and Tissue Quality Quantification

The development of pathologist-directed scoring systems for biopsy tumor content and tissue quality (Section 8.3.4) is an important but still incomplete step toward establishing a high-precision method for quantifying these factors. An ideal tissue quality monitoring system would entail use of a tumor-specific marker that is robust and detectable in both microscopy- and tissue extract-based analyses. While proteins such as MUC1 and CEA are currently used as tumor markers for microscopy-based analysis in some tumor histologies [10,11], these are not universal tumor markers and are often not useful for extract-based assays due to their expression in nonmalignant tissues. Laser capture microdissection can be used to separate malignant from nonmalignant tissue in paraffin-embedded sections prior to an extract-based assay, but large proteins are

often difficult to extract from fixed tissue [42]. Thus the identification of a universal tumor marker with very low levels of nonmalignant expression would be ideal both for masking tumor regions in microscopy-based assays and for normalizing PD biomarker measurements to viable tumor content in extract-based assays.

Because many biomarkers are susceptible to artifacts resulting from tissue handling and other preanalytic variables, there is also a need for combining measurements for markers of environmental stressors to yield an overall tissue quality index (TQI). Though there have been promising efforts to construct TQIs for microscopy assays [43], a framework for extract-based assays is lacking; both types of TQI may be developed and further refined as proteome-wide analyses reveal new, robust biomarkers of cold ischemia [22] and other stressors.

8.6.3 Methodology That Combines Specificity and Tissue Geography

An ideal biomarker assay would provide the molecular specificity afforded by a two-antibody-based sandwich assay of tumor lysates coupled with the detailed histological-geographical information that is obtained through microscopy-based approaches. One such technique is mass spectrometry imaging (MSI), particularly, matrix-assisted laser desorption ionization-MSI, which creates a "chemical microscope" in which molecules within a slide-mounted tissue section are extracted, desorbed, and ionized for label-free detection by a mass spectrometer; additionally, the ability to examine drug distribution geography using this approach could allow for cellular-resolution PK–PD analyses [44]. However, MSI is currently limited by protein molecular weight, and precise identification of proteins and posttranslational modification states can be challenging. High-specificity molecular visualization might also be achievable by combining multiplex imaging with a multiple-antibodies-per-molecule approach [2], as in NanoString's high-plex digital immunohistochemistry microscopy platform, which uses DNA bar codes for simultaneous detection of hundreds of analytes on a single slide [45].

8.7 CONCLUSION

Given the importance of demonstrating clinical PoM for facilitating successful passage of new targeted therapies from early- to late-phase trials and into their proper roles in combination therapies, understanding of how and when to implement various PD biomarker analyses in the clinic is key. Furthermore, in light of the 21st Century Cures Act, PD biomarker endpoints for clinical trials are poised to become increasingly valuable, as surrogate endpoints alone may suffice for accelerated FDA approval of new agents. We hope this chapter has provided useful details regarding considerations for biomarker and assay development, applications for biomarker assays, constructing clinical protocols with PD endpoints, and possibilities for expanding the scope of knowledge that can be gained through PD biomarker studies.

Acknowledgment

This project has been funded in part with federal funds from the National Cancer Institute, National Institutes of Health, under Contract No. HHSN261200800001E. The content of this publication does not necessarily reflect the views or policies of the Department of Health and Human Services, nor does mention of trade names, commercial products, or organizations imply endorsement by the U.S. Government.

References

[1] 21st Century Cures Act, Pub. L. No. 114-255; 2016.

[2] Parchment RE, Doroshow JH. Pharmacodynamic endpoints as clinical trial objectives to answer important questions in oncology drug development. Semin Oncol 2016;43(4):514−25.

[3] Do K, Wilsker D, Ji JP, et al. Phase I Study of Single-Agent AZD1775 (MK-1775), a Wee1 Kinase Inhibitor, in Patients With Refractory Solid Tumors. J Clin Oncol 2015;33(30):3409−15.

[4] Arrowsmith J. Phase II failures: 2008-2010. Nat Rev Drug Discov 2011;10(5):1.

[5] Morgan P, Van der Graaf PH, Arrowsmith J, et al. Can the flow of medicines be improved? Fundamental pharmacokinetic and pharmacological principles toward improving Phase II survival. Drug Discov Today 2012;17(9−10):419−24.

[6] U.S. Department of Health and Human Services Food and Drug Administration Center for Drug Evaluation and Research (CDER). Guidance for Industry, Investigators, and Reviewers: Exploratory IND Studies, <http://www.fda.gov/downloads/drugs/guidancecomplianceregulatoryinformation/guidances/ucm078933.pdf>; 2006 [accessed 27.11.15].

[7] Doroshow JH, Parchment RE. Oncologic phase 0 trials incorporating clinical pharmacodynamics: from concept to patient. Clin Cancer Res 2008;14(12):3658−63.

[8] Kummar S, Kinders R, Gutierrez ME, et al. Phase 0 clinical trial of the poly (ADP-ribose) polymerase inhibitor ABT-888 in patients with advanced malignancies. J Clin Oncol 2009;27(16):2705−11.

[9] Kinders RJ, Hollingshead M, Khin S, et al. Preclinical modeling of a phase 0 clinical trial: qualification of a pharmacodynamic assay of poly (ADP-ribose) polymerase in tumor biopsies of mouse xenografts. Clin Cancer Res 2008;14(21):6877−85.

[10] Painter JT, Clayton NP, Herbert RA. Useful immunohistochemical markers of tumor differentiation. Toxicol Pathol 2010;38(1):131−41.

[11] Duffy MJ. Role of tumor markers in patients with solid cancers: a critical review. Eur J Intern Med 2007;18(3):175−84.

[12] Parchment RE, Doroshow JH. Theory and practice of clinical pharmacodynamics in oncology drug development. Semin Oncol 2016;43(4):427−35.

[13] Kinders RJ, Hollingshead M, Lawrence S, et al. Development of a validated immunofluorescence assay for gammaH2AX as a pharmacodynamic marker of topoisomerase I inhibitor activity. Clin Cancer Res 2010;16(22):5447−57.

[14] Srivastava AK, Hollingshead MG, Weiner J, et al. Pharmacodynamic response of the MET/HGF-receptor to small molecule tyrosine kinase inhibitors examined with validated, fit-for-clinic immunoassays. Clin Cancer Res 2016;22(14):3683−94.

[15] Srivastava AK, Jaganathan S, Stephen L, et al. Effect of a Smac mimetic (TL32711, Birinapant) on the apoptotic program and apoptosis biomarkers examined with validated multiplex immunoassays fit for clinical use. Clin Cancer Res 2016;22(4):1000–10.

[16] Marrero A, Lawrence S, Wilsker D, et al. Translating pharmacodynamic biomarkers from bench to bedside: analytical validation and fit-for-purpose studies to qualify multiplex immunofluorescent assays for use on clinical core biopsy specimens. Semin Oncol 2016;43(4):453–63.

[17] LoRusso PM, Li J, Burger A, et al. Phase I safety, pharmacokinetic, and pharmacodynamic study of the Poly (ADP-ribose) Polymerase (PARP) inhibitor Veliparib (ABT-888) in combination with irinotecan in patients with advanced solid tumors. Clin Cancer Res 2016;22 (13):3227–37.

[18] Kummar S, Do K, Coyne GO, et al. Establishing proof of mechanism: assessing target modulation in early-phase clinical trials. Semin Oncol 2016;43(4):446–52.

[19] Dancey JE, Dobbin KK, Groshen S, et al. Guidelines for the development and incorporation of biomarker studies in early clinical trials of novel agents. Clin Cancer Res 2010;16(6):1745–55.

[20] Ferry-Galow KV, Makhlouf HR, Wilsker DF, et al. The root causes of pharmacodynamic assay failure. Semin Oncol 2016;43(4):484–91.

[21] Rapisuwon S, Vietsch EE, Wellstein A. Circulating biomarkers to monitor cancer progression and treatment. Comput Struct Biotechnol J 2016;14:211–22.

[22] Mertins P, Yang F, Liu T, et al. Ischemia in tumors induces early and sustained phosphorylation changes in stress kinase pathways but does not affect global protein levels. Mol Cell Proteomics 2014;13 (7):1690–704.

[23] Baker AF, Dragovich T, Ihle NT, et al. Stability of phosphoprotein as a biological marker of tumor signaling. Am Assoc Cancer Res 2005;11(12):4338–40.

[24] Wang LH, Balasubramanian P, Chen AP, et al. Promise and limits of the CellSearch platform for evaluating pharmacodynamics in circulating tumor cells. Semin Oncol 2016;43(4):464–75.

[25] Kummar S, Ji J, Morgan R, et al. A phase I study of veliparib in combination with metronomic cyclophosphamide in adults with refractory solid tumors and lymphomas. Clin Cancer Res 2012;18(6):1726–34.

[26] Kummar S, Oza AM, Fleming GF, et al. Randomized trial of oral cyclophosphamide and veliparib in high-grade serous ovarian, primary peritoneal, or fallopian tube cancers, or BRCA-mutant ovarian cancer. Clin Cancer Res 2015;21(7):1574–82.

[27] Reiss KA, Herman JM, Zahurak M, et al. A Phase I study of veliparib (ABT-888) in combination with low-dose fractionated whole abdominal radiation therapy in patients with advanced solid malignancies and peritoneal carcinomatosis. Clin Cancer Res 2015;21 (1):68–76.

[28] Wang LH, Pfister TD, Parchment RE, et al. Monitoring drug-induced gammaH2AX as a pharmacodynamic biomarker in individual circulating tumor cells. Clin Cancer Res 2010;16(3):1073–84.

[29] Postel-Vinay S, Arkenau HT, Olmos D, et al. Clinical benefit in Phase-I trials of novel molecularly targeted agents: does dose matter? Br J Cancer 2009;100 (9):1373–8.

[30] Sachs JR, Mayawala K, Gadamsetty S, et al. Optimal dosing for targeted therapies in oncology: drug development cases leading by example. Clin Cancer Res 2016;22(6):1318–24.

[31] Srivastava AK, Hollingshead MG, Govindharajulu JP, et al. Abstract 3691: Met target inhibition-guided efficacy in preclinical models. Cancer Res 2014;74 (Suppl. 19):3691.

[32] He Q, Zhu J, Dingli D, et al. Optimized treatment schedules for chronic myeloid leukemia. PLOS Comput Biol 2016;12(10):e1005129.

[33] Liu SL, Chen G, Zhao YP, et al. Optimized dose of imatinib for treatment of gastrointestinal stromal tumors: a meta-analysis. J Dig Dis 2013;14(1):16–21.

[34] Wong SF. New dosing schedules of dasatinib for CML and adverse event management. J Hematol Oncol 2009;2:10.

[35] Jones S, Zhang X, Parsons DW, et al. Core signaling pathways in human pancreatic cancers revealed by global genomic analyses. Science 2008;321 (5897):1801–6.

[36] Engelman JA, Zejnullahu K, Mitsudomi T, et al. MET amplification leads to gefitinib resistance in lung cancer by activating ERBB3 signaling. Science 2007;316 (5827):1039–43.

[37] U.S. Department of Health and Human Services Food and Drug Administration. Principles for codevelopment of an in vitro companion diagnostic device with a therapeutic product, Draft Guidance, <http://www.fda.gov/ucm/groups/fdagov-public/@fdagov-meddev-gen/documents/document/ucm510824.pdf>; 2016 [accessed 14.12.16].

[38] Sweis RF, Drazer MW, Ratain MJ. Analysis of impact of post-treatment biopsies in Phase I clinical trials. J Clin Oncol 2016;34(4):369–74.

[39] Parchment RE, Voth AR, Doroshow JH, et al. Immuno-pharmacodynamics for evaluating mechanism of action and developing immunotherapy combinations. Semin Oncol 2016;43(4):501–13.

[40] Sheth RA, Heidari P, Esfahani SA, et al. Interventional optical molecular imaging guidance during percutaneous biopsy. Radiology 2014;271(3):770–7.

[41] Spliethoff JW, Prevoo W, Meier MA, et al. Real-time in vivo tissue characterization with diffuse reflectance spectroscopy during transthoracic lung biopsy: a clinical feasibility study. Clin Cancer Res 2016;22(2):357–65.

[42] Datta S, Malhotra L, Dickerson R, et al. Laser capture microdissection: big data from small samples. Histol Histopathol 2015;30:1255–69.

[43] Neumeister VM, Parisi F, England AM, et al. A tissue quality index: an intrinsic control for measurement of effects of preanalytical variables on FFPE tissue. Lab Invest 2014;94(4):467–74.

[44] van Hove ERA, Smith DF, Heeren RMA. A concise review of mass spectrometry imaging. J Chromatogr A 2010;1217(25):3946–54.

[45] NanoString Technologies. NanoString launches Technology Access Program (TAP) for transformative platform for high-plex digital spatial profiling, <http://investors.nanostring.com/releasedetail.cfm?ReleaseID = 998136>; 2016 [accessed 13.01.17].

Can Early Clinical Trials Help Deliver More Precise Cancer Care?

Joline S.J. Lim[1,2], Jessica S. Brown[1,3] and Johann S. De Bono[1,3]

[1]Royal Marsden Hospital, London, United Kingdom [2]National University Cancer Institute of Singapore, Singapore, Singapore [3]The Institute of Cancer Research, London, United Kingdom

9.1 INTRODUCTION

Phase I studies have traditionally been carried out in eligible patients with molecularly uncharacterized treatment-refractory cancers. The advent of targeted therapies in cancer therapeutics, however, shifted trial enrollment from an "all-comers" approach to a more "precise" strategy whereby specific tumor genomic aberrations are sought out through various methods of genomic analysis in ethically-driven efforts to increase the likelihood of clinical benefit while minimizing toxicities. The initial success of imatinib in patients with chronic myeloid leukemia harboring the BCL-ABL translocation and gastrointestinal stromal tumors with KIT or PDGFR mutations, followed quickly with evidence for benefit from trastuzumab in patients with HER2-positive cancers, PARP inhibitors for DNA homologous recombination repair defective cancers especially BRCA1/2-defective tumors, and targeted agents for treating non-small-cell lung cancers (NSCLC) with a myriad of aberrations including epidermal growth factor receptor (EGFR) mutations, anaplastic lymphoma kinase (ALK) translocations, and ROS-1 fusions. These significant successes, many fueled through pioneering Phase I trials, have brought precision medicine and molecular profiling of tumors to the front line. Nonetheless, there is increasing awareness that this precision medicine strategy has its limitations, including technical challenges in molecular characterization, tumor factors including disease genomic instability and heterogeneity resulting in clonal evolution, and limitations in anticancer drug design. Increasingly, questions have been raised about whether personalized medicine strategies are frequently imprecise. In this chapter, we endeavor to give an overview of the concept of precision medicine and review current evidence of its feasibility and ability to improve patient outcomes. We also discuss challenges in molecular profiling, its current role in an institutional compared to a third party commercial setting, and its value in a Phase I setting. Finally, we conclude by outlining how we think molecular profiling can be optimally implemented and used in a clinical setting, and envision its role in the ever changing landscape of cancer therapeutics.

9.2 WHAT IS PRECISION MEDICINE?

The National Institutes of Health defined precision medicine as "an approach to disease treatment and prevention that seeks to maximize effectiveness by taking into account individual variability in genes, environment, and lifestyle" [1]. In a broader perspective, precision medicine endeavors to measure individual factors that potentially contribute to a disease in an attempt to improve understanding of the disease history, treatment response, and patient outcome. In the context of cancer therapeutics, the concept of precision medicine is largely linked to molecular profiling of an individual's tumor sample to personalize a treatment strategy based on specific putative mutations that may be found in tumor tissue.

While DNA sequencing was first reported in 1970 [2], it was the Sanger sequencing technique, based on a primer-extension method developed by Frederick Sanger, that became widely adopted in research studies [3] and eventually formed the basis of sequencing for the human genome project. With more advanced sequencing technologies allowing more refinement, higher throughput and better efficiency, while simultaneously becoming more affordable, these methods have paved the way for routine clinical utilization. Technological platforms now allow molecular profiling of tumors based on various "omic" approaches, including genomics, proteomics, and transcriptomics.

In parallel to this sequencing technological revolution, and partly as a result of its impact on target selection, drug discovery and development has been increasingly guided by deeper understanding of molecular oncology.

The hallmarks of cancer, first described by Hanahan and Weinberg in 2000 was updated a decade later in 2011 to accommodate the growing knowledge of pathways and processes involved in carcinogenesis [4,5]. In a similar fashion, cancer therapeutics has evolved from a "one size fits all" approach for cytotoxic chemotherapy to include molecular targeted agents designed to act against specific molecular subtypes of cancers, such as oncogene addicted cancers, to improve efficacy while decreasing drug toxicities. Molecular profiling of individual tumors prior to treatment provides a roadmap of potential "actionable" putative genetic aberrations that may be amenable to treatment with specific targeted agents. Additionally, in the early phase clinical setting, this provides a "line of sight" to drug approval for a selected indication, whereby predictive biomarkers identifying patients acquiring substantial benefit support expedited regulatory approval [6].

The concept behind precision medicine, simply stated, is therefore an attempt to seek out the root cause(s) (or early/truncal event) behind the transformation of a normal cell into a cancerous entity, in order to find the most compatible drug or drugs that may eliminate this cell type with minimal collateral damage to normal surrounding tissue. Nonetheless, the successful implementation of this in a clinical setting has multiple challenges, including technical limitations in molecular profiling methods, intrinsic properties of tumor biology such as tumor evolution and cellular heterogeneity, and drug-related issues such as drug specificity and concerns regarding off-target activity. Ultimately, a sound understanding of cancer genomics, coupled with acknowledgements of the strengths and weakness of these precision medicine therapeutic strategies will be required to critically appraise the results of tumor profiling and apply it to the individual patient and provide better care both within and outside clinical trials.

9.3 EVIDENCE FOR IMPLEMENTATION OF MOLECULAR PROFILING

While the concept behind precision medicine is in theory sound, critics continue to question whether the broad application of this therapeutic strategy in a clinical context is feasible, and whether it will lead to improved patient outcomes. Despite these valid criticisms, it is nevertheless clear that in some cancers (probably genomically more stable tumors), such strategies have had a major impact as we will describe below. This strategy is, however, much less likely to be impactful in genomically unstable and highly heterogeneous cancers.

Arguably, a major success of precision medicine has been improving the treatment of NSCLC with molecular targeted agents (MTA), with multiple effective drugs designed against specific pathway aberrations like EGFR, ALK, and ROS1. Riding on the success of these drugs, the lung cancer mutation consortium has employed "Basket" or "Umbrella" trial approaches, whereby patients enrolled are tested for a panel of genes through multiplex genotyping for mutation detection to demonstrate that a particular targeted drug benefits patients with matched actionable detected oncogenic drivers. This genotype-match treatment was reported to improve median overall survival (OS) compared to patients receiving genotype-unmatched treatment (hazard ratio 0.69, $P = 0.006$) [7] (Table 9.1). Several collaborative groups are looking into similar trial designs using next-generation sequencing (NGS) methods such as the Lung Matrix Trial (NCT026647935) and LUNG-MAP study (NCT02154490) which may yield more insight into the role of molecular profiling for lung cancer treatment.

Other trials have focused on patients with advanced tumors of various origins; a study examining patients with advanced cancers undergoing molecular profiling by targeted hotspot mutation analysis showed that implementation of such profiling techniques is feasible. Of the 2000 consecutive patients included, 39% had one or more potentially actionable mutations, of which 11% eventually went on a genotype-match trial that was specifically targeting the genetic aberration identified. Within a focused group of 230 patients with PIK3CA/AKT1/PTEN/BRAF mutations, 50% were able to receive a genotype-matched drug, either on trial or in an off-trial setting. The authors concluded that implementation of targeted molecular testing is feasible, although successful matching to trials may be limited by various reasons included issues with drug(s) access, patient preference, and performance status [8]. Another similar study from the Princess Margaret Hospital looked at the use of molecular profiling in an academic center and community oncology setting. In this study, 15% of 1640 patients who were tested were successfully enrolled onto therapeutic clinical trials, although only 5% eventually enrolled onto a genotype-matched trial. Patients treated on a genotype-matched trial had, however, an improved response rate compared to those treated on a genotype-unmatched trial (overall response rate 19% vs 9%, $P < 0.026$) [9], providing further evidence of improved patient outcomes with molecular profiling. Conversely, the SHIVA study, an open-label, randomized Phase II study comparing the use of MTA with chemotherapy of physician choice in patients whose cancers had actionable mutations in at least one of three pathways (hormone receptor, PI3K/AKT/mTOR, and Raf/Mek pathways) [10] demonstrated no improvement in progression-free survival (PFS) (2.3 vs 2.0 months, $P = 0.41$) from this patient selection strategy, although this study was reported to have multiple limitations, including an overall poor PFS, the use of monotherapy MTA targeting pathways that

TABLE 9.1   Clinical Studies Evaluating Personalized Cancer Medicine With Published Results

Trial	Methods	Molecular Targets	Targeted Agents	Primary Endpoint
FEASIBILITY STUDIES				
M.D Anderson feasibility study (8)	Feasibility of allocating targeted treatment based on molecular profile	11−50 gene platform	Not stated	Potentially actionable mutations identified in 39% of patients, of which 11% received genotype-matched trials
Cleveland precision oncology study (56)	Feasibility of allocating targeted treatment based on molecular profile	Foundation 1 platform	Not stated	Potentially actionable mutations identified in 49% of patients. 11% patients received genotype-matched trials
INTERVENTION STUDIES				
SHIVA (10)	Randomized molecularly targeted agent vs conventional therapy	Hormone receptor, PI3K/AKT/MTOR and RAF/MEK pathway	Abiraterone, letrozole, tamoxifen, erlotinib, imatinib, dasatinib, everolimus, sorafenib, vemurafenib	No PFS benefit of experimental vs control group
ONCO-T-PROFILE (57)	Targeted treatment allocation based on molecular profile	DNA repair, Wnt signalling, RAS/RAF/ MEK, HER2, PI3K/ AKT/MTOR, MAPK	Chemotherapy (multiple regimens), exemestane + everolimus, regorafinib	PFS ratio $\geq$ 1.3 achieved in 42% patients (=PFS upon treatment according to the molecular profile/PFS upon the last prior therapy)
IMPACT/COMPACT trial (9)	Trial allocation based on molecular profile	Aberrations in: *PIK3CA, BRAF, KRAS, NRAS, EGFR, FGFR2, PTEN, KIT*	Inhibitors of: EGFR, PI3K, BRAF, VEGF, MEK, IGF1R, MTOR, WEE1, HER2, FGFR, HER3, VEGF, ANG2	Overall response rate higher in genotype matched trials (19%) compared with genotype-unmatched trials (9%; $P < 0.026$)
Lung cancer mutation consortium (7)	Targeted treatment allocation based on molecular profile in lung adenocarcinoma	*KRAS, EGFR, ALK* rearrangement, *HER2, BRAF, PIK3CA, MET* amplification, *NRAS, MEK, AKT1* mutations	Inhibitors of: EGFR, ALK, HER2, others not specified	mOS 3.5 years in patients allocated treatment based on molecular profile vs 2.4 years ($P < 0.01$) in patients allocated treatment irrespective of molecular profile
SAFIR01 / UNICANCER (58)	Targeted treatment allocation based on molecular profile in breast cancer	Mutations in *PIK3CA* or *AKT*. Amplifications of: *CCND1, FGFR1, FRS2, EGFR, RPTOR, MDM2, PIK3CA, FGFR2, AKT2, IGFR1, ALK, BRAF, FGFR3, MET*		9% objective response rate
Japanese study (59)	Phase I trial allocation based on molecular profile	Aberrations in *PIK3CA, ERBB2, BRCA2, CCND1, BRCA1, EGFR, AKT, MDM2, FGFR1, ROS1*	FGFR inhibitor, PI3K inhibitor, PARP inhibitor, AKT inhibitor, MTOR inhibitor	RR 33% in patients receiving "matched" trial and 6% in unmatched trials

can lead to hyper-activation of reciprocal pathways and the use of hormonal therapy in heavily pretreated patients where response was unlikely [11–13]. A subsequent meta-analyses, looking at the utility of genotype-matching, showed that patients with genotype-matched treatment can have a high median RR and longer median PFS and OS compared to genotype-unmatched treatment [14,15].

Studies have also been done specifically in the Phase I setting to examine the role of molecular profiling. Retrospective analyses of patients with triple negative breast cancer referred to a Phase I unit at MD Anderson Cancer Centre reported that patients with matched MTA therapy had improved PFS compared to those receiving nonmatched MTA therapy [16]. A study in our institution looking at all breast cancer patients treated in the Royal Marsden Drug Development Unit showed that patients treated on genotype-matched trials had a significantly higher likelihood of clinical benefit compared to patients treated on genotype-unmatched studies (60% vs 33%, $P = 0.004$) [17]. More recently, the interim analysis of the MOSCATO1 trial, a prospective trial looking at "on-purpose" tumor biopsy carried out from patients with metastatic cancers referred for a Phase I trial, showed that 49% of patients with clinically significant molecular alterations were able to be matched to a targeted therapy or dedicated Phase I trial, providing further support of the feasibility of carrying out molecular profiling in the Phase I trial setting [18].

9.4 TECHNOLOGICAL PLATFORMS FOR PRECISION MEDICINE

9.4.1 Genomics

Genomic sequencing for molecular profiling frequently employs NGS techniques whereby massively parallel DNA sequencing is carried out, then subsequently aligned to reference genomes during data analysis to obtain whole sequences of genes of interest [19]. Targeted sequencing techniques, where a panel of specific genes, either preselected or custom designed, is used are by far most commonly employed for molecular profiling currently (Table 9.2). This method allows for high throughput, deep coverage, of such genes at a relatively affordable price, an important criterion for implementation of molecular profiling more broadly. Nonetheless, while targeted sequencing is able to detected specific genetic mutations with good sensitivity and specificity, detection of genomic rearrangements like fusions or copy number changes is more challenging to detect [20]. With increased economic efficiency in sequencing, the use of whole-exome sequencing (WES) and whole-genome sequencing (WGS) have been gaining momentum in such molecular profiling. Comparing WES and hotspot mutation analysis in a cohort of lung cancer sufferers showed that WES identified actionable genomic alterations in 65% of patients thought to be negative for driver mutations [21]. While the ability to obtain more information from an individual tumor sample is attractive, this increased information can come at a price of either increased costs or decreased depth or coverage, limiting the confidence in confirming that the identified genetic aberrations are a true biological finding instead of artifact. Additionally, larger datasets from WES or WGS require greater bioinformatic resources, resulting not only in longer turnaround time, but also challenges in accurate interpretation of the clinical significance of the molecular findings [22].

9.4.2 Other Molecular Profiling Strategies

While DNA may be a major roadmap to studying cancer genomics, there has been increased interest in evaluating RNA. RNA studies have resulted in a deeper understanding

TABLE 9.2   Selected Technology Platforms for Precision Medicine

Strategy	Method	Advantage	Limitations
Genomics	Whole-exome sequencing	− Allows simultaneous detection of sequences − Allows assessment of copy number changes − Use of FFPE samples to give reasonable data	− Need for bioinformatics support − Results limited to protein-coding regions of genome
	Whole-genome sequencing	− Allows study of genomic rearrangements − Allows assessment of noncoding regions	− Longer readout time required due to large size of data generated − Increased cost
Transcriptomics	Microarrays	− Specific assay developed allow for quick read out of transcription levels of genes of interest − lower cost	− Limited to smaller number of genes of interests − Higher background noise − Larger amounts of RNA required
	RNA sequencing	− Transcriptome size smaller than genome size, allowing for a shorter readout time − Allows detection of RNA splice variant	− Unable to study untranscribed regions − Need for bioinformatics support

of cancer biology, including the roles of RNA editing, microRNA (miRNA), and noncoding RNAs. For example, RNA sequencing was utilized to detect the EML-ALK fusion protein in NSCLC [23,24], and miRNA signatures have also been shown to help elucidate primary origins sites for patients with tumor of unknown origin [25]. The routine study of RNA, either through targeted analyses or RNASeq evaluation, empowers any DNA analyses and in particular has utility for the detection of not only altered target expression but specifically identifying genomic rearrangements.

Ultimately, the human genome is translated into proteins, with amino acids. Arguably, proteomic studies may end up yielding the most precise molecular characterization of any molecular aberration occurring at the genomic level. Post-translational profiling of the PI3K pathway, for example, has been extensively studied with identification of a putative biomarker for PI3K pathway overactivity which predicts for sensitivity to AKT inhibition [26].

Like the human genome project, the proteome is actively being studied, despite current technology limitations, with the human protein atlas likely to further support anticancer drug development and target identification [27].

9.5 TUMOR EVOLUTION AND HETEROGENEITY AND ITS IMPACT ON MOLECULAR PROFILING

Regardless of the technology platform used for molecular profiling, the basis of such analyses ultimately lies in the source tissue available for testing. Frequently, patients considered for early clinical trials give consent for archival tumor samples (acquired at diagnosis and usually stored as formalin-fixed, paraffin-embedded, material) from previous surgery or biopsies for molecular profiling. Whether such tissue material used for molecular profiling is representative of the tumor composition at the time of trial screening is a subject of concern and much debate stemming from concerns that at least a subset of cancers are genomically highly unstable. These studies indicate that tumor growth and progression is often not a static state of cell multiplication, but instead can involve a constant evolution of genomic aberrations. This concept of a clonal evolution model of tumor carcinogenesis was first proposed by Nowell back in 1976 with the hypothesis that selection pressures from external factors like the tumor cell microenvironment and prior therapies will cause susceptible clonal populations to perish while resistant cell populations emerge and proliferate [28]. This was hypothesized to lead to the natural selection of resistant and more robust subclonal populations, with changes in the course of tumor growth being at least in part dependent on previous treatments [29]. This concept was supported by studies demonstrating evaluating tumor biopsies from multiple sites, both primary and metastatic, from patients with renal cell carcinoma. The construction of phylogenetic trees provided evidence of a branching pattern in mutational heterogeneity [30]. Genomic aberrations found through molecular profiling efforts can therefore be interpreted by where they are found in the phylogenetic tree, to either be neutral passenger mutations that do not impact functionality, or truncal pathogenic mutations that are important drivers to oncogenesis. The analyses of large databases such as The Cancer Genome Atlas and International Cancer Genome Consortium [31,32], with the implementation of complex bioinformatics and computational methods to determine driver mutational status have supported these efforts [33]. Studies are underway to analyze the functional roles of the molecular aberrations identified across various tumor types to allow for deeper understanding of how therapies designed for one tumor type may be potentially extended into others with similar genomic profiles to provide patient benefit [34].

In a Phase I setting, the issue of tumor evolution and disease heterogeneity merits careful scrutiny since patients reviewed in a Phase I setting are usually heavily pretreated. It is therefore likely that in genomically unstable cancers, the plasticity of these cancer genomes can lead to dynamic changes in these genomic aberrations during the course of the disease. This supports the acquisition of further tumor material for molecular profiling at the time of consideration of trial participation. Furthermore, other than differentiating between passenger and pathogenic mutations, it can be also challenging to determine if the identified mutations represent a truncal clonal driver mutation or a subclonal aberration present only in a small percentage of the total tumor burden [35]. Additionally, the use of archival tumor tissue is unlikely to reflect the current genomic make-up of tumor tissue, with a single tumor biopsy sample likely to underestimate intratumor heterogeneity. A key question that needs addressed for such genomically unstable tumors is whether we are able to obtain tumor control by chopping the trunk down by targeting driver mutations, or whether pruning branches of subclonal mutations can still have an impact on overall tumor growth? [36].

To overcome this issue of tumor evolution and heterogeneity, there is an increased advocacy for fresh tumor biopsies to be pursued, and also serial monitoring of tumor tissue samples to identify changes in molecular aberrations that may indicate merging resistance to treatment [37]. Prospective studies are currently underway to explore the role of subclonal driver mutations in therapeutic outcomes, including the TRACERx (TRAcking non-small-cell lung cancer Cancer Evolution through therapy, NCT01888601) and DARWIN II (Deciphering Antitumor Response With INtratumor Heterogeneity; NCT02183883) studies in lung cancer.

As tumor tissue is not always available and serial biopsies of tumor samples may be logistically challenging or unsafe, studies have looked into studying other available material such as circulating cell-free DNA (cfDNA) or circulating tumor cells. In a Phase I setting, the use of serial NGS of cfDNA to evaluate tumor clone response to MTA has been studied, and shown to be feasible, with monitoring of mutational allele frequency in consecutive plasma samples during treatment demonstrating treatment-associated clonal responses [38]. In another subgroup of patients enrolled prospectively on the MOSCATO trial previously described (Table 9.1), cfDNA extracted from blood samples was analyzed by targeted NGS for 50 genes and compared against tumor samples from matched patients. The specificity of the cfDNA in the detection of mutation when compared to tissue sample was 95%, with a sensitivity of 55%. Sensitivity of detection improved when a prediction score based on clinical parameters were applied, with sensitivity increasing to 83% in patients with a high score of 8 and above [39]. While this is an exploratory study that will need further validation, it provides preliminary evidence that circulating material may have major utility for the disease molecular characterization of patients enrolling onto early clinical trials even if tumor tissue is available.

9.6 THE IMPORTANCE OF ON-TARGET INHIBITION OF DRUG ACTION

While identification of molecular aberrations is a vital first step in precision medicine, an accurate understanding of the MTA and its mechanism of action is also crucial to ensure the success of precision medicine. The cautionary tale of iniparib has illustrated the importance of demonstrating on-target inhibition, as precision medicine can only be as precise as we are at hitting the target [40]. Iniparib was said to be designed to target poly(ADP-ribose) polymerase (PARP), an important player in DNA damage repair (DDR). PARP inhibition

has been shown to lead to synthetic lethality in cancers with homologous recombination DDR pathway defects such as deleterious loss of function *BRCA1 or BRCA2* mutations. The first-in-man trial of iniparib did not pursue sufficiently rigorous pharmacodynamic testing, but this drug was deemed successful in a randomized Phase II study in triple negative breast cancer where patients with iniparib with carboplatin and gemcitabine appeared to have a better outcome with a statistically significant extension of PFS (3.6 vs 5.9 months, $P = 0.01$) and OS (7.7 vs 12.3 months, $P = 0.01$) [41] compared to patients receiving the chemotherapy alone. However, studies by independent researchers reported that iniparib did not inhibit PARP at clinically relevant doses, raising concerns [42]. The Phase III study of iniparib with combination chemotherapy eventually failed to recapitulate the Phase II findings, and other Phase II trials involving iniparib in other tumor types were also prematurely terminated for futility [43]. Retrospective analysis of the molecular chemistry of iniparib showed that iniparib was the only molecule, among the PARP inhibitor class, that did not target the NAD + binding site of PARP1 or PARP2. Indeed, preclinical studies in cell lines and xenograft models suggested that the effects of iniparib are not mediated by PARP, but other mechanisms linked to reactive oxygen species [44,45].

Tivantinib, an MTA designed to target MET and reported to have promising results in patients with hepatocellular carcinoma (HCC) failing first-line systemic therapy [46], has been reported to have similar concerns. Preclinical studies have reported that the cytotoxic activity of tivantinib may not be solely attributable to c-MET inhibition [47–49] but that at higher doses this agent also binds tubulin, although Phase III trials to confirm the role of tivantinib in HCC are underway (NCT01755767).

Overall, therefore, the ability to demonstrate target inhibition at pharmacologically active

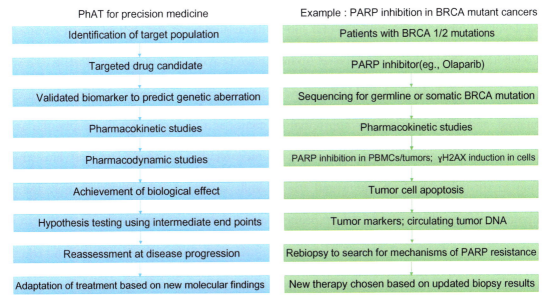

FIGURE 9.1   The pharmacological audit trial in the context of precision medicine (Adapted from ref. [6]).

drug doses and pharmacokinetic exposures in animal models, followed by confirmation of target engagement and downstream pathway modulation in early phase studies cannot be overemphasized. The use of frameworks like the Pharmacological Audit Trail can help to provide a structure for drug discovery and development of novel compounds undergoing evaluation, and also allow for critical appraisal to assist in making "go" or "no-go" drug development decisions (Fig. 9.1) [6].

9.7 MOLECULAR PROFILING IN ACADEMIC AND COMMERCIAL SETTINGS

Molecular profiling is currently widely pursued both in academic settings by institutions or collaborative groups, and in commercial settings by various companies that offer NGS facilities for tumor samples provided by oncologists. There is undoubtedly a wealth of information available, but the optimal ways to

harness these data and ensure that they are implemented appropriately in clinical settings are still controversial.

At an institutional level, multiple academic cancer centers have set up individual programs to allow large-scale sequencing efforts of either archival or fresh biopsy tissue. As discussed earlier, various reports of such studies have shown feasibility of implementation of such molecular profiling programs, although detection rates are variable and clinical utility and impact patient outcome largely unknown [8,10,50]. Nonetheless, systematic profiling of tumor material allows for a framework through which patients can be optimally matched to studies with MTAs also allowing the retrospective analyses of databases that may further yield insight into the molecular characteristics of other tumor types. What is still lacking, however, is the determination of the degree of genomic instability in such tumors; ongoing circulating biomarker studies may allow the dissection of this key issue. Overall, however, it is likely that the application of molecular profiling at an institutional level will improve the outcome of a subset of patients.

Collaborative groups have also been set up in efforts to optimize trial allocation for patients. "Basket" studies include the NCI-MATCH and the Lung Matrix Trial, where tumor samples are sequenced and then matched to appropriate trials based on the driver mutations identified. Besides collaborative groups, large pharmaceuticals have also started to run similar trial designs, hoping to streamline trial allocation and trial enrollment for patients receiving multiple novel compounds that may be available in the pipeline portfolio. These include the "signature" trial from Novartis and the "My Pathway" trial from Genentech. In a community setting, The French Cooperative Thoracic Intergroup (IFCT) conducted a nationwide molecular profiling study, screening more than 18,000 molecular samples collected from patients with advanced NSCLC over a year for six routinely screened genes (*EGFR, ALK, HER2, KRAS, BRAF*, and *PIK3CA*) and found that about 50% of patients had at least one genomic aberration detected, with this associating with a significant improvement in the proportion of patients achieving a response to treatment. This was the first study to show that nationwide molecular profiling of patients is feasible, with acceptable turnaround times and a translatable improvement in patient outcome [51].

While molecular profiling was initially practiced primarily in an academic setting, there has been a rise of commercial companies set up to provide similar molecular profiling services to oncologists keen to sequence their patient's tumors but with limited access to molecular profiling facilities. Third-party companies like Foundation Medicine and Myriad Diagnostics provide tumor sample sequencing services with various targeted sequencing panels, providing a summary sheet of findings with a brief description of likely significance and possible clinical applications that is then sent to the oncologist for further review and discussion with the patient. Such commercial companies providing such sequencing assays have provided oncologists and patients a route to molecular profiling, and potentially more precise trial enrollment and clinical care. Such commercial sequencing generally, however, comes at a high cost fiscally despite the uncertain benefits. There are also concerns about the interpretation of such data and how this is eventually provided to the patient. Moreover, while each molecular alteration may theoretically have similar effects on a pathway, its actual functional implication may differ in various biological backgrounds. For example, *BRAF* mutations in melanoma are functionally active and BRAF inhibitors like vemurafinib have antitumor activity [52], whereas BRAF inhibitors in BRAF mutated colorectal cancer have been disappointing [53]. As such, the results of molecular profiling need to be carefully interpreted in the context of the patient and tumor type prior to making recommendations to patients with regards to treatment implications in the absence of definitive trials.

9.8 THE VALUE OF MOLECULAR PROFILING FOR EARLY CLINICAL TRIALS

Tumor molecular profiling for patients being considered for an early clinical trial overall therefore merits consideration, as long as the related caveats are kept in mind and this is used in an appropriate hypothesis-testing experimental context. For the patient, the detection of potentially actionable mutation in genomically more stable tumors may open new opportunities for trial options. In the absence of any other evidence-based treatment options, enrollment onto such trials with a genotype-matched treatment remains an attractive option to patients. This is best done on clinical trials.

From a drug discovery perspective, molecular profiling also provides a platform to better understand the mechanisms of action of drugs in a clinical context. While the majority of patients may not respond to treatment, the occasional patient with an exceptional response can be hugely valuable as the molecular characteristics of that tumor can be studied in detail in attempts to delineate possible reasons for the profound response. In cases of exceptional responses, more extensive sequencing including WES or WGS and RNASeq are recommended as these may provide further insight to patient selection for responders. The identification of a response biomarker can then impact patient selection and accelerate drug approval [54].

Ultimately, the aim of such molecular profiling efforts is to complement drug development and trial design to accelerate the improvement of patient outcomes. The integration of molecular profiling into trial design is vital in this process and the TOPARP study which incorporates a multi-part adaptive design attempting to identify predictive biomarkers utilizing test and validation sets. An initial "test-set" cohort of patients suffering from metastatic prostate cancer were treated with olaparib; targeted NGS was carried out to assess for mutations in genes commonly associated with DNA damage repair and compared responding and nonresponding patients. NGS studies of tumor acquired from these patients revealed that almost all responding patients had deleterious DNA repair defects, with most nonresponders having tumors without such aberrations and providing the first clinical data to support molecular stratification for the treatment of advanced prostate cancer. Molecular profiling for these deleterious DNA repair gene aberrations through panel based next generation sequencing is now being pursued in a validation second cohort on this same study, and will provide further insight into the feasibility of such a trial design [55].

9.9 CONCLUSIONS

In conclusion, molecular profiling is becoming more widely adopted in the practice of oncology as a tool to optimize early clinical trial conduct and patient care. In specialized centers with appropriate expertise, molecular profiling can provide invaluable information about tumor characteristics and help direct trial selection that frequently otherwise involves a random choice of available options. Nonetheless, there are still many challenges remaining, and continued discussion between the various stakeholders will be necessary to develop consensus statements and guidelines to allow for the optimal implementation of molecular profiling to guide patient care in clinical trials.

References

[1] Hudson K, Lifton R. The precision medicine initiative cohort program—building a research foundation for 21st century medicine; 2015.
[2] Wu R. Nucleotide sequence analysis of DNA. I. Partial sequence of the cohesive ends of bacteriophage lambda and 186 DNA. J Mol Biol 1970;51:501−21.
[3] Sanger F, Nicklen S,, Coulson AR. DNA sequencing with chain-terminating inhibitors. Proc Natl Acad Sci USA 1977;74:5463−7.
[4] Hanahan D,, Weinberg RA. The hallmarks of cancer. Cell 2000;100:57−70.
[5] Hanahan D,, Weinberg RA. Hallmarks of cancer: the next generation. Cell 2011;144:646−74.
[6] Yap TA, Sandhu SK, Workman P,, De bono JS. Envisioning the future of early anticancer drug development. Nat Rev Cancer 2010;10:514−23.
[7] Kris MG, Johnson BE, Berry LD, Kwiatkowski DJ, Iafrate AJ, Wistuba II, et al. Using multiplexed assays of oncogenic drivers in lung cancers to select targeted drugs. JAMA 2014;311:1998−2006. Available from: http://jama.jamanetwork.com/article.aspx?articleid=1872815.
[8] Meric-Bernstam F, Brusco L, Shaw K, Horombe C, Kopetz S, Davies MA, et al. Feasibility of large-scale genomic testing to facilitate enrollment onto genomically matched clinical trials. J Clin Oncol 2015;33:2753−62.

[9] Stockley TL, Oza AM, Berman HK, Leighl NB, Knox JJ, Shepherd FA et al. Molecular profiling of advanced solid tumors and patient outcomes with genotype-matched clinical trials: the Princess Margaret IMPACT/ COMPACT trial. Genome Med 2016; 8: 109 [Internet] Available from: http://www.ncbi.nlm.nih.gov/ pubmed/27782854\n Available from: http://www.pub-medcentral.nih.gov/articlerender.fcgi? artid = PMC5078968.

[10] Le tourneau C, Delord JP, Goncalves A, Gavoille C, Dubot C, Isambert N, et al. Molecularly targeted therapy based on tumour molecular profiling versus conventional therapy for advanced cancer (SHIVA): a multicentre, open-label, proof-of-concept, randomised, controlled phase 2 trial. Lancet Oncol 2015;16:1324–34.

[11] Hahn AW, Martin MG. Precision medicine: lessons learned from the SHIVA trial. Lancet Oncol 2015;16: e580–1.

[12] Miyata M, Albini B, Kreis H, Milgrom F,, Dausset J. IgG rheumatoid factor in human and rabbit transplantation sera. Int Arch Allergy Appl Immunol 1989;89:191–6.

[13] Tsimberidou AM,, Kurzrock R. Precision medicine: lessons learned from the SHIVA trial. Lancet Oncol 2015;16:e579–80.

[14] Jardim DL, Schwaederle M, Wei C, Lee JJ, Hong DS, Eggermont AM, et al. Impact of a biomarker-based strategy on oncology drug development: a meta-analysis of clinical trials leading to FDA approval. J Natl Cancer Inst 2015;107(11).

[15] Schwaederle M, Zhao M, Lee JJ, Eggermont AM, Schilsky RL, Mendelsohn J, et al. Impact of precision medicine in diverse cancers: a meta-analysis of phase II clinical trials. J Clin Oncol 2015;33:3817–25.

[16] Ganesan P, Moulder S, Lee JJ, Janku F, Valero V, Zinner RG, et al. Triple-negative breast cancer patients treated at MD Anderson Cancer Center in phase I trials: improved outcomes with combination chemotherapy and targeted agents. Mol Cancer Ther 2014;13:3175–84.

[17] O'carrigan B, Jalil A, Papadatos-Pastos D, Harris SJ, Lopez JS, Banerji U, et al. Target-based therapeutic matching of phase I trials in patients with advanced breast cancer (BC pts) in the Royal Marsden Hospital Drug Development Unit (RMH DDU). J Clin Oncol 34, no. 15_suppl (2016) 11508-11508 (18). Annals of Oncology 2015;26(2) Pages ii4 (44) Mol Cancer Ther Volume 10, Issue 11.

[18] Massard C. Enriching phase I trials with molecular alterations: interim analysis of 708 patients enrolled in the MOSCATO 01. Ann Oncol 2015;26.

[19] Shendure J, Ji H. Next-generation DNA sequencing. Nat Biotechnol 2008;26:1135–45.

[20] Metzker ML. Sequencing technologies - the next generation. Nat Rev Genet 2010;11:31–46.

[21] Drilon A, Wang L, Arcila ME, Balasubramanian S, Greenbowe JR, Ross JS, et al. Broad, hybrid capture-based next-generation sequencing identifies actionable genomic alterations in lung adenocarcinomas otherwise negative for such alterations by other genomic testing approaches. Clin Cancer Res 2015;21:3631–9.

[22] Gagan J, Van allen EM. Next-generation sequencing to guide cancer therapy. Genome Med. 2015;7:80.

[23] Moskalev EA, Frohnauer J, Merkelbach-Bruse S, Schildhaus HU, Dimmler A, Schubert T, et al. Sensitive and specific detection of EML4-ALK rearrangements in non-small cell lung cancer (NSCLC) specimens by multiplex amplicon RNA massive parallel sequencing. Lung Cancer 2014;84:215–21.

[24] Fernandez-Cuesta L, Sun R, Menon R, George J, Lorenz S, Meza-Zepeda LA, et al. Identification of novel fusion genes in lung cancer using breakpoint assembly of transcriptome sequencing data. Genome Biol 2015;16:7.

[25] Pentheroudakis G, Pavlidis N, Fountzilas G, Krikelis D, Goussia A, Stoyianni A, et al. Novel microRNA-based assay demonstrates 92% agreement with diagnosis based on clinicopathologic and management data in a cohort of patients with carcinoma of unknown primary. Mol Cancer 2013;12:57.

[26] Andersen JN, Sathyanarayanan S, Di bacco A, Chi A, Zhang T, Chen AH, et al. Pathway-based identification of biomarkers for targeted therapeutics: personalized oncology with PI3K pathway inhibitors. Sci Transl Med 2010;2 43ra55.

[27] Uhlen M, Fagerberg L, Hallstrom BM, Lindskog C, Oksvold P, Mardinoglu A, et al. Proteomics. Tissue-based map of the human proteome. Science 2015;347:1260419.

[28] Nowell PC. The clonal evolution of tumor cell populations. Science 1976;194:23–8.

[29] Gerlinger M,, Swanton C. How Darwinian models inform therapeutic failure initiated by clonal heterogeneity in cancer medicine. Br J Cancer 2010;103:1139–43.

[30] Gerlinger M, Rowan AJ, Horswell S, Larkin J, Endesfelder D, Gronroos E, et al. Intratumor heterogeneity and branched evolution revealed by multiregion sequencing. N Engl J Med 2012;366:883–92.

[31] International Cancer Genome Consortium, Hudson TJ, Anderson W, Artez A, Barker AD, Bell C, et al. International network of cancer genome projects. Nature 2010;464:993–8.

[32] Cancer Genome Atlas research Network. Comprehensive genomic characterization defines human glioblastoma genes and core pathways. Nature 2008;455:1061–8.

[33] Pavlopoulou A, Spandidos DA,, Michalopoulos I. Human cancer databases (review). Oncol Rep 2015;33:3−18.

[34] Cancer Genome Atlas research Network, Weinstein JN, Collisson EA, Mills GB, Shaw KR, Ozenberger BA, et al. The Cancer Genome Atlas Pan-Cancer analysis project. Nat Genet 2013;45:1113−20.

[35] Van allen EM, Wagle N,, Levy MA. Clinical analysis and interpretation of cancer genome data. J Clin Oncol 2013;31:1825−33.

[36] Mcgranahan N,, Swanton C. Biological and therapeutic impact of intratumor heterogeneity in cancer evolution. Cancer Cell 2015;27:15−26.

[37] Jamal-Hanjani M, Quezada SA, Larkin J,, Swanton C. Translational implications of tumor heterogeneity. Clin Cancer Res 2015;21:1258−66.

[38] Frenel JS, Carreira S, Goodall J, Roda D, Perez-Lopez R, Tunariu N, et al. Serial next-generation sequencing of circulating cell-free DNA evaluating tumor clone response to molecularly targeted drug administration. Clin Cancer Res 2015;21:4586−96.

[39] Jovelet C, Ileana E, Le deley MC, Motte N, Rosellini S, Romero A, et al. Circulating cell-free tumor DNA analysis of 50 genes by next-generation sequencing in the prospective MOSCATO trial. Clin Cancer Res 2016;22:2960−8.

[40] Mateo J, Ong M, Tan DS, Gonzalez MA,, De bono JS. Appraising iniparib, the PARP inhibitor that never was—what must we learn? Nat Rev Clin Oncol 2013;10:688−96.

[41] O'shaughnessy J, Osborne C, Pippen JE, Yoffe M, Patt D, Rocha C, et al. Iniparib plus chemotherapy in metastatic triple-negative breast cancer. N Engl J Med 2011;364:205−14.

[42] Patel AG, De lorenzo SB, Flatten KS, Poirier GG, Kaufmann SH. Failure of iniparib to inhibit poly(ADP-Ribose) polymerase in vitro. Clin Cancer Res 2012;18:1655−62.

[43] O'shaughnessy J, Schwartzberg L, Danso MA, Miller KD, Rugo HS, Neubauer M, et al. Phase III study of iniparib plus gemcitabine and carboplatin versus gemcitabine and carboplatin in patients with metastatic triple-negative breast cancer. J Clin Oncol 2014;32:3840−7.

[44] Licht S, Cao H, Li Z, Zhang J, Liu F, Brittain S, et al. Mechanism of action of iniparib: stimulation of reactive oxygen species (ROS) production in an iniparib-sensitive breast cancer cell line. Mol Cancer Ther 2011;10.

[45] Liu X, Shi Y, Maag DX, Palma JP, Patterson MJ, Ellis PA, et al. Iniparib nonselectively modifies cysteine-containing proteins in tumor cells and is not a bona fide PARP inhibitor. Clin Cancer Res 2012;18:510−23.

[46] Santoro A, Rimassa L, Borbath I, Daniele B, Salvagni S, Van laethem JL, et al. Tivantinib for second-line treatment of advanced hepatocellular carcinoma: a randomised, placebo-controlled phase 2 study. Lancet Oncol 2013;14:55−63.

[47] Katayama R, Aoyama A, Yamori T, Qi J, Oh-Hara T, Song Y, et al. Cytotoxic activity of tivantinib (ARQ 197) is not due solely to c-MET inhibition. Cancer Res 2013;73:3087−96.

[48] Basilico C, Pennacchietti S, Vigna E, Chiriaco C, Arena S, Bardelli A, et al. Tivantinib (ARQ197) displays cytotoxic activity that is independent of its ability to bind MET. Clin Cancer Res 2013;19:2381−92.

[49] Calles A, Kwiatkowski N, Cammarata BK, Ercan D, Gray NS,, Janne PA. Tivantinib (ARQ 197) efficacy is independent of MET inhibition in non-small-cell lung cancer cell lines. Mol Oncol 2015;9:260−9.

[50] Tsimberidou AM, Iskander NG, Hong DS, Wheler JJ, Falchook GS, Fu S, et al. Personalized medicine in a phase I clinical trials program: the MD Anderson Cancer Center initiative. Clin Cancer Res 2012;18:6373−83.

[51] Barlesi F, Mazieres J, Merlio JP, Debieuvre D, Mosser J, Lena H, et al. Routine molecular profiling of patients with advanced non-small-cell lung cancer: results of a 1-year nationwide programme of the French Cooperative Thoracic Intergroup (IFCT). Lancet 2016;387:1415−26.

[52] Chapman PB, Hauschild A, Robert C, Haanen JB, Ascierto P, Larkin J, et al. Improved survival with vemurafenib in melanoma with BRAF V600E mutation. N Engl J Med 2011;364:2507−16.

[53] Kopetz S, Desai J, Chan E, Hecht JR, O'dwyer PJ, Maru D, et al. Phase II pilot study of vemurafenib in patients with metastatic BRAF-mutated colorectal cancer. J Clin Oncol 2015;33:4032−8.

[54] Yap TA, Sandhu SK, Carden CP,, De bono JS. Poly (ADP-ribose) polymerase (PARP) inhibitors: exploiting a synthetic lethal strategy in the clinic. CA Cancer J Clin 2011;61:31−49.

[55] Mateo J, Carreira S, Sandhu S, Miranda S, Mossop H, Perez-Lopez R, et al. DNA-repair defects and olaparib in metastatic prostate cancer. N Engl J Med 2015;373:1697−708.

[56] Sohal DPS, Rini BI, Khorana AA, Dreicer R, Abraham J, Procop GW, et al. Prospective clinical study of precision oncology in solid tumors. J Natl Cancer Inst 2016;108:10−12.

[57] Seeber A, Gastl G, Ensinger C, Spizzo G, Kocher F, Leitner I, et al. Treatment of patients with refractory metastatic cancer according to molecular profiling on tumor tissue in the clinical routine: an interim-analysis of the ONCO-T-PROFILE project. Genes and Cancer 2016;7:9−10.

[58] André F, Bachelot T, Commo F, Campone M, Arnedos M, Dieras V, et al. Comparative genomic hybridisation array and DNA sequencing to direct treatment of metastatic breast cancer: a multicentre, prospective trial (SAFIR01/UNICANCER). Lancet Oncol. 2014;15:267−74.

[59] Tanabe Y, Ichikawa H, Kohno T, Yoshida H, Kubo T, Kato M, et al. Comprehensive screening of target molecules by next-generation sequencing in patients with malignant solid tumors: guiding entry into phase I clinical trials. Mol Cancer 2016;15:73. Available from: http://molecular-cancer.biomedcentral.com/articles/10.1186/s12943-016-0553-z.

Role of Imaging in Early-Phase Trials

Lacey Greene, Shyam Srinivas, Sonya Park, Negin Hatami,
Tomomi Nobashi, Lucia Baratto, Akira Toriihara
and Sanjiv S. Gambhir

Stanford University, Stanford, CA, United States

10.1 APPLICATION OF NOVEL IMAGING PROBES IN EARLY DRUG DEVELOPMENT: BENEFITS AND CHALLENGES

Today the quest for new diagnostic and therapeutic agents is a fervent search akin to the gold miners and prospectors of the gold rush in the mid-1800s: the hope of discovering genuine gold nuggets kept these prospectors motivated. Discovering novel diagnostic or therapeutic agents is a similar process as vast resources and time are spent synthesizing and testing tens of thousands of potential candidate molecules from preclinical discovery through the US Food and Drug Administration (FDA) approval process. It is, however, a process that can be streamlined if trialists efficiently manage and leverage all available resources at strategic stages of the clinical trial [1,2].

Molecular imaging has traditionally played a significant role in understanding and tracking of disease pathophysiology and progression in vivo [3]. When applied in the initial stages of drug development, it can provide evidence of biological activity (biodistribution, pharmacokinetics (PK)), confirm on-target drug effects (pharmacodynamics (PD)), and select patients who are more likely to benefit from treatment [2]. Nontargeted radiopharmaceuticals (e.g., ^{18}F FDG) reveal metabolic and cellular processes vital to tumor growth and survival (e.g., glucose metabolism, angiogenesis) allowing investigators to image the effect of drugs on cellular metabolism [2]. Molecular imaging using ^{18}F FDG also has demonstrated prognostic value in a breadth of oncologic settings both at interim analysis and posttreatment [4–16]. The standardized uptake values (SUVs) mathematically derived from the images have provided reliable data about tumor burden and aggressiveness sometimes irrespective of changes in tumor size [2]. Evidence further shows that ^{18}F FDG lesion uptake at varying intervals of therapy can be used to redirect or reevaluate courses of treatment [4,15,17]. This also allows an earlier evaluation of drug efficacy rates, which may

Novel Designs of Early Phase Trials for Cancer Therapeutics
DOI: https://doi.org/10.1016/B978-0-12-812512-0.00010-5

129

subsequently highlight areas where novel drugs are needed [2].

Cancer therapeutics have evolved from a generalized regimen (e.g., surgery, radiation, chemotherapy) to a more customized approach with the advent of agents that target-specific molecular characterizational changes, for example, receptor upregulation or antigen expression on a tumor [18]. One example is immunotherapy, where a certain aspect of a patient's own immune system is "targeted" to treat cancer. Though immunotherapy drugs such as pembrolizumab and nivolumab have demonstrated significantly longer progression-free survival rates in the treatment of metastatic melanoma (the driving force behind recent FDA approval), the objective response rate is only 29% and 31%, respectively [19]. Importantly, patient prognosis and therapy effectiveness are often dependent upon procuring an accurate tumor molecular profile [20].

This situation highlights that more precise treatments require highly specific methods of selecting favorable patients who will most benefit from therapy. Molecular imaging using positron emission tomography/computed tomography (PET/CT) [21] and PET/magnetic resonance imaging [18] has shown promise in this area [3] with the design and synthesis of "companion diagnostic probes" (e.g., radiolabeled monoclonal antibodies or fragments, natural peptide ligands or analogues, tyrosine kinase inhibitors or analogues, or high-affinity peptides) [18]. These probes are designed to mimic the investigational drug's behavior(s) so as to better stratify patients at earlier time points.

Evidence suggests that molecular imaging is most valuable when implemented early in the clinical development stage (Fig. 10.1), though challenges to its incorporation (i.e., addressing the significant time and cost associated with

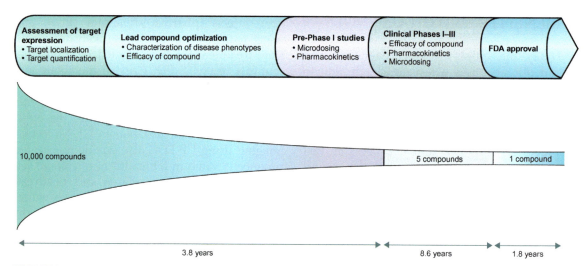

FIGURE 10.1   On average, for approximately 10,000 compounds evaluated in preclinical studies, about five compounds enter clinical trials and about one compound finally receives regulatory approval by the US Food and Drug Administration (FDA) [22,23]. The mean time from synthesis of a new compound to marketing approval in the United States is 14.2 years [24]. Molecular imaging can be used at various stages in the drug development process, as illustrated here, which may help reduce attrition rates and allow the selection of the most promising drug candidates early on in development. *Reprinted with permission from Willmann JK, van Bruggen N, Dinkelborg LM, Gambhir SS. Molecular imaging in drug development. Nat Rev Drug Discov 2008;7(7):591–607.*

preclinical testing (FDA exploratory investigational new drug (eIND), Section 10.6); ensuring the clinical protocol and techniques are appropriately written and executed with minimal deviation (Sections 10.3 and 10.4); improving collaboration within multidisciplinary teams (Section 10.3)) to its incorporation should be addressed [2,22]. Given the paradigm shift toward targeted therapies [18,25–27], the numerous available PET radionuclides [28], and the substantial innovations in imaging equipment [18,21], molecular imaging is a prime modality to streamline clinical use of current FDA-approved drugs and fast-track the translation of new drugs from bench-to-bedside [3]. The following sections explore key areas where molecular imaging can assist drug development and elucidates opportunities to cater suitable methods for structuring early-phase clinical trials in translational research.

10.2 DESIGNING IMAGING TRIALS: EARLY PHASE I AND BEYOND

Molecular and functional imaging are likely to have the greatest impact on the initial stages of drug development by providing evidence of biological activity, confirming on-target drug effects, and identifying patients who are more likely to benefit from the drug. Once a specific target is validated, molecular imaging allows detection of specific targets in vivo, including assessment of the presence of the targets as well as quantification of their spatial and temporal distribution.

Ideally an imaging agent is codeveloped with an exploratory drug candidate. Because this is more feasible when trace amounts of an imaging agent are required, novel imaging agents are often PET based. PET also allows assessment of parameters such as drug absorption, biodistribution, metabolism, delivery, and

dose determinations and can guide in planning later-phase clinical trials [2].

The following sections illustrate imaging trials with novel PET tracers.

10.2.1 ^{64}Cu-DOTA-B-Fab PET/CT Imaging in Breast and Ovarian Cancer

Some of the most promising advances in recent cancer research involve immunotherapy with antibodies targeting specific antigens. The tumor-associated mucin-1-sialoglycotope CA6 is overexpressed in a number of epithelial cancers with demonstrated poor patient prognosis. In particular the CA6 antigen is found in a high percentage of ovarian (70% with threshold of more than 30% with intensity staining $2+/3+$ by immunohistochemistry and 89% with more than one positive cell, $n = 187$) and breast (29%–35% with threshold of more than 30% cells with intensity staining $2+/3+$ and 78%–86% with more than one positive cell, $n = 359$) cancers [29,30]. SAR566658 is an antibody-drug conjugate currently in phase I clinical development by the French pharmaceutical company Sanofi S.A. (NCT01156870) in patients who have received a diagnosis of CA6-positive ovarian, pancreatic, and breast tumors [30]. It is composed of a humanized monoclonal antibody (huDS6) specifically targeting CA6, and upon antibody and/or antigen binding and internalization, SAR566658 releases DM4, the cytotoxic component maytansinoid analogue that inhibits microtubule polymerization [30,31].

Molecular imaging using the companion diagnostic probe ^{64}Cu-DOTA-B-Fab assists physicians in distinguishing CA6-positive from CA6-negative tumors to noninvasively stratify patients who will most benefit from SAR566658 therapy (Fig. 10.2) [31]. Additionally, because the immunoglobulin fragment B-Fab is derived from huDS6, quantifying CA6 density and affinity using SUV measurements may offer

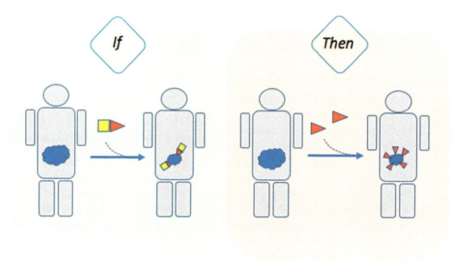

Administration of radioactive labeled drug   **Administration of drug at therapeutic dose**
at diagnostic dose

FIGURE 10.2   Role of imaging in targeted cancer therapeutics. When used in conjunction with a therapeutic agent, the companion diagnostic imaging probe demonstrates evidence of biological activity, confirms on-target localization, and selects patients who are more likely to benefit from treatment. Yellow box on agent indicates radionuclide.

investigators a means at early evaluation of therapeutic effectiveness. Preclinical studies showed high affinity for CA6-positive WISH cells (Kd of xx nM), with superior results in radiosynthesis, serum stability, and biodistribution profiles [30].

In designing the first-in-human ^{64}Cu-DOTA-B-Fab study (IND# 118493), the availability of either biopsy or surgical specimen(s) was required for correlation with serial imaging. Chemotherapy and radiation therapy naïve participants with bulky disease were favored to increase the likelihood of CA6 expression and potential ^{64}Cu-DOTA-B-Fab signal.

10.2.1.1 Image Analysis

Antibodies are larger (~150 kDa) and slower than most imaging agents and thus the plasma half-life of the radiopharmaceutical is longer. Statistical image analysis must therefore be performed at least 24 hours after tracer administration when target-to-background ratio is highest (Fig. 10.3) [32]. Regions of

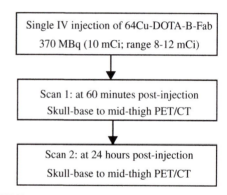

FIGURE 10.3   Imaging schema for first-in-human ^{64}Cu-DOTA-B-Fab PET/CT in ovarian and breast cancer.

interest were drawn around areas of visually increased uptake of ^{64}Cu DOTA B-Fab compared to background. Lesions identified on each ^{64}Cu DOTA B-Fab PET/CT scan were correlated with immunohistochemistry testing of the biopsy or surgical specimen to determine the affinity of ^{64}Cu-DOTA-B-Fab to localize to antigen CA6-positive breast or ovarian cancer lesions.

10.2.2 ^{18}F-FP-R01-MG-F2 PET/CT Imaging in Idiopathic Pulmonary Fibrosis

Idiopathic pulmonary fibrosis (IPF) is a devastating, progressive disease of the lung that presents a major challenge in clinical management because of its unpredictable clinical course and the lack of an easily reproducible surrogate endpoint, e.g., biomarkers [33,34]. Drug studies focused on specific, yet difficult to reproduce clinical end-points can be time-consuming and costly, so imaging of selective biomarkers that provide early indications of potential diagnosis, measurement of disease severity, and/or monitoring of response to therapy is attractive, especially for chronic diseases such as IPF.

Integrin $\alpha_v\beta_6$ is a cell surface receptor that is upregulated on alveolar epithelial cells in the fibrotic foci of IPF, while its expression remains relatively low in the healthy adult lung [33,34]. Integrin $\alpha_v\beta_6$ in turn activates transforming growth factor-b (TGF-b), a potent inducer of alveolar epithelial-to-mesenchymal transition [35]. TGF-b also contributes to the upregulation of $\alpha_v\beta_6$ thereby promoting a positive amplification loop that initiates, maintains, and even increases the rate of pulmonary fibrogenesis [36]. Paralleling the drug development process (e.g., development of a humanized monoclonal antibody directed against $\alpha_v\beta6$ integrin) with noninvasive imaging and quantification of integrin $\alpha_v\beta_6$ expression levels in vivo initially help investigators demonstrate the potential feasibility of the drug at the earliest stage. Imaging also improves patient stratification throughout the trial. Longitudinal efficacy of anti-integrin $\alpha_v\beta_6$ therapeutic drugs may also be determined using molecular imaging.

The first-in-human study of ^{18}F-FP-R$_0$1-MG-F2 (exploratory IND#: 126379) demonstrated high synthetic yield, high and prolonged $\alpha_v\beta_6$ uptake and retention, and increased integrin $\alpha_v\beta_6$-to-normal tissue ratios with low uptake in the cardiopulmonary region of healthy volunteers, which was an expected biodistribution based on immunohistochemical staining of healthy lung tissue [36]. To confirm the presence of the specific target under pathologic conditions, i.e., uptake in the receptor integrin $\alpha_v\beta_6$, patients with diagnosed IPF were recruited.

10.2.2.1 Image Analysis

The primary aim of this collaborative effort is assessing the presence of integrin $\alpha_v\beta_6$ using ^{18}F-FP-R0 1-MG-F2 in patients with diagnosed IPF. To that end, image interpretation (Fig. 10.4) is as follows: *Scan 1*: Initial ^{18}F-FP-R0 1-MG-F2 uptake and PK measurements during the 60-minute dynamic scan over the lung field of view. Blood samples were collected at 1, 3, 5, 10, 30, and 60 minutes after tracer injection for tracer kinetic analysis, which describe the changes in radiopharmaceutical disposition in the body compartments over time.

Scans 2 and 3: Regions of interest were drawn to contour entire lung fields in both the images of healthy volunteers and patients with

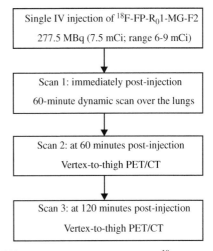

FIGURE 10.4 Imaging schema for ^{18}F-FP-R$_0$1-MG-F2 PET/CT in IPF.

known IPF. Maximum and mean SUV measurements of each contoured lung were calculated to analyze the uptake values of ^{18}F-FP-R$_0$ 1-MG-F2 within the lung. Maximum and mean SUV values obtained from healthy volunteers (control) were compared to the SUV values for patients with known IPF to determine if ^{18}F-FP-R$_0$ 1-MG-F2 can accurately detect lung expression of integrin $\alpha v \beta 6$ in patients with IPF.

10.2.3 ^{64}Cu-DOTA-Pembrolizumab PET/CT Imaging in Metastatic Non-Small-Cell Lung Cancer and Metastatic Melanoma

Immune checkpoint blockade strategies that induce an anticancer immune response are a promising new area of targeted cancer therapy [37]. Immune checkpoints refer to a negative feedback loop that prevents autoimmunity during normal physiologic conditions and limits collateral tissue damage during an immune response [37–40]. One checkpoint of interest is the programmed cell death receptor protein 1 (PD1) widely expressed on immune cells (e.g., CD4 and CD8 T-cells, activated T-cells (within 24 hours of activation), B-cells, monocytes, natural killer cells, etc.) and its ligands (PD-L1 and PD-L2 [PD-L's]) expressed on various cells, including cancer cells [38].

Pembrolizumab (KEYTRUDA) is an FDA approved, highly selective anti-PD1 monoclonal antibody indicated for the treatment of various cancers, including unresectable or metastatic melanoma and metastatic non-small-cell lung cancer (mNSCLC). Pembrolizumab blocks the interaction between the PD1 receptor and its ligands stimulating the immune system to trigger a T-cell response within the tumor microenvironment. Many studies reported clinically meaningful tumor regression, progression-free survival, and overall survival in patients with metastatic melanoma [19,41–45] and mNSCLC

[46—49], further demonstrating the success of targeted immunotherapy and suggesting the PD1 pathway could be used as a biomarker to guide and monitor therapy.

Molecular imaging permits noninvasive visualization of drug biodistribution and quantification of PD1 receptor uptake in patients with metastatic melanoma or mNSCLC to accurately predict which patients will most benefit from anti-PD1-pathway immunotherapy (Fig. 10.3) [50,51]. The broad expression of PD1 and its ligands suggest that this immune checkpoint pathway regulates a wide spectrum of immune response [38] and would be an excellent conduit to stratify patients who would best respond to pembrolizumab immunotherapy among these cohorts.

10.2.3.1 *Image Analysis*

The primary objectives of this study were to investigate whether ^{64}Cu-DOTA-pembrolizumab was suitable for clinical use as a predictive biomarker for pembrolizumab immunotherapy and to detect and quantify PD1 receptor uptake (direct measure of activated T-cells) in these two cohorts. Scan 2 (Fig. 10.5) was used for interpretation since ^{64}Cu-DOTA-pembrolizumab is an antibody. Regions of interest (ROI) were drawn around areas of visually increased uptake of ^{64}Cu-DOTA-pembrolizumab both pre- and mid-pembrolizumab therapy. Maximum and mean SUV measurements of each lesion were calculated to analyze the uptake values compared to background. Comparison of ^{64}Cu-DOTA-pembrolizumab and ^{18}F FDG PET/CT uptake was also performed in both cohorts pre- and mid-pembrolizumab therapy.

10.3 PARTICIPANT RECRUITMENT AND SELECTION

Successful clinical translation of imaging probes relies heavily on designing clinical trials that balance research objectives with the

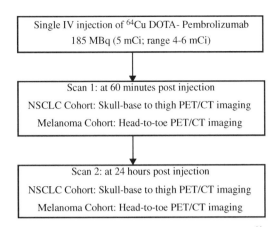

| Single IV injection of ^{64}Cu DOTA- Pembrolizumab 185 MBq (5 mCi; range 4-6 mCi) |
| Scan 1: at 60 minutes post injection
NSCLC Cohort: Skull-base to thigh PET/CT imaging
Melanoma Cohort: Head-to-toe PET/CT imaging |
| Scan 2: at 24 hours post injection
NSCLC Cohort: Skull-base to thigh PET/CT imaging
Melanoma Cohort: Head-to-toe PET/CT imaging |

FIGURE 10.5 Imaging schema for first-in-human ^{64}Cu-DOTA-pembrolizumab PET/CT in mNSCLC and metastatic melanoma.

realities of patient care. Fewer deviations from routine standard-of-care increase both support from physician and/or surgeon partners and participant compliance.

10.3.1 Participant Recruitment and Selection

Participant recruitment and retention is often the most challenging aspect of a clinical trial [52,53]. It is vital that sponsors and collaborators design protocols with number of subjects, eligibility criteria, and study procedures that are feasible and realistic [53], otherwise conducting a clinical trial may become an exercise in futility. Many frequently encountered recruitment issues among participants (e.g., complexity of the protocol, lack of awareness, fear of side effects) [53] can be overcome when investigators seek physician and/or surgeon partners early on (pre-FDA and IRB approval) since garnering their support increases trial awareness, interest, and positive attitudes for the trial [1]. Patient selection may begin once patients are identified under suitable eligibility criteria.

Eligibility criteria are specifically designed to ensure participant safety [54] and create a representative sample that will meet the scientific objectives of the study [55]. Strict adherence to eligibility criteria is necessary to standardize enrollment so as to minimize trial bias in the selection process and increase the generalizability of study results. Trialists are encouraged to clearly define the methodology used to determine eligibility in early-phase trials for these reasons [1,55].

10.4 CLINICAL WORKFLOW

10.4.1 Informed Consent

The FDA has published guidelines that outline the mandatory content and appropriate language used in a consent form and the proper conduct of an effective informed consent process [56]. This process must occur under circumstances that minimize the possibility of coercion (e.g., threat of harm) or undue influence (e.g., excessive participation compensation; minimization of risks; overestimation of benefits). Informed consent documents must clearly notate that the drug used in the clinical trial is investigational (not FDA approved) and outline all potential risks associated with its administration, i.e., listing radiation exposures for ionizing radiopharmaceuticals or x-rays, or outlining potential contrast agent reactions [56].

10.4.2 Standard Clinical Safety Testing

Standard clinical safety evaluations should include serial assessments of patient symptoms, physical signs (e.g., vitals), clinical laboratory tests (e.g., blood chemistry, hematology, coagulation profiles, urinalyses), other tests (e.g., electrocardiograms as appropriate), and adverse events [57]. Additional specialized evaluations may be necessary (e.g., immunological or toxicology evaluations) if there is the potential for organ toxicity based on preclinical trials with known pharmacological properties of the medical imaging agent [57].

Safety testing of imaging probes used for in vivo diagnosis or monitoring is classified by the FDA as contrast agents or diagnostic radiopharmaceuticals [57]. FDA guidance on safety testing for therapeutic agents is out of the scope of this chapter.

FDA defines a contrast agent (e.g., iodinated compounds; paramagnetic metallic ions; microparticles; microbubbles; and related microparticles) as an imaging probe used to enhance the visualization of tissues, organs, and physiologic processes by increasing the signal intensity of one region relative to an adjacent region [57]. Diagnostic radiotracers (used in nuclear medicine or PET) utilize the spontaneous emission(s) of an unstable nucleus (coupled to a pharmaceutical) to diagnose or monitor a disease or a manifestation of a disease. Medical imaging agents are characterized as Group 1 and Group 2 agents based on their special characteristics [57].

Group 1 agents are not biological products (e.g., radiolabeled cells, monoclonal antibodies or fragments, see 21CFR600.3(h)) and do not predominantly emit alpha or beta particles. Group 1 agents must meet either the *preclinical safety-margin* or the *clinical-use* considerations outlined by the FDA in the guideline. If one criterion is met, a less extensive clinical safety assessment plan is recommended by the FDA for Group 1 agents. All agents that do not meet these criteria default to Group 2 (unless the Group 2 agent demonstrates that its product lacks immunogenicity) including Group 1 agents that present safety concerns during the clinical trial. Group 1 agents may follow a reduced safety monitoring plan, such as monitoring of toxicity and recording adverse events, whereas Group 2 agents should follow the standard clinical safety evaluations and other tests as appropriate (e.g., immunological or toxicology evaluations) [57]. Creating an efficient safety monitoring plan based on FDA recommendations should be a key element when designing early-phase clinical trials to avoid extending resources toward unnecessary monitoring and also potentially alleviating subject fears about participation risks.

10.4.3 Patient Preparation, Imaging Agent Administration, and Imaging Protocol

All patient preparations related to the clinical trial (e.g., medication reconciliation, height/weight recording, safety assessments, IV placement(s)) should be described in the research protocol and performed prior to tracer administration. Some radiopharmaceuticals require predosing with an unlabeled or "cold" compound to block source organ uptake [27,50,51] This both increases the availability of the probe to reach the target and decreases organ toxicity to prevent unwanted medical side effects (e.g., hypothyroidism). For example, "cold" rituximab is given to block splenic uptake of ^{90}Y-ibritumomab tiuxetan (^{90}Y-Zevalin) in the treatment of non-Hodgkin's lymphoma. Introducing an unlabeled agent to saturate the source organ allows more antibody-based radiolabeled tracer to target CD20 receptors overexpressed on circulating B-cells [50]. Similarly, administering potassium iodide, super-saturated potassium iodide, or Lugol's solution prevents hypothyroidism by blocking thyroid accumulation of free radioactive iodine during ^{131}I metaiodobenzylguanidine treatment [27].

The protocol should outline the dose, route, and duration of probe administration, define the imaging protocol, and outline all safety assessments to be performed during the scan. First-in-man clinical trials with healthy volunteers will likely have a more robust imaging protocol in order to obtain biodistribution, PK and/or PD, and dosimetry information, which requires dynamic imaging and whole-body static serial imaging [58,59]. Whenever possible, dynamic imaging should begin at least

1 minute prior to radiopharmaceutical injection, with blood draws accurately timed and documented to acquire the most precise input functions for kinetic modeling [58]. For cohorts other than healthy volunteers, imaging protocols should align optimal imaging times based on PK data with research goals. Eliminating scans that will not provide usable research data reduces study cost, increases efficiency at various stages of the trial, and improves overall patient experience.

10.4.4 Follow-Up

Participant safety (including adverse event reporting) and/or medical assessment follow-up(s) may be performed by various members of the research team via phone interview(s) or clinic visit(s) at time intervals outlined in the protocol. A schematic of a clinical workflow is illustrated in Fig. 10.6.

10.5 DRUG PHARMACOKINETICS AND INTERNAL DOSIMETRY USING POSITRON EMISSION TOMOGRAPHY/COMPUTED TOMOGRAPHY

10.5.1 Drug Pharmacokinetics

PK (e.g., absorption, distribution, metabolism, excretion) effects can be measured using continuous, dynamic PET imaging, where investigators gather information about the drug effects in tissues, receptors, or compartments of interest in humans beyond the spatial domain and in real-time [58,60–64]. Incorporating temporal information allows researchers to answer meaningful quantitative questions such as the receptor concentration in a volume of tissue, or the rate of influx/efflux from (or to) the intravascular space or trapping of the probe within the tissue [63]. Regulatory framework is less stringent since the

radiopharmaceutical is administered in microdose amounts (defined as equal to or less than $100\ \mu g$ for imaging agents and 30 nmol for protein products) [22,65–67]. Given the significance of identifying the presence or absence of these properties, PK data using the microdose approach in early-phase clinical trials may arguably be the most pivotal aspect of predicting the success of a drug for sponsors and collaborators [61].

PK effects are derived from compartmental modeling, which is the most common method used in PET to illustrate the many possible transformations of the probe across the many potential physical spaces and/or the chemical state of the probe (e.g., intravascular or extracellular, bound to plasma proteins or receptors, or metabolized, respectively) in vivo at a given time postinjection [58,60–64]. The simplest model is depicted as a one-tissue, irreversible compartment model with no tracer efflux back to blood, as in the example of radioactive microspheres (Fig. 10.7) [62]. A three-tissue compartment model for a receptor-binding ligand is more complex where the three compartments represent "free" tracer, tracer bound to a specific receptor, and tracer nonspecifically bound to other tissue elements, a proportion of which at any time and/or under any physiologic condition(s) could move between compartments (Fig. 10.7) [62–64].

Once a an ROI is drawn on an image, the measured tissue time-activity curve (TAC) is estimated by a compartmental model which uses the arterial plasma TAC as its "input function." The input function represents the concentration of unchanged (non-metabolized) probe that is transported in arterial plasma to the site of interest as a function of time [58,62,63]. Since the probe is delivered to versus carried away from the area of interest, input functions are best obtained using arterial blood sampling at distinct time points collected during dynamic imaging (though mixed or venous blood sampling would suffice provided

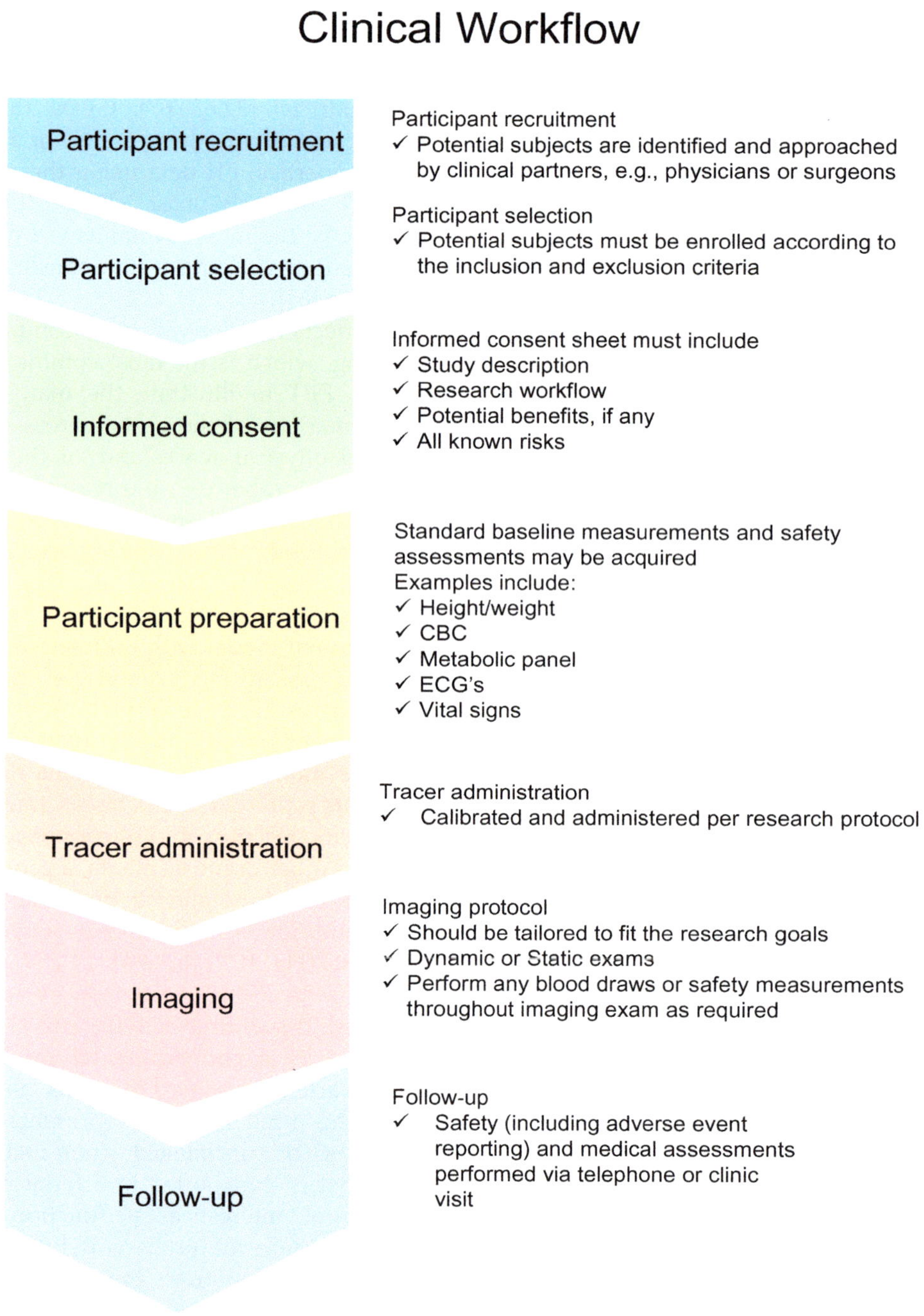

Clinical Workflow

Participant recruitment

Participant recruitment
✓ Potential subjects are identified and approached by clinical partners, e.g., physicians or surgeons

Participant selection

Participant selection
✓ Potential subjects must be enrolled according to the inclusion and exclusion criteria

Informed consent

Informed consent sheet must include
✓ Study description
✓ Research workflow
✓ Potential benefits, if any
✓ All known risks

Participant preparation

Standard baseline measurements and safety assessments may be acquired
Examples include:
✓ Height/weight
✓ CBC
✓ Metabolic panel
✓ ECG's
✓ Vital signs

Tracer administration

Tracer administration
✓ Calibrated and administered per research protocol

Imaging

Imaging protocol
✓ Should be tailored to fit the research goals
✓ Dynamic or Static exams
✓ Perform any blood draws or safety measurements throughout imaging exam as required

Follow-up

Follow-up
✓ Safety (including adverse event reporting) and medical assessments performed via telephone or clinic visit

FIGURE 10.6   Clinical workflow schematic.

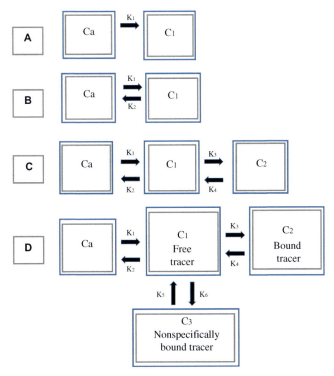

FIGURE 10.7 (A) One-tissue compartment model illustrating irreversible uptake of tracer, e.g., microspheres. (B) One-tissue compartment model illustrating reversible uptake of tracer, e.g., a diffusible tracer such as ^{13}N-ammonia used in cardiac rest/stress imaging. (C) Two-tissue compartment model demonstrating reversible tracer from arterial compartment to tissue, e.g., F18-FDG. This model represents a tracer that enters tissue (C_1, unmetabolized) from blood, is either metabolized to a form that is trapped in the tissue (C_2, metabolized) at a rate defined by k_3, or returns to blood at a rate defined by k_2. (D) Three-compartment model illustrating a receptor-binding ligand. Ca is the tracer concentration (activity/volume, usually in MBq/ml) in arterial blood while C_1, C_2, C_3 represent the tracer concentrations in each compartment listed; K_1 is initial rate of exchange of the radiotracer from the arterial compartment to the first compartment and the only rate constant denoted with an upper case and having units of mL plasma/cm^3 tissue/min, which is related to perfusion; k_x denotes the rate of tracer exchange between compartments.

that the difference in the arteriovenous concentrations are not too large) [62]. The blood TAC can also be obtained from PET images of blood pool. ROI's drawn within the left ventricle, left atrium, carotids, or other available arteries near the target tissue may be used so long as partial volume [68] and spillover effects are corrected for [58,64] (e.g., due to the partial volume effect and spillover of activities between the myocardium and left ventricle blood pool, the measured radioactivity concentration for the input function may be contaminated with tissue signal). When superimposing "simple" compartmental models upon complex biological systems, one must make certain assumptions, namely that each compartment houses a uniform tracer concentration and that rates of physiologic change with respect to imaging time are balanced [58,62,63].

So as to overcome the inherent limitations of the tracer, the patient population, and the equipment, it is important to provide the research team with explicitly defined protocols when incorporating PK in early-phase clinical trials. The acquisition protocol must outline precisely the time intervals for blood collections if they are to be used for the input function. A synchronized clock system is an excellent way to ensure radiotracer activity measurements are accurately documented (and decay corrected) at initial dose calibration, injection, imaging start/stop time, blood-draw timing measurements, and residual-dose calibration across many sites since these measurements are critical to the kinetic analysis equations. Nuclear medicine physicians must clearly define the spatial and temporal parameters for PET dynamic imaging and attenuation correction (CT or rod-source) that correspond to the desired PK plan. Collaboration with PK analysis experts will ensure all aspects of the clinical protocol are appropriately built to properly gather the data necessary to examine the quantitative questions set forth in the clinical trial. In-depth mathematics for kinetic modeling can be accessed here [62–64].

10.5.2 Internal Dosimetry

Radiation dosimetry is the method used to convert the amount of ionizing radiation deposited in tissue to its effect in tissue, which is influenced by the "damage potential" of the radiation type (e.g., energy, size, charge, half-life, etc.), the administered dose, and the dose rate [69–71]. The quantities obtained from dosimetry calculations are fundamental to estimating radiation protection, risk assessment, diagnostic dose estimates, and treatment planning [72].

Internal dosimetry in drug development is primarily used from two perspectives [72]. For early-phase I or phase I clinical trials, dosimetry is performed after radiopharmaceutical administration to provide standard diagnostic procedural dose estimates and define dose-limiting organs in a limited number of healthy volunteers. A second type of dosimetry is used to guide treatment and thus performed prior to the therapeutic drug administration for all patients undergoing treatment. Organ-specific (target and source organs) and total effective dose equivalent dosimetry estimates are calculated in diagnostic studies, whereas in treatment planning, dosimetry estimates are focused regionally that correspond to the treatment area [69,71,72].

Since radiation dose calculations include many factors [73,74] and are lengthy, tedious, and error-prone when performed manually, the FDA strongly recommends using dosimetry code software when submitting dosimetry estimates for new radiopharmaceuticals that are or will be administered to humans for experimental or clinical use (Table 10.1) [59]. Dosimetry software such as Medical Internal Radiation Dose (MIRDose) [75] or Organ Level Internal Dose Assessment Exponential Modeling

TABLE 10.1 Advantages to Using Dosimetry Code Software [71]

1. Provides a standardized framework and methodology for automated dosimetry calculations in the user community
2. Minimal user input data required to generate radiation dose estimates
3. Most standard and up-to-date models for internal dosimetry are incorporated (i.e., software already includes quantities effective dose equivalent and effective dose derived from the most recent tissue weighting factors and quality factors recommended by the International Commission on Radiological Protection (ICRP) and the MIRD of the Society of Nuclear Medicine and Molecular Imaging (SNMMI))
4. Greatly facilitates difficult dose calculations that can be tedious to complete manually
5. The same output quantities are reproduced by all users when inputting the same data
6. Can be used to make theoretical calculations for existing radiopharmaceuticals, teaching, and other purposes
7. FDA readily accepts the dosimetry calculations when reviewing new IND applications, thereby speeding up the approval process

(OLINDA/EXM, successor to MIRDose, FDA 510(k)-approved device) [71] offer users a variety of phantoms that permit calculating radiation doses for individuals at various ages and sizes, and for women at different stages of pregnancy.

To create radiation dose estimates for the reference population (Table 10.2), the user inputs the radionuclide, chooses the anthropomorphic model, and inputs the integral values (that demonstrate cumulated percent activity) derived from the PK time—activity curve data from the patient's images [59].

Currently, dosimetry estimates assume uniform distributions of absorbed radiation energy across the entire organ and do not provide dosing gradients at tissue boundaries or direct tumor dose correlations [59,71]. While standardized dose estimates using these phantoms are sufficient for diagnostic imaging because the dose/exposures are relatively low and justifiable, dose estimates prior to radiolabeled therapy (e.g., dosimetry-guided radiotherapy using ^{177}Lu) [76—79] must be more precise so as to better predict toxicity in dose-limiting organs, namely bone marrow (most radiosensitive organ) and kidneys (most common method of radionuclide excretion) [72,76,77,79—83]. One method to address these limitations includes incorporating an organ-specific tomographic activity distribution data map from the patient's SPECT/CT or PET/CT scan [76,78,80,84—87]. Access to 3D voxel data would maximize tumor dose while minimizing toxicity to surrounding tissues [76]. Additionally, blood collections (timing and quantity of samples) must match the PK properties of the radiotracer and be precisely recorded by the research team during imaging [80].

10.6 REGULATORY PERSPECTIVE

Bench-to-bedside probe translation relies heavily on the efficient use of current regulatory avenues to reduce product attrition early in the development phase [88]. Traditionally, once a specific target is identified (via genomics or proteomics) [89] and the imaging probe is designed, synthesized, and validated as functional in vitro, the most promising probe is selected to undergo a myriad of costly and resource-intensive pharmacologic and toxicological safety tests to support one IND application for safe introduction into human subjects. Statistically however, a small percentage of probes actually produce acceptable human profiles and progress beyond the investigational stage [22,65]. High probe attrition can often be attributed to the limitations associated with animal research, such as poor experimental designs and failure of animal physiology to accurately mimic the indication or disease-state being tested. The growing concern for the high clinical failure rate led the FDA to release the Critical Path Report [90] in March 2004, which outlined modern product-development toolkits that offered ways to improve the current system early-on in the developmental pathway, while maintaining important regulatory safety requirements for human testing. Thus it is crucial that translational scientists understand the available early-phase I regulatory avenues to leverage the pathway best-suited to their research objectives and goals.

In compliance with the FDA Modernization Act [91], every novel imaging probe and/or any imaging probe postearly phase I necessitates filing an IND for human studies. An IND is also required for investigators who wish to initiate and conduct research studies of approved drugs for new indications or in new patient populations [67]. For clinical studies performed in academic institutions in which investigational radiopharmaceuticals (e.g., SPECT or PET probes) are used, researchers may utilize two early-phase I regulatory pathways: the Radioactive Drug Research Committee (RDRC) [92] and an eIND [22]

TABLE 10.2   Radiation Dosimetry Calculated Using OLINDA Code

Organ	Adult Female Total Dose (rem/mCi)	Adult Male Total Dose (rem/mCi)
Adrenals	8.84E − 02	6.94E − 02
Brain	2.57E − 02	2.10E − 02
Breasts	7.17E − 02	5.70E − 02
Gallbladder wall	8.63E − 02	7.16E − 02
LLI wall	8.81E − 02	6.90E − 02
Small intestine	8.37E − 02	7.32E − 02
Stomach wall	8.55E − 02	6.86E − 02
ULI wall	9.00E − 02	7.19E − 02
Heart wall	1.33E − 01	1.03E − 01
Kidneys	3.03E − 01	2.76E − 01
Liver	1.13E − 01	8.52E − 02
Lungs	5.39E − 02	4.28E − 02
Muscle	4.03E − 02	3.01E − 02
Ovaries	8.67E − 02	NR
Pancreas	8.96E − 02	7.19E − 02
Red marrow	6.66E − 02	5.46E − 02
Osteogenic cells	1.65E − 01	1.25E − 01
Skin	6.62E − 02	5.23E − 02
Spleen	8.55E − 02	6.83E − 02
Testes	NR	6.00E − 02
Thymus	7.97E − 02	6.17E − 02
Thyroid	7.46E − 02	6.05E − 02
Urinary bladder wall	7.48E − 02	6.75E − 02
Uterus	8.62E − 02	NR
Total body	8.47E − 02	6.60E − 02
Effective dose (rem/mCi)	8.09E − 02	6.57E − 02

Dosimetry in 5 Healthy Human Volunteers Imaged at Stanford University. Dosimetry values were based on the average percent injected activity (%IA) in the kidney, stomach, small intestine, bladder, pancreas, liver, lung, heart, muscle and whole body remainder. The average area under the curve (AUC) of the %IA was determined by ROI analysis of static ^{18}F-FP-R0 1-MG-F2 PET scans acquired immediately upon tracer injection, 1 hour and 2 hours after injection. These values were entered into OLINDA to determine the radiation dosimetry to each of the organs listed in the table. The kidneys were determined to be the dose limiting organ at 0.0490 mSV/MBq in an adult male. (manuscript entitled "A First-in-Human Study of Integrin avb6 Cystine Knot Positron Emission Tomography (PET) Tracers "submitted for review by Kimura, R, Wang, L, Shen, B, Huo, L, Tummers, W, Filipp, F, Abou-Elkacem, L, Baratto, L, Habte, F, Devulapally, R, Witney, T, Cheng, Y, Haywood, T, Tikole, S, Chakraborti, S, Nix, J, Bonagura, C, Hatami, N, Visser, B, Poultsides, G, Norton, J, Natarajan, A, Ilovich, O, Srinivas, S, Srinivasan, A, Paulmurugan, R, Willmann, J, Chin, F, Cheng, Z, Iagaru, A, Li, F, Gambhir, S)".

TABLE 10.3 Comparison Between RDRC, eIND, and IND

	RDRC	eIND	IND
May perform first-in-man studies	No	Yes	Yes
Radiochemistry published in the literature	Usually	No	Perhaps
Number of mammalian species required for toxicity studies	None	1	2
Preclinical testing requirements	Complete series of toxicology testing either performed by self or referenced	Reduced risk of testing the molecule = reduced requirements for toxicology testing	Complete series of toxicology testing either performed by self or referenced
Number of molecules studied per application	1	Up to five structurally related molecules	1

eIND: Exploratory Investigational New Drug; *RDRC*: Radioactive Drug Research Committee.

before choosing to file an IND application (Table 10.3) [93]. Investigators should also consider the advantages of IND sharing by a letter of right of reference to decrease the burden of preclinical costs [3].

10.6.1 Radioactive Drug Research Committee

The RDRC provides an efficient pathway for investigators interested in conducting basic science research of radioactive drugs in up to 30 subjects when the probe is not a novel radiopharmaceutical (i.e., prior dosing in humans has been previously demonstrated) [65,88,92,94]. Research is conducted for the purpose of advancing scientific knowledge to obtain basic information about the metabolism (including kinetics, distribution, and localization) of a radioactively labeled drug and/or for human physiology, pathophysiology, or biochemistry, but is not intended for immediate diagnostic purposes [92,94]. As such, studies conducted under RDRC oversight are considered as initial (feasibility, early phase I) studies. While the information obtained during these investigations may have eventual diagnostic or therapeutic implications, basic research studies are not classified as applicable clinical trials according to the FDA.

Additional conditions as outlined in 21CFR361.1 [94] must be satisfied and justified when investigating a radiopharmaceutical under RDRC oversight. To ensure the administered radioactive drug is considered safe and effective, the following limits on pharmacologic dose, radiation dose, and radiation exposure must be met:

1. *Limit on pharmacologic dose:* The active ingredient(s) of the radioactive drug to be administered (exclusive of the radionuclide) must display no clinically detectable pharmacologic effect in humans at the intended mass dose [94]. Researchers should refer to the package insert or search the literature to determine if the chemical structure of the radiopharmaceutical poses undue risk to human subjects at the

recommended mass dose [67]. An IND must be filed when sufficient evidence describing the pharmacologic effect in humans at the proposed mass dose cannot be established.

2. *Limit on radiation dose:* The amount of administered radioactivity should be the lowest possible dose to reasonably perform the study without jeopardizing the primary aims of the study. Researchers should consider radiopharmaceutical characteristics (e.g., biodistribution, binding potential, method of localization, etc.), specifics of the protocol (e.g., imaging equipment, indication), and previously conducted clinical studies when determining the lowest possible dose for their study.

3. *Limit on radiation exposure:* Limits to the radiation dose from all procedures (including x-ray procedures and potentially any follow-up procedures as part of the study) apply to the whole body, active blood-forming organs, lens of the eye, and gonads of an adult research subject from a single study or cumulatively from multiple studies conducted within 1 year; and for research subjects under 18 years of age shall not exceed 10% of those limits [94].

The RDRC is an institutional-based FDA-sanctioned committee consisting of at least five individuals, of which each committee must include the following three individuals: (1) a physician recognized as a specialist in nuclear medicine, (2) a person qualified by training and experience to formulate radioactive drugs, and (3) a person with special competence in radiation safety and radiation dosimetry [94]. Remaining committee membership shall consist of individuals qualified in various disciplines relevant to the field of nuclear medicine. The committee is responsible for monitoring RDRC-approved studies and filing detailed annual reports to the FDA per 21CFR 361.1 FDA regulation [94].

10.6.2 Exploratory Investigational New Drug

The eIND mechanism is aimed specifically at reducing prohibitive preclinical expenditures for novel imaging probes and thus is most appropriate for first-in-man studies where investigators have no diagnostic intent as an immediate objective [22,90]. The ultimate goal of an eIND is to corroborate preclinical experimental data of a new probe in humans earlier in drug development. Examples of early phase I testing include determination of OLINDA (organ level internal dose assessment) dosimetry, normal biodistribution, mechanism-of-action, dose, optimal imaging time, PK, and PD. Furthermore, sponsors may utilize the eIND as a screening approach to evaluate two to five structurally related probes and select the most promising lead candidate to then pursue an IND [22,65−67,88−90].

The FDA is able to provide more regulatory flexibility for studies conducted under an eIND because the imaging probe is to be administered at a microdose level, defined as equal to or less than 100 µg for imaging agents and 30 nmol for protein products [22,65−67]. Microdose studies involve limited human exposure and thus present fewer risks [67] to participants so FDA requirements for preclinical safety testing are less burdensome. Sponsors filing an eIND need only perform one mammalian toxicity study per drug candidate compared to two species for the traditional IND, which is a significant budget reduction given a single toxicology study costs around $70,000−$100,000 [66]. So as to reduce the number of nonessential studies and enable sponsors to efficiently advance the clinical development of promising candidates [22], researchers should discuss with the FDA the extent of nonclinical testing required to safely administer the drug to human subjects during the pre-eIND meeting [66]. To advance the radiopharmaceutical into phases I−III clinical trials the investigative team must withdraw the eIND and verify that all toxicity assessments (i.e., use of human toxicity data derived from the eIND may be used in conjunction with pre-clinical animal toxicology data for a total of two species) are sufficient to support filing a traditional IND [67].

10.7 MOLECULAR PROBE REIMBURSEMENT

10.7.1 Research and Development Reimbursement

Pharmaceutical companies use molecular imaging agents to ensure participants have the condition under study and assess potential responses to the investigational drug prior to trial enrollment. For feasibility studies, collaborators may add a new indication to a sponsor's existing eIND/IND (IND sharing). This is a highly effective method for potentially fast-tracking FDA approval of their therapeutic drugs [3].

Sponsors may request permission from the FDA to charge for an investigational drug if (1) the investigational drug demonstrates potential clinical advantage over other available products; (2) it is necessary for establishing safety and efficacy and obtaining initial drug approval; and (3) conducting the trial is cost-prohibitive without charging for the investigative agent [95].

10.7.2 Insurance Reimbursement

Reimbursement of imaging probe costs by insurance following FDA approval is a critical component to its widespread adoption [89]. To accomplish this, adequate evidence must effectively demonstrate that the probe both improves current clinical practice (when compared to existing alternatives) and patient management in a meaningful way [3].

10.8 SUMMARY

Predicting the success of an imaging probe hinges on determining in vivo characteristics in man at the earliest stage of development. Academic facilities should develop a tailored, collaborative, and cost-effective molecular probe IND submission strategy to best streamline the regulatory process for their institutions.

References

[1] Farrell B, Kenyon S, Shakur H. Managing clinical trials. Trials 2010;11:78.
[2] Willmann JK, van Bruggen N, Dinkelborg LM, Gambhir SS. Molecular imaging in drug development. Nat Rev Drug Discov 2008;7(7):591−607.
[3] Liu CH, Sastre A, Conroy R, Seto B, Pettigrew RI. NIH workshop on clinical translation of molecular imaging probes and technology—meeting report. Mol Imaging Biol 2014;16(5):595−604.
[4] Adams HJ, Kwee TC. Prognostic value of interim FDG-PET in R-CHOP-treated diffuse large B-cell lymphoma: systematic review and meta-analysis. Crit Rev Oncol Hematol 2016;106:55−63.
[5] Adams HJ, Nievelstein RA, Kwee TC. Systematic review and meta-analysis on the prognostic value of complete remission status at FDG-PET in Hodgkin lymphoma after completion of first-line therapy. Ann Hematol 2016;95(1):1−9.
[6] Ghooshkhanei H, Treglia G, Sabouri G, Davoodi R, Sadeghi R. Risk stratification and prognosis determination using (18)F-FDG PET imaging in endometrial cancer patients: a systematic review and meta-analysis. Gynecol Oncol 2014;132(3):669−76.
[7] Hassanzadeh-Rad A, Yousefifard M, Katal S, Asady H, Fard-Esfahani A, Moghadas Jafari A, et al. The value of (18) F-fluorodeoxyglucose positron emission tomography for prediction of treatment response in gastrointestinal stromal tumors: a systematic review and meta-analysis. J Gastroenterol Hepatol 2016;31(5):929−35.
[8] Huang Y, Feng M, He Q, Yin J, Xu P, Jiang Q, et al. Prognostic value of pretreatment 18F-FDG PET-CT for nasopharyngeal carcinoma patients. Medicine (Baltimore) 2017;96(17):e6721.
[9] Kubo T, Furuta T, Johan MP, Ochi M. Prognostic significance of (18)F-FDG PET at diagnosis in patients with soft tissue sarcoma and bone sarcoma; systematic review and meta-analysis. Eur J Cancer 2016;58:104−11.

[10] Liu J, Dong M, Sun X, Li W, Xing L, Yu J. Prognostic value of 18F-FDG PET/CT in surgical non-small cell lung cancer: a meta-analysis. PLoS One 2016;11(1) e0146195.

[11] Na F, Wang J, Li C, Deng L, Xue J, Lu Y. Primary tumor standardized uptake value measured on F18-fluorodeoxyglucose positron emission tomography is of prediction value for survival and local control in non-small-cell lung cancer receiving radiotherapy: meta-analysis. J Thorac Oncol 2014;9(6):834–42.

[12] Pak K, Cheon GJ, Nam HY, Kim SJ, Kang KW, Chung JK, et al. Prognostic value of metabolic tumor volume and total lesion glycolysis in head and neck cancer: a systematic review and meta-analysis. J Nucl Med 2014;55(6):884–90.

[13] Peare R, Staff RT, Heys SD. The use of FDG-PET in assessing axillary lymph node status in breast cancer: a systematic review and meta-analysis of the literature. Breast Cancer Res Treat 2010;123(1):281–90.

[14] Sheikhbahaei S, Ahn SJ, Moriarty E, Kang H, Fakhry C, Subramaniam RM. Intratherapy or posttherapy FDG PET or FDG PET/CT for patients with head and neck cancer: a systematic review and meta-analysis of prognostic studies. Am J Roentgenol 2015;205(5):1102–13.

[15] Sun N, Zhao J, Qiao W, Wang T. Predictive value of interim PET/CT in DLBCL treated with R-CHOP: meta-analysis. BioMed Res Int 2015;2015 648572.

[16] Xia Q, Liu J, Wu C, Song S, Tong L, Huang G, et al. Prognostic significance of (18)FDG PET/CT in colorectal cancer patients with liver metastases: a meta-analysis. Cancer Imaging 2015;15:19.

[17] Zhu Y, Lu J, Wei X, Song S, Huang G. The predictive value of interim and final [18F] fluorodeoxyglucose positron emission tomography after rituximab-chemotherapy in the treatment of non-Hodgkin's lymphoma: a meta-analysis. BioMed Res Int 2013;2013:275805.

[18] Huo E, Wilson DM, Eisenmenger L, Hope TA. The role of PET/MR imaging in precision medicine. PET Clin 2017;12(4):489–501.

[19] Ribas A, Hamid O, Daud A, Hodi FS, Wolchok JD, Kefford R, et al. Association of pembrolizumab with tumor response and survival among patients with advanced melanoma. JAMA 2016;315(15):1600–9.

[20] Heidari P, Deng F, Esfahani SA, Leece AK, Shoup TM, Vasdev N, et al. Pharmacodynamic imaging guides dosing of a selective estrogen receptor degrader. Clin Cancer Res 2015;21(6):1340–7.

[21] Slomka PJ, Pan T, Germano G. Recent advances and future progress in PET instrumentation. Semin Nucl Med 2016;46(1):5–19.

[22] US Food and Drug Administration. In: U.S. Department of Health and Human Services CfDEaRC, editor. Guidance for industry, investigators, and

reviewers: exploratory IND studies. Silver Spring, MD: US Food and Drug Administration; 2006.

[23] Zambrowicz BP, Sands AT. Knockouts model the 100 best-selling drugs—will they model the next 100? Nat Rev Drug Discov 2003;2(1):38–51.

[24] Dimasi JA. New drug development in the United States from 1963 to 1999. Clin Pharmacol Ther 2001;69(5):286–96.

[25] Basu S. The scope and potentials of functional radio-nuclide imaging towards advancing personalized medicine in oncology: emphasis on PET-CT. Discov Med 2012;13(68):65–73.

[26] Basu S, Alavi A. PET-based personalized management in clinical oncology: an unavoidable path for the foreseeable future. PET Clin. 2016;11(3):203–7.

[27] Subramaniam R. Molecular imaging and precision medicine, Part 1. An issue of PET clinics, E-Book. Elsevier Health Sciences; 2016. https://play.google.com/store/books/details?id = HvkTDgAAQBAJ&rdid = book-HvkTDgAAQBAJ&rdot = 1&source = gbs_vpt_read.

[28] Cherry S, Sorenson J, Phelps M. Positron emission tomography. Physics in nuclear medicine. 4th ed. Amsterdam: Elsevier; 2012. p. 307–43.

[29] Smith NL, Halliday BE, Finley JL, Wennerberg AE. The spectrum of immunohistochemical reactivity of monoclonal antibody DS6 in nongynecologic neoplasms. Appl Immunohistochem Mol Morphol 2002;10(2):152–8.

[30] Ilovich O, Natarajan A, Sathirachinda A, Hori S, Kimura R, Srinivasan A, et al. Development and validation of an immuno-PET tracer for patient stratification and therapy monitoring of antibody-drug conjugate therapy. J Clin Oncol 2013;31(15):110006.

[31] Carrigan C, Suany-Amorim C, Mayo M, et al. Preclinical evaluation of SAR566658 (huDS6-DM4) in mice bearing human tumor xenografts of breast, ovarian, lung, cervical and pancreatic cancer. EJC Suppl 2008;6(12):166.

[32] Warram JM, de Boer E, Sorace AG, et al. Antibody-based imaging strategies for cancer. Cancer Metastasis Rev 2014;33(2-3):809–22.

[33] Raghu G, Collard HR, Anstrom KJ, Flaherty KR, Fleming TR, King Jr TE, et al. Idiopathic pulmonary fibrosis: clinically meaningful primary endpoints in phase 3 clinical trials. Am J Respir Crit Care Med 2012;185(10):1044–8.

[34] Raghu G, Collard HR, Egan JJ, Martinez FJ, Behr J, Brown KK, et al. An official ATS/ERS/JRS/ALAT statement: idiopathic pulmonary fibrosis: evidence-based guidelines for diagnosis and management. Am J Respir Crit Care Med 2011;183(6):788–824.

[35] Aschner Y, Downey GP. Transforming growth factor-beta: master regulator of the respiratory system in

health and disease. Am J Respir Cell Mol Biol 2016;54 (5):647−55.

[36] Horan GS, Wood S, Ona V, Li DJ, Lukashev ME, Weinreb PH, et al. Partial inhibition of integrin alpha (v)beta6 prevents pulmonary fibrosis without exacerbating inflammation. Am J Respir Crit Care Med 2008;177(1):56−65.

[37] Pardoll DM. The blockade of immune checkpoints in cancer immunotherapy. Nat Rev Cancer 2012;12 (4):252−64.

[38] Jin HT, Ahmed R, Okazaki T. Role of PD-1 in regulating T-cell immunity. Curr Top Microbiol Immunol 2011;350:17−37.

[39] Keir ME, Butte MJ, Freeman GJ, Sharpe AH. PD-1 and its ligands in tolerance and immunity. Ann Rev Immunol 2008;26:677−704.

[40] Tumeh PC, Harview CL, Yearley JH, Shintaku IP, Taylor EJ, Robert L, et al. PD-1 blockade induces responses by inhibiting adaptive immune resistance. Nature 2014;515(7528):568−71.

[41] Robert C, Ribas A, Wolchok JD, Hodi FS, Hamid O, Kefford R, et al. Anti-programmed-death-receptor-1 treatment with pembrolizumab in ipilimumab-refractory advanced melanoma: a randomised dose-comparison cohort of a phase 1 trial. Lancet 2014;384(9948):1109−17.

[42] Hua C, Boussemart L, Mateus C, Routier E, Boutros C, et al. Association of vitiligo with tumor response in patients with metastatic melanoma treated with pembrolizumab. JAMA Dermatol 2016;152(1):45−51.

[43] Bagcchi S. Pembrolizumab for treatment of refractory melanoma. Lancet Oncol 2014;15(10):e419.

[44] Robert C, Schachter J, Long GV, et al. Pembrolizumab versus ipilimumab in advanced melanoma. N Eng J Med 2015;372(26):2521−32.

[45] Hamid O, Robert C, Daud A, Hodi FS, Hwu WJ, Kefford R, et al. Safety and tumor responses with lambrolizumab (anti-PD-1) in melanoma. N Eng J Med 2013;369(2):134−44.

[46] Hui R, Garon EB, Goldman JW, Leighl NB, Hellmann MD, Patnaik A, et al. Pembrolizumab as first-line therapy for patients with PD-L1-positive advanced non-small cell lung cancer: a phase 1 trial. Ann Oncol 2017;28(4):874−81.

[47] Garon EB, Rizvi NA, Hui R, et al. Pembrolizumab for the treatment of non-small-cell lung cancer. N Eng J Med 2015;372(21):2018−28.

[48] Reck M, Rodriguez-Abreu D, Robinson AG, Hui R, Csőszi T, Fülöp A, et al. Pembrolizumab versus chemotherapy for PD-L1-positive non-small-cell lung cancer. N Eng J Med 2016;375(19):1823−33.

[49] Herbst RS, Baas P, Kim DW, Felip E, Pérez-Gracia JL, Han JY, et al. Pembrolizumab versus docetaxel for previously treated, PD-L1-positive, advanced non-small-cell lung cancer (KEYNOTE-010): a randomised controlled trial. Lancet 2016;387(10027): 1540−50.

[50] Natarajan A, Gambhir SS. Radiation dosimetry study of [(89)Zr]rituximab tracer for clinical translation of B cell NHL imaging using positron emission tomography. Mol Imaging Biol 2015;17(4):539−47.

[51] Natarajan A, Mayer A, Reeves R, Nagamine C, Gambhir S. Development of novel immunoPET tracers to image human PD-1 checkpoint expression on tumor-infiltrating lymphocytes in a humanized mouse model. Mol Imaging Biol 2017;19(6):903−14.

[52] Sygna K, Johansen S, Ruland CM. Recruitment challenges in clinical research including cancer patients and their caregivers. A randomized controlled trial study and lessons learned. Trials 2015;16:428.

[53] Kadam RA, Borde SU, Madas SA, Salvi SS, Limaye SS. Challenges in recruitment and retention of clinical trial subjects. Perspect Clin Res 2016;7(3):137−43.

[54] Department of Health and Human Services. CFR Title 45 public welfare, Part 46 protection of human subjects. Washington, DC; 2009.

[55] Guyatt G, Rennie D, Meade M, Cook D. Users' guides to the medical literature: a manual for evidence-based clinical practice. 2nd ed. New York City, NY: The McGraw-Hill Companies Inc; 2008.

[56] Food and Drug Administration. In: U.S. Department of Health and Human Services Office of Good Clinical Practice, Center for Drug Evaluation and Research (CDER), Center for Biologics Evaluation and Research (CBER), Center for Devices and Radiological Health (CDRH), editors. Informed consent information sheet. Guidance for IRBs, clinical investigators, and sponsors. Rockville, MD: Food and Drug Administration; 2014.

[57] Food and Drug Administration. In: U.S. Department of Health and Human Services. Center for Drug Evaluation and Research (CDER), Center for Biologics Evaluation and Research (CBER), editor. Guidance for industry: developing medical imaging drug and biological products. Part 1: Conducting safety assessments. Rockville, MD: Food and Drug Administration; 2004.

[58] Bentourkia M, Zaidi H. Tracer kinetic modeling in PET. PET Clin 2007;2(2):267−77.

[59] Stabin MG, Sparks RB, Crowe E, Crowe E. OLINDA/ EXM: the second-generation personal computer software for internal dose assessment in nuclear medicine. J Nucl Med 2005;46(6):1023−7.

[60] Bergstrom M, Grahnen A, Langstrom B. Positron emission tomography microdosing: a new concept with application in tracer and early clinical drug development. Eur J Clin Pharmacol 2003;59(5−6): 357−66.

[61] Burt T, Yoshida K, Lappin G, Vuong L, John C, de Wildt SN, et al. Microdosing and other phase 0 clinical

trials: facilitating translation in drug development. Clin Transl Sci 2016;9(2):74–88.

[62] Carson R. Tracer kinetic modeling in PET. In: Valk P, Bailey D, Townsend D, Maisey MN, editors. Positron emission tomograpy: basic science and clinical practice. London: Springer-Verlag; 2003. p. 147–79.

[63] Morris E, Endres C, Schmidt K, Christian B, Muzic R, Fisher R. Kinetic modeling in positron emission tomography Revised edition In: Wernick MN, Aarsvold JN, editors. Emission tomography: the fundamentals of PET and SPECT. Cambridge, MA: Academic Press; 2004. p. 499–540.

[64] Nelissen N, Warwick J, D'upont P. Kinetic modelling in human brain imaging. Positron emission tomography—current clinical and research aspects. Europe: InTech; 2012. p. 55–84.

[65] Mosessian S, Duarte-Vogel SM, Stout DB, Roos KP, Lawson GW, Jordan MC, et al. INDs for PET molecular imaging probes-approach by an academic institution. Mol Imaging Biol 2014;16(4):441–8.

[66] Schwarz SW, Oyama R. The role of exploratory investigational new drugs for translating radiopharmaceuticals into first-in-human studies. J Nucl Med 2015;56(4):497–500.

[67] Harapanhalli RS. Food and Drug Administration requirements for testing and approval of new radiopharmaceuticals. Semin Nucl Med 2010;40(5):364–84.

[68] Soret M, Bacharach SL, Buvat I. Partial-volume effect in PET tumor imaging. J Nucl Med 2007;48(6):932–45.

[69] Paquet F, Bailey MR, Leggett RW, Harrison JD. Assessment and interpretation of internal doses: uncertainty and variability. Ann ICRP 2016;45(Suppl. 1):202–14.

[70] Spielmann V, Li WB, Zankl M, Oeh U, Hoeschen C. Uncertainty quantification in internal dose calculations for seven selected radiopharmaceuticals. J Nucl Med 2016;57(1):122–8.

[71] Stabin MG, Sparks RB, Crowe E. OLINDA/EXM: the second-generation personal computer software for internal dose assessment in nuclear medicine. J Nucl Med 2005;46(6):1023–7.

[72] Stabin MG, Sharkey RM, Siegel JA. RADAR commentary: evolution and current status of dosimetry in nuclear medicine. J Nucl Med 2011;52(7):1156–61.

[73] Bolch WE, Eckerman KF, Sgouros G, Thomas SR. MIRD pamphlet No. 21: a generalized schema for radiopharmaceutical dosimetry–standardization of nomenclature. J Nucl Med 2009;50(3):477–84.

[74] Howell RW, Wessels BW, Loevinger R, Watson EE, Bolch WE, Brill AB, et al. The MIRD perspective 1999. Medical Internal Radiation Dose Committee. J Nucl Med 1999;40(1):3S–10S.

[75] Stabin MG. MIRDOSE: personal computer software for internal dose assessment in nuclear medicine. J Nucl Med 1996;37(3):538–46.

[76] Chalkia MT, Stefanoyiannis AP, Chatziioannou SN, Round WH, Efstathopoulos EP, Nikiforidis GC. Patient-specific dosimetry in peptide receptor radionuclide therapy: a clinical review. Australas Phys Eng Sci Med 2015;38(1):7–22.

[77] Kabasakal L, AbuQbeitah M, Aygun A, Yeyin N, Ocak M, Demirci E, et al. Pre-therapeutic dosimetry of normal organs and tissues of (177)Lu-PSMA-617 prostate-specific membrane antigen (PSMA) inhibitor in patients with castration-resistant prostate cancer. Eur J Nucl Med Mol Imaging 2015;42(13):1976–83.

[78] Ljungberg M, Celler A, Konijnenberg MW, Eckerman KF, Dewaraja YK, Sjögreen-Gleisner K, et al. MIRD Pamphlet No. 26: joint EANM/MIRD guidelines for quantitative 177Lu SPECT applied for dosimetry of radiopharmaceutical therapy. J Nucl Med 2016;57(1):151–62.

[79] Sundlov A, Sjogreen-Gleisner K, Svensson J, Ljungberg M, Olsson T, Bernhardt P, et al. Individualised 177Lu-DOTATATE treatment of neuroendocrine tumours based on kidney dosimetry. Eur J Nucl Med Mol Imaging 2017;44(9):1480–9.

[80] Hindorf C, Glatting G, Chiesa C, Linden O, Flux G, Committee ED. EANM Dosimetry Committee guidelines for bone marrow and whole-body dosimetry. Eur J Nucl Med Mol Imaging 2010;37(6):1238–50.

[81] Vicini P, Brill AB, Stabin MG, Rescigno A. Kinetic modeling in support of radionuclide dose assessment. Sem Nucl Med 2008;38(5):335–46.

[82] Huang SY, Bolch WE, Lee C, et al. Patient-specific dosimetry using pretherapy [(1)(2)(4)I]m-iodobenzyl-guanidine ([(1)(2)(4)I]mIBG) dynamic PET/CT imaging before [(1)(3)(1)I]mIBG targeted radionuclide therapy for neuroblastoma. Mol Imag Biol 2015;17(2):284–94.

[83] Svensson J, Ryden T, Hagmarker L, Hemmingsson J, Wangberg B, Bernhardt P. A novel planar image-based method for bone marrow dosimetry in (177)Lu-DOTATATE treatment correlates with haematological toxicity. EJNMMI Phys 2016;3(1):21.

[84] Dewaraja YK, Frey EC, Sgouros G, Brill AB, Roberson P, Zanzonico PB, et al. MIRD pamphlet No. 23: quantitative SPECT for patient-specific 3-dimensional dosimetry in internal radionuclide therapy. J Nucl Med 2012;53(8):1310–25.

[85] Song YS, Paeng JC, Kim HC, Chung JW, Cheon GJ, Chung JK, et al. PET/CT-based dosimetry in 90Y-microsphere selective internal radiation therapy: single cohort comparison with pretreatment planning on (99m)Tc-MAA imaging and correlation with treatment efficacy. Medicine 2015;94(23):e945.

[86] Schwartz J, Humm JL, Divgi CR, Larson SM, O'Donoghue JA. Bone marrow dosimetry using 124I-PET. J Nucl Med 2012;53(4):615—21.

[87] Ao EC, Wu NY, Wang SJ, Song N, Mok GS. Improved dosimetry for targeted radionuclide therapy using nonrigid registration on sequential SPECT images. Med Phys 2015;42(2):1060—70.

[88] Hung JC. Bringing new PET drugs to clinical practice — a regulatory perspective. Theranostics 2013;3(11): 885—93.

[89] Hoffman JM, Gambhir SS, Kelloff GJ. Regulatory and reimbursement challenges for molecular imaging. Radiology 2007;245(3):645—60.

[90] US Food and Drug Administration. In: Services USDoHaH, editor. Innovation or stagnation: challenge and opportunity on the critical path to new medical products. Silver Spring, MD: US Food and Drug Administration; 2004. p. 1—31.

[91] Congress US. Food and Drug Administration Modernization Act of 1997. Washington, DC: Congress US; 1997.

[92] US Food and Drug Administration. In: U.S. Department of Health and Human Services CfDEaRCCfBEaR, editor. Guidance for industry and researchers: the radioactive drug research committee: human research without an investigational new drug application. Silver Spring, MD: US Food and Drug Administration; 2010.

[93] US Food and Drug Administration. In: U.S. Department of Health and Human Services CfDEaRC, editor. Guidance: investigational new drug applications for positron emission tomorgraphy (PET) drugs. Silver Spring, MD: US Food and Drug Administration; 2012.

[94] US Food and Drug Administration. In: Services DoHaH, editor. 21CFR361.1: prescription drugs for human use generally recognized as safe and effective and not misbranded: Drugs used in research. Silver Spring, MD: US Food and Drug Administration; 2016.

[95] US Food and Drug Administration. In: Services USDoHaH, editor. 21CFR312.8: charging for investigational drugs under an IND. Silver Spring, MD: US Food and Drug Administration; 2017.

Clinical Trial Design in Immuno-Oncology

Houssein A. Sater[1,2], John Janik[3] and Samir N. Khleif[4]

[1]National Cancer Institute, Bethesda, MD, United States [2]Johns Hopkins Medicine, Bethesda, MD, United States [3]Incyte Corporation, Chadds Ford, PA, United States [4]Georgetown University Medical School, Washington DC, United States

11.1 INTRODUCTION

A clinical trial is the investigation of humans' response to a medication or intervention. The design of any clinical trial should take into consideration fundamental principles of respect for persons, beneficence, and justice [1]. The decision of answering who, how, and why we test, implicitly follows these principles to shape meaningful endpoints. A clear understanding of how a medication or intervention could impact the natural history of a disease is essential. Chemotherapy has relatively well-understood kinetics and limitations. Over the last two decades, immunotherapy emerged as a new hope for many cancer patients. Despite our relatively limited understanding of its effect in human biology, immunotherapy differs substantially from chemotherapy in mechanism of action, target, response, and safety profile. Drugs or interventions used in immunotherapy mainly enhance immune cells to recognize and kill cancer cells with high specificity. The sequence of examination continues to involve the three standard phases of clinical development, Phases I, II, and III, that evaluate safety, efficacy, and a specific endpoint [2], respectively. Current clinical trials continue to study similar endpoints since late 1960s mainly time to an event (death, first relapse, metastasis, disease recurrence, or death from a particular cause). Certainly, improved survival and cure are the ultimate goal of interest for all researchers and their patients. Since this endpoint is not always achievable in a time frame that permits rapid drug development, other endpoints such as progression free survival or objective response might be more relevant. Response Evaluation Criteria In Solid Tumors (RECIST) were developed and updated between 2000 and 2009 by an international collaboration between the European Organization for Research and Treatment of Cancer (EORTC), National Cancer Institute of the United States, and the National Cancer Institute of Canada Clinical Trials Group to define objective responses in solid tumors [3]. The modern era of immuno-therapy presents a number of major challenges in the design of early phase clinical trials, including Phase 1 trials with more than thousand patients, the proliferation of over 800 ongoing clinical trials, and many additional experimental medications yet to come. In this chapter, we discuss these challenges and the need for adopting new designs for early phase clinical trials of Immuno-Oncology agents. We also highlight the current clinical experience with immune therapy.

11.2 CHALLENGES OF CONDUCTING EARLY PHASE CLINICAL TRIALS WITH IMMUNE-THERAPIES

11.2.1 General Challenges

A major challenge to clinical trial design stems from the fact that we are moving into an era of personalized medicine. Most cancers are now recognized to comprise a multitude of subtypes due to identification of novel molecular markers. Tumors with relatively similar histology are subdivided into distinct tumor subtypes by specific mutations or overexpression of certain proteins. Examples include epithelial growth factor receptor family [4], Anaplastic lymphoma kinase (ALK), ROS proto-oncogene 1 (ROS), and Rat sarcoma (RAS) gene mutations typically seen in lung adenocarcinoma. The ability to study any specific subtype using the traditional 3 + 3 Phase I clinical trial design followed by Phase II and Phase III studies over 5- to 10-year period is not practical anymore. In response to this, researchers in the field have shifted to either biomarker enrichment, early drug switch

strategy, or a basket design permitting many different cancer types to be entered in the same trial. Indeed with the recognition that common mutations may be present in entirely distinct tumors, the same targeted drug may have significant or no activity. BRAF mutation first identified and targeted in melanoma is associated with colon cancer where there is little or no activity and hairy cell leukemia where many responses have been observed.

Another major difficulty in the development of immunotherapy is the fact that tumor response and progression free survival may not correlate with overall survival. Sipuleucel-T, the only approved vaccine for cancer, demonstrated no improvement in progression free survival and few objective responses but in two randomized trials demonstrated a 4 month improvement in survival. In contrast to the effects of chemotherapy where there are few if any long term survivors immunotherapy produces cures in a small percentage of patients and combination studies have yielded response rates that approach 50% in some tumor types. The majority of patients receiving immunotherapy can work and go about their daily life activities more freely when compared to patients receiving chemotherapy although fatigue is a major side effect of most immunotherapies. Yet the use of experimental agents is limited to fit patients with a Karnofsky Performance Status of 0 to 1 in most trials. The inclusion of less fit patients who might benefit from these trials is likely to be explored with continued respect for persons, beneficence, and justice as the outcomes of therapy continue to improve. The other challenges are due to the mechanism of action of novel therapies and the shift from traditional chemotherapy effect. This is reflected on the traditional endpoints, and statistical analysis used which do not meet the observations noticed particularly in immune therapies.

Immunotherapy has a mode of action and adverse event (AE) profile that is different from traditional chemotherapy. This AE profile, shown to be correlated with response in some studies, could still be fatal in some patients or have permanent effects [5]. In most cases, it is a form of autoimmune process that involves the skin, lungs, gastro-intestinal track, liver, thyroid, or pituitary gland. These reactions are typically delayed and unpredictable, but immediate institution of immunosuppression is key to avoid further damage. In its worst form, a cytokine storm syndrome has been observed with chimeric antigen receptor T cell therapies and remain a major challenge [6]. Infusion related reactions occur with many of these agents but are usually limited to the initial weeks of dosing and are readily managed with antipyretics, antihistamines, intravenous fluid and occasionally steroids. Importantly, many immunotherapies employ monoclonal antibodies that fail to reach a maximally tolerated dose (MTD) and have therapeutic benefit at relatively low dose levels. An increase in the dose does not predict more benefit but adds significantly to the cost compared to [7] lower dose levels. Tumor responses are similarly unpredictable. Delayed response after a progressive or stable disease is not uncommon and may be observed in about 10% of patients treated with immunotherapy agents. Classically, chemotherapy leads to either stable disease, no response (progressive disease), or response (partial response, or complete response) based on radiologic RECIST criteria. This pattern has a direct clinico-radio-pathologic correlation to validate it. In contrast, immunotherapy can lead to what appears as a progressive disease radiologically, yet the patient is clinically stable and the increase in size is driven by tumor infiltration with immune cells that, when biopsied, can show necrotic tumor cells, which has be defined as "pseudoprogression." Absolute proof of pseudoprogression requires a confirming biopsy at the time of initial progression but if subsequent tumor shrinkage occurs after early signs of progression, its occurrence can be inferred. It not only positions a treating physician in a dilemma between changing therapy and waiting for potential benefit, but also creates a challenge for physicians treating patients on clinical trials. This has led to many clinical trials that use RECIST response criteria to allow for continued treatment provided there is no worsening of clinical symptoms when faced with initial tumor progression. Continued treatment for 1−2 months allows for the resolution of this quandary and it is usually sufficient to resolve the issue. Patients with pseudoprogression usually demonstrate clinically improvement whereas patients with true progression can show decreased performance status and other signs of advancing cancer.

Despite a plethora of preclinical data, immune driven anticancer effect is not equally translated from mice into humans. Deeper understanding of cancer driven resistance to immune therapy led to combinatorial strategies that might yield synergistic antitumor effect. In addition, a burst of immunotherapeutic agents over the last 5−10 years created a vast potential for different combinations with other immune modulatory agents or chemotherapy, radiation, etc. There are currently more than 800 clinical trials testing these combinations (listed on clinicaltrials.gov website). They all have at least one common goal: curing cancer efficiently. This diversified list of combinations not only yielded a huge excitement but also a big challenge at different levels in early clinical trial design: number of patients needed, enrollment criteria, treatment schedules and sequencing, time of follow up, response criteria, and meaningful endpoints. Given the multiple experimental options available, and immunotherapy drugs not reaching MTDs, some Phase I clinical trials ended up with enrolling more than 1000 patients as they follow the traditional 3 + 3 Phase I design with expansion cohorts [8].

The response rates in these trials are still mandated by the Food and Drug Administration (FDA) to be reported based on RECIST criteria. Unfortunately, these criteria do not reflect the new natural history of disease in the setting of immunotherapy. Wolchock et al. suggested a new dynamic tumor volume assessment, called immune related RECIST or irRECIST criteria. The goal is to recognize the volume change of different tumors through the summation of perpendicular diameters of target and new lesions. The new criteria helps with clinical trials but not day to day clinical decisions. In addition, it remains a non FDA approved measurement parameter.

These reasons and others highly mandate serious revision of current design in early phase clinical trials to meet all these challenges. In addition, designs need to be adapted to the setting of treatment. The use of immunotherapy in early [9] versus late phases (therapeutic) post a different challenge by itself. Failure of achieving significant responses by vaccine therapy in adjuvant setting is an example. Many of these clinical trial questions aim to better understand the human biology which remains the fundamental challenge. In the following paragraphs, we discuss each point individually

11.2.2 Number of Patients Needed

In early phase trials, primary endpoints are traditionally safety and efficacy along with pharmacokinetics (PK) and pharmacodynamics (PD) in case of a novel agent. To achieve these endpoints, a number of patients should be tested. This number is calculated based on the clinical trial design. In Phase I as described in Chapter 2, Requirements for Filing an Investigational New Drug Application, a $3 + 3$ approach is commonly used where three patients at same dose level are treated with

monitoring for a disease limiting toxicity (DLT) is noticed [10]. In this study design, up to six patients are treated at each dose levels, which would typically imply a maximum number of patients (6 multiplied by the number of dose levels tested) in the range of 20–80. With immunotherapy agents not reaching MTD, as toxicity do not seem to be dose dependent, the number of unknown variables increased (more new agents being tested), the dose levels in some studies might be as high as above 80 patients might just be tested in a Phase I trial. In a review of early clinical trials by Khleif et al., only 3 out of 127 cancer vaccine (CV) trials (2987 patients) had reported a DLT [7]. In addition, dose escalation strategy has no predictive role in terms of bioactivity. Similarly, immune check-point inhibitors which are another form of immunotherapy had a DLT in the range of 17%–33% of patients although combination trials produce DLT toxicity in over half of the patients. The question whether Phase I study need to be omitted or modified especially with CV was formally discussed in "Cancer Immunotherapy Clinical Trials: Concepts & Challenges" program at the Society of Immune therapy of Cancer (SITC) in 2013 and continues to be open. Alternative Phase I designs have been suggested but none is officially accepted yet. Monoclonal antibodies are in general safe with the expectation of infusional reactions, particularly if there are circulating cells in the blood that express the receptor and expected immune related events in a fraction of patients, notable exceptions are known. The anti-CD28 antibody was associated with severe toxicity in its initial evaluations that unfortunately allowed for the treatment of multiple patients with a dose that was expected to be safe in normal volunteers. The IRB responsible for review of this trial did not provide adequate protections and the FDA has instituted guidelines for these first in human trials. Another example is the antibody directed at CD137 that produced hepatic toxicity at higher doses albeit not with the first dose but upon repeated dosing. These examples provide pause for the rapid escalation of these agents. These include strategies to reduce cohorts to one patient at a time, decreasing the DLT threshold, and combining Phase I and Phase II data for safety measures. Despite these suggestions, most trials continue to use the $3 + 3$ design with some variations. The limits of what can be acceptable for trials of immuno-therapy agents is also distinct. Immune related AEs would in many cases be considered dose limiting under standard criteria but these events are not considered to be dose limiting in most trials if they resolve within 4 weeks with administration of immunosuppressive doses of steroids. The need for additional immunosuppressive agents such as anti-TNF for colitis, mycophenolate mofetil for hepatic toxicity or immune events that do not resolve in 4 weeks would be dose limiting.

In the old paradigm of drug development, once a safe recommended Phase 2 dose (RP2D) is determined, a new trial is written for patients efficacy testing or Phase II. In the current drug development model where higher response rates are anticipated the addition of multiple cohorts of patients with various tumor histologies are typically entered. The numbers of patients entered in these trials approaches that in large Phase III trials with thousands of patients sometimes treated. The number of patients examined in Phase II (traditionally $100-300$) is statistically calculated based on endpoint with clear assumptions of changes in hazard ratio, statistical power, margin of error (Type I) and confidence interval. Since most of these agents were new to researchers, and their effect on anticipated endpoint is unpredictable, a smaller anticipated HR change demanded a very high number of patients to achieve statistical significance. As there are multiple tumor subtypes being tested, many studies adopted expansion phases into their Phase II designs. This was meant to detect early signals of efficacy, and biomarker development to enrich studies based on discovered biomarkers [11]. Unfortunately, there was no valid biomarkers when these studies have started and hence we witnessed studies with cohorts of total 1000 patients in Phase 1/Ib expansion. In addition, the response rates seen with traditional RECIST criteria tend to be delayed with immunotherapy compared to chemotherapy. To see a significant difference based on number of events needed, studies would need to enroll bigger number of patients in Phase II compared to traditional therapy. Alternative studies that are potentially adaptive in design helped bypass the strict statistical requirements for the sake of biomarker evaluation and enrichment. While umbrella design focuses on one histologic type, it screens for various biomarkers. In contrast, a basket design screens for large group of different tumor subtypes based on molecular or biomarkers signatures. NCI-Molecular Analysis for Therapy Choice (MATCH NCI) [12] is a great example of this clinical trial design. It is expected to screen up to 6000 patients with various malignancies and enroll 35 patients in 25 treatment groups based on mutations for which a drug exists. Many of the early stage immunotherapy trials used this design.

With the significant benefit associated with immunotherapy another major difficulty in new drug development is the requirement for incorporation of the newly approved agents targeting PD-1, PD-L1, and CTLA4 in combination studies to permit adequate patient participation and understand the toxicity profile of the new agents.

In addition to being a challenge by itself, higher number poses another challenge which is accrual in a timely fashion. In one study by the National Cancer Institute (NCI) Cancer Therapy Evaluation Program, 135 corrective action plans (CAP) for slow-accruing Phase I (69) and II (66) trials were analyzed. Safety/ toxicity, design/protocol concerns, and eligibility criteria were found to be primary reasons for slow accrual [2]. More than two thirds of Phase I and Phase II trials met their primary objectives after corrective actions (adding more institutions, protocol, and design amendments), but still required three times longer than anticipated. The challenge created by increased number needed to treat translates into Phase II with delayed response as progression free survival seen in immune check point inhibitors (ICI). It also extends into Phase III trials especially in CV trials in adjuvant setting where much more patients and longer follow up is needed to reach a meaningful difference between groups treated.

11.2.3 Eligibility Criteria

These are the inclusion and exclusion criteria by which a study subject is deemed fit for a clinical trial. In Immunotherapy trials, patients follow the same pattern as chemotherapy trials with modifications based on AE profile seen with similar agents tested before. These agents typically rely on an intact immune system to function and lead to immune-related AEs in addition to some other traditional side effects seen with chemotherapy. For this reason, patients with underlying autoimmune disorders or on chronic immunosuppressive agents are typically excluded. Common exclusion criteria are listed on Cancer Research Institute (CRI) website (http://www.cancerresearch.org/cancer-immunotherapy/about-clinical-trials).

Eligibility criteria remain strict with immunotherapy despite a different AE profile seen with these agents. In the case of CVs and many ICIs, the patient performance status is not altered as seen with chemotherapy. Yet, enrollment of patients with poor performance status that are not candidates for palliative/therapeutic chemotherapy remains not considered. We wonder if this could be open for discussion at some point between researchers. The design of early clinical trials in immunotherapy shifted

into enrichment/biomarker strategy. Hence, patients harboring different tumors with particular mutational loads, or specific genetic mutations are mostly enrolled in a basket design into groups or arms with specific treatments/combinations. Examples include patients with RAS, RAF mutations or tumors with microsatellite instability (colon, pancreas). In addition, there is a potential shift from traditional hierarchy of treatment lines. In the world of chemotherapy, patients are offered a first line of therapy upon diagnosis of cancer, followed by second or third line upon progression of disease. This holds true in the case of chemotherapy because of class/regimen resistance. In other words, it is not likely that a patient who progressed on a specific drug to respond to a similar regimen or drug from same family. In the era of immunotherapy, these assumptions may not be valid. Patients that fail an ICI could still respond to same ICI alone or in combination with other drugs. This is reflected in trial designs which allow re-challenge with same treatment and as an example is the ipilimumab trial with successful rechallenge in two patients with BRAF-V600-mutant melanoma who experienced previous progression during treatment with a selective BRAF inhibitor [13]. Also, the fact that the immune therapeutic agents are not fully explored yet, in terms of proper sequencing, combinations, and dosing continues to give researchers a hope of their unexplored potentials. This is certainly a challenge where treating a patient in standard of care setting remains in the gray zone with these agents. Properly designed clinical trials will address these questions over time.

11.2.4 Treatment Schedules and Sequencing

There is a tremendous optimism among immune therapy researchers that the proper sequence and combination of agents will improve cure rates for cancer patients. The way that immune therapy agents work relies mostly on the responses mounted by immune system· elements. In the case of CVs, immunogenicity is determined by drug factors as vaccine structure itself (peptide, cell, vehicle), adjuvants used, site of injection, time of injection (if used with other agents), constituent doses, and host factors (early or late disease, suppressed or intact immune system, major histocompatibility complex, etc.). Similarly, CPIs indirect effect on tumor rely on drug and host properties. Priming of the immune system involves steps like introduction of antigen by specialized antigen presenting cells, creating a synapse like signals with costimulatory or co-inhibitory secondary signals, followed by multiplication or differentiation of immune cells all orchestrated with chemicals as cytokines, growth factors, enzymes, and other signaling molecules. Interfering with any of these steps yields results that are very time dependent. Preclinical models primarily test these effects in mice to draw conclusions that might help translational scientists develop better treatment designs. Since these data are not well translated into humans, hundreds of trials are currently open for enrollment. These should offer over time some insight on human biology. As expected, many trials have several arms with different combinations, and we are seeing more trials addressing the sequencing in humans. As we learn more, designs should focus more evidence rather than expectations. Sequencing is so important in CV with check-point inhibitors. There have been cases where vaccine therapy has worsened outcome [14]. Resistance mechanisms are thought to be due to check-point inhibitors overexpression by tumor although multiple mechanisms of immune-evasion exit. Using CPIs before, with or after vaccine remains an open question.

As for treatment schedules, it should be straightforward based on PK/PD studies. Monoclonal antibodies as cytotoxic lymphocyte antigen-4 (CTLA-4) and programmed death-1 (PD-1) inhibitors have been tested in different schedules and doses. An important factor in this consideration is the side effect profile difference in different combinations and schedules. CV schedules are mostly straightforward, and do not need pharmacokinetic studies, but when in combination, sequencing becomes critical. Sequencing is not only important when combining with another immune agent, but also when another modality of treatment is used, such as radiation therapy, surgery, and chemotherapy. All three interventions have direct or indirect effect on the immune system development. Cancer Vaccine Clinical Trial Working Group (CVCTWG) defined the following differences in CVs mandating a switch in design in early clinical trials

1. Lack of serious toxicity risks or proof of a linear dose-potency relationship for CV.
2. Dose and schedule are not determined through escalation based on toxicity.
3. CV usually do not get metabolized: no need for conventional pharmakokinetics.
4. Many CV are designed to address one tumor type.
5. RECIST criteria are not well applicable to CV and historical control comparisons on RR are not useful: proof-of-principle endpoints should reflect biologic activity including immunogenicity.

The working group suggested a two-step design:

1. Proof-of-Principle/Exploratory Trials (>20 patients) from a well-defined population.
2. Efficacy Trial(s) (Randomized Trials) with prospective adaptive designs.

11.2.5 Time of Follow-Up

Patients treated in Phase I studies are followed for a period that allows researchers to detect any dose-limiting toxicity (DLT) in addition to further follow up if treatment continues.

The follow-up time commonly used to determine a DLT is a one cycle although with many immunotherapies the time course of onset of these events is prolonged and it is not uncommon for particularly toxic combinations to have DLT periods of up to three cycles. Toxicities occurring in subsequent cycles of therapy are used to determine the recommended Phase II dose. Treatment with immunotherapy agents differs from chemotherapy by having a delayed and unpredictable AE profile. Researchers in the field adapted quickly to this fact by increasing the monitoring period following last administered dose of immunotherapy. Phase I studies typically last several months and last patient follow up would go up to 120 days after last dose given. As for Phase II studies the follow up remains as several months to 2 years. Another challenge to immunotherapy is due to lack of tumor response with only the presence of long-term stable disease as the best tumor response and delayed response patterns associated with a survival benefit. This is one of the reasons to suggest fusion of Phase I and Phase II into "proof of principle phase" leaving phase three as confirmatory phase with longer follow up. Although Phase I and Phase II emphasis are on safety and efficacy relatively, both phases are interchangeably used to draw conclusions on both endpoints. Some ICIs Phase II studies sensed the need for longer follow ups with endpoints as survival extending to 3 years. Trials of CVs have an even greater need for long follow-up. The nine valent vaccine was launched into Phase III after the four valent vaccine proved safe [15]. In such a design, patients in Phase IIB gained longer follow up and added to statistical power of final data analysis.

11.2.6 Response Criteria

The FDA continues to recommend the use of RECIST in clinical trials. These criteria were developed and updated between 2000 and 2009 by an international collaboration between the European Organization for Research and Treatment of Cancer (EORTC), National Cancer Institute of the United States, and the National Cancer Institute of Canada Clinical Trials Group to define objective responses in solid tumors [3]. Computed tomography (CT) scan was considered by the collaboration to be the best available and reproducible method for response assessment. The approach includes baseline assessment of disease by measuring at most 5 total target lesions (maximum two per organ involved) and follow up of same lesions overtime. Target lesions could be nodal (Lymph nodes with shortest axis diameter ≥ 15 mm) or nonnodal (lesions with longest axis diameter ≥ 10 mm). Measurement of disease at any point in time is the sum of diameters of target lesions (short axis for nodal lesions and long axis for nonnodal lesions). Baseline sum and the smallest sum on study are used as references to determine type of responses as shown in Table 11.1 below.

In addition to existing lesions at diagnosis, new lesions might occur during therapy. These are counted into overall response as shown in Table 11.2. These criteria reflect the natural history of disease in the era of chemotherapy. The update in 2009 with lessening the total number of target lesions to measure from 10 to 5 speaks of this trend that is reproducible with less measured lesions [3]. While a tumor response to chemotherapy goes in one direction (either progression or regression), response to immunotherapy agents is more dynamic. After a period of stable disease or initial progression (increase in preexisting tumor or appearance of new lesions), shrinkage of tumor is seen with immune therapy [16,17]. This initial progression would be considered a progressive disease based on RECIST criteria and hence patient will be subject to change in therapy if he/she was treated with traditional chemotherapy. This new pattern of progression seen with immunotherapy, has been noticed early on by

TABLE 11.1 Response Evaluation Criteria in Solid Tumors (RECIST V1.1)

Complete response (CR)	Target lesions	Disappearance of all target lesions. Any pathological lymph nodes (whether target or nontarget) must have reduction in short axis to <10 mm.
	Nontarget lesions	Disappearance of all nontarget lesions and normalization of tumor marker level. All lymph nodes must be nonpathological in size (<10 mm short axis).
Partial response (PR)	Target lesions	At least a 30% decrease in the sum of diameters of target lesions, taking as reference the baseline sum diameters.
Non-CR/non-PD	Nontarget lesions	Persistence of one or more nontarget lesion(s) and/or maintenance of tumor marker level above the normal limits.
Progressive disease (PD)	Target lesions	At least a 20% increase in the sum of diameters of target lesions, taking as reference the smallest sum on study (this includes the baseline sum if that is the smallest on study). In addition to the relative increase of 20%, the sum must also demonstrate an absolute increase of at least 5 mm. (Note: the appearance of one or more new lesions is also considered progression).
	Nontarget lesions	Unequivocal progression (see comments below) of existing nontarget lesions. (Note: the appearance of one or more new lesions is also considered progression).
Stable disease (SD)	Target lesions	Neither sufficient shrinkage to qualify for PR nor sufficient increase to qualify for PD, taking as reference the smallest sum diameters while on study

TABLE 11.2 One Time Point Response Evaluation in Patients With Nontarget (+/− Target) Disease

Target Lesions	Nontarget Lesions	New Lesions	Overall Response
CR	CR	No	CR
CR	Non-CR/non-PD	No	PR
CR	Not evaluated	No	PR
PR	Non-PD or not all evaluated	No	PR
SD	Non-PD or not all evaluated	No	SD
Not all evaluated	Non-PD	No	NE
PD	Any	Yes or No	PD
Any	PD	Yes or No	PD
Any	Any	Yes	PD
No target lesions	CR	No	CR
	Non-CR/non-PD	No	Non-CR/non-PD
	Not all evaluated	No	NE
	Unequivocal PD	Yes or No	PD
	Any	Yes	PD

CR, complete response; NE, inevaluable; PD, progressive disease; PR, partial response; SD, stable disease.

TABLE 11.3   Immune-Related Response Criteria (irRC) 2009

irComplete response (irCR)	Complete disappearance of all lesions (whether measurable or not, and no new lesions)[a]
irPartial response (irPR)	Decrease in tumor burden ≥50% relative to baseline[a]
irProgressive disease (irPD)	Increase in tumor burden ≥25% relative to nadir (minimum recorded tumor burden)[a]
irStable disease (irSD)	Not meeting criteria for irCR or irPR, in absence of irPD

[a] *Confirmation by a repeat, consecutive assessment no less than 4 week from the date first documented.*

experts in the field and flagged it as "pseudo-progression." Efforts did not stop here, but just around the time RECIST was updated, a more dynamic criteria was suggested by Wolchok et al. team [18] based on a Phase II clinical trial of ipilimumab in patients with advanced melanoma. This set of criteria were called immune-related response criteria irRC has been criticized for possible measurement variability [19].

To capture the dynamic nature of tumor response to immunotherapy, irRC focused on the overall burden of disease at any point in time (Tables 11.3). This implies the measurement of preexisting and new lesions bi-dimensionally (the sum of the products of the two largest perpendicular diameters (SPD)). All index lesions (five lesions per organ, up to 10 visceral lesions and five cutaneous index lesions) are measurable if 5×5 mm or more on helical CT scans. The formula is as follows:

$$\text{Tumor Burden} = \text{SPD(index)} + \text{SPD}$$
$$\text{(new measurable)}$$

Immune-related RECIST or irRECIST criteria is another approach with unidimensional irRC. It combines standardized methods used in RECIST with important features of irRC (confirmation of progression and new lesion assessment). IrRECIST is expected to decrease measurement variability and more accurately capture the "pseudoprogression" phenomenon. It is not approved by FDA yet and immune therapy trials continue to use RECIST for tumor response as primary endpoint, and

explore irRECIST in secondary endpoints (Table 11.4).

Early "pseudoprogression" is typically seen around the third month of therapy with immune therapeutic agents. In one study a retrospective review of 356 patients cohort enrolled in Phase I/II at Harvard Cancer Center network from 2008 to 2015 showed a pseudoprogression rate of 6% using irRC compared to 2% using RECIST criteria [20]. Interestingly the drugs used in these patients included the monoclonoal antibodies anti-PD1 (57%), anti-PDL1 (23%), and anti-CTLA4 (16%). New lesions were commonly seen in Nodes (35%), Lungs (24%), Peritoneum (18%), Liver (6%), Bone (6%), subcutaneous (6%), and Kidney (5%) while pseudoprogressive lesions were seen in Nodes (31%), Lung (31%), Peritoneum (12%), Subcutaneous (12%), Intramuscular/body wall (7%), Liver (4%), and Adrenal (3%). Similarly, Stephen Hodi et al. [21] showed that among 592 patients with advanced melanoma treated with pembrolizumab 15 patients (4.6%) had early pseudoprogression defined as less than 12 weeks of therapy, and 9 patients (2.8%) had delayed pseudoprogression (>12 weeks).

11.2.7 Biomarker Evaluation

A biomarker is defined by NCI dictionary as a biological molecule found in blood, other body fluids, or tissues that is a sign of a normal or abnormal process, or of a condition or

TABLE 11.4   One Time irRC Overall Responses

Measurable Response	Nonmeasurable Response		Overall Response
Index and new, measurable lesions (tumor burden),[a] %	Nonindex lesions	New, nonmeasurable lesions	irRC
↓100	Absent	Absent	irCR[b]
↓100	Stable	Any	irPR[b]
↓100	Unequivocal progression	Any	irPR[b]
↓ ≥50	Absent/stable	Any	irPR[b]
↓ ≥50	Unequivocal progression	Any	irPR[b]
↓ <50 to <25↑	Absent/stable	Any	irSD
↓ <50 to <25↑	Unequivocal progression	Any	irSD
≥25?	Any	Any	irPD[b]

[a] Decreases assessed relative to baseline, including measurable lesions only (>5 × 5 mm).
[b] Assuming response (irCR) and progression (irPD) are confirmed by a second, consecutive assessment at least 4 week apart.

disease. A biomarker may be used to see how well the body responds to a treatment for a disease or condition. In a personalized medicine era and immune therapy of cancer a biomarker is perhaps the most needed measure. A reproducible biomarker helps achieve clinical and nonclinical endpoints as it:

1. Identifies patients that are likely to respond and benefit (predictive and prognostic). This proves useful for clinical trial enrichment and exclusion of patients less likely to benefit.
2. Predicts who will have toxicity to the drugs used among treated patients.
3. Understand mechanism of action and resistance in human biology through correlation with therapeutic intervention (e.g., immune response).

As immune therapies work primarily on the immune system and not on the cancer itself, it was clear from the beginning the importance of studying biologic measures as endpoints in

clinical trials in addition to clinical endpoints. Since 2004, several initiatives were launched, supported by the Cancer Immunotherapy Consortium of the Cancer Research Institute (CIC-CRI) in collaboration with the Association for Cancer Immunotherapy (C-IMT) in Europe and the International Society for Biological Therapy of Cancer in the United States [22]. The major challenge in studying these biomarkers is consistency. These cultivated in 2008 with efforts to establish cellular immune response as a reproducible biomarker through assay harmonization (to minimize T-cell assay variability of results) and subsequently investigating its relationship with clinical outcomes [23]. Hoos et al. and other working groups identified bioassays for immune monitoring [22,24]. Detailed discussion of these assays is beyond the scope of this chapter. It suffices to say that there have are challenges pertaining to the specimen being examined (Peripheral Blood vs tumor, heterogeneity even within a single patient, etc.), validation process (different antibodies for same target as PD-L1 antibodies), and collaboration among different trials. These assays and their use include: Enzyme-linked immunosorbent spot assay, Cytometry-based tests, HLA-peptide multimer staining, Carboxyfluorescein succinimidyl ester assay, Whole exome sequencing, Gene signature, Epigenetic modification, Protein microarray, B/T cell receptor repertoire, and Multicolor or multiplex Immunohistochemistry (IHC)/Fluorescence. Three broad types of biomarkers could be generated from these assays: (1) Immunologic—e.g., PD-L1 expression, (2) Genetic—e.g., Tumor Mutation Burden, Mismatch Repair Deficiency or Microsatellite Instability (MSI), and (3) Viral—e.g., Human Papilloma Virus (HPV).

The most updated review by Society of Immunotherapy of Cancer (SITC) Biomarker Task force considers biomarkers identifiable from these technologies can help differentiate tumors by the mutation load, gene/protein/antibody signature profile, phenotype and function of immune cells, and can also provide clinical strategies for personalized cancer immunotherapies [24]. In addition, the Cancer Vaccine Clinical Trial Working Group [25], proposed that immunoassays in clinical trials should be performed at least at three different time points throughout any study (at baseline and two follow-up time points). It also confirmed assays should be reproducible, and technically (not clinically) validated in the respective laboratories with at least two assays run in parallel to demonstrate the same findings (e.g., ELISPOT and HLA-peptide multimer staining). This is important for reliable and efficient move of a new agent from early into more late trials testing. Moreover, cutoff values and changes leading to an immune response determine the number of study patients needed for a positive trial outcome. This should be identified early on to get proper validation in a timely fashion. Among all the immunotherapy drugs available today, only

two have an approved companion assays with validated biomarkers (see Table 11.5).

Dako PD-L1 IHC 22C3 (Anti-PD-L1, CD274) was the first FDA-approved companion diagnostics for selecting NSCLC patients for treatment with pembrolizumab. This approval was based on results of two randomized, controlled trials that demonstrated statistically significant improvements in PFS and overall survival (OS) for patients randomized to pembrolizumab compared with chemotherapy. In one trial, frontline use of pembrolizumab in patients with PD-L1 expression (expressed in $\geq 50\%$ tumor cells) had a significant improvement in PFS versus chemotherapy [26]. In a second trial, patients with previously treated metastatic NSCLC and expressed PD-L1 (in $\geq 1\%$ tumor cells) had an improved OS with pembrolizumab compared with patients receiving chemotherapy [27]. **VENTANA PD-L1** (SP142) Assay is a complimentary diagnostic approved by the FDA for selecting urothelial carcinoma patients for treatment with Atezolizumab. In the trial leading to this approval, patients with PD-L1 expression ($\geq 5\%$ tumor infiltrating immune cells) compared to those PD-L1 expression ($<5\%$ tumor infiltrating immune cells), had a significant improvement in tumor response (26% vs to 9.5%) [28].

Other examined biomarkers like ICOS + CD4 T cells found to identify melanoma patients who are more likely to respond to ipilimumab in one study [29], are not FDA approved. Data from last ASCO in June 2016, showed potential biomarkers that could predict response to immunotherapy in a variety of cancers. There were no good data to support PD-L1 expression for biomarker candidacy. KEYNOTE-021 study showed improved efficacy of Keytruda combined with different chemotherapy regimens regardless of PD-L1 expression in advanced NSCLC patients [30]. Tumor mutation burden (TMB), calculated as the number of synonymous and nonsynonymous variants from a series of 236–315 genes determined by HC NGS, was

TABLE 11.5   FDA Approved Immune Check Point Inhibitors, Cancer Vaccines, Their Indication, And Biomarkers

ICI PD-1/-L1	Indication	FDA Approved Biomarkers
Keytruda (pembrolizumab, Merck & Co.)	Nonsmall cell Lung Cancer (PDL-1 $\geq$ 50% first line and $\geq$ 1% second line) or first line in combination with pemetrexed and carboplatin.	Dako PD-L1 IHC 22C3 (Anti-PD-L1, CD274): companion diagnostics for selecting NSCLC patients
	HNSCC (second line)	
	Advanced Melanoma (first line)	
	Advanced or metastatic urothelial carcinoma (second line)	
	Relapsed/refractory classical Hodgkin lymphoma (cHL) (second line or more)	
Opdivo (nivolumab, Bristol Myers-Squibb/Ono Pharmaceuticals)	Advanced urothelial carcinoma (second line)	NA
	Relapsed urothelial carcinoma (first line)	
	SCCHN (second line)	
	Hodgkin Lymphoma (second line)	
	RCC (second line)	
	Advanced Melanoma (second Line $\pm$ Yervoy)	
Tecentriq (atezolizumab, Genentech/Roche)	Advanced urothelial carcinoma	VENTANA PD-L1 (SP142): complimentary diagnostic for selecting urothelial carcinoma patients
	NSCLC (second Line)	
Avelumab (BAVENCIO, EMD Serono, Inc.)	Advanced urothelial carcinoma (second line)	
	Metastatic Merkel cell carcinoma (MCC) (first line)	
Durvalumab (IMFINZI, AstraZeneca UK Limited)	Advanced urothelial carcinoma (second line)	
CTLA-4		
Ipilimumab (Yervoy, Bristol-Myers Squibb Company)	Advanced Melanoma (first line)	NA
	Melanoma (Adjuvant)	
Vaccines		NA
Treatment		
Sipuleucel-T (PROVENGE, Dendreon Corporation)	Asymptomatic or minimally symptomatic metastatic castrate-resistant (hormone refractory) prostate cancer	NA
Talimogene laherparepvec (T-VEC, or Imlygic) by Amgen	Unresectable Melanoma	NA
Prevention		NA
Gardasil, Gardasil 9, and Cervarix	HPV	NA
Engerix-B and Recombivax HB	HBV	NA
Other: peginterferon alfa-2b (Sylatron)	Advanced melanoma	NA

evaluated as a possible predictor of immuno-therapy response in 3 studies of NSCLC [31], melanoma [32], and urothelial carcinoma [33] patients. The three studies had 3 different cut-offs for TMB (15, 23.1, 16 mutations/Mb or more, respectively). These studies suggest that a high TMB is correlated with clinical response to immunotherapy setting TMB as a potential bio-marker. The challenge again is to use similar cut-off or deduct results by consensus. Mismatch Repair testing has the strongest evidence sup-porting its predictive behavior for response to Keytruda in metastatic colorectal cancer patients [34]. There were no responses in MMR-proficient colorectal tumors, compared to 57% ORR in MMR deficient colorectal tumors both treated with Keytruda. This need to be con-firmed in other Phase II/III trials. Meanwhile different trials already started to enrich for MSI-Hi tumors.

11.2.8 Trial Setting: Neoadjuvant, Adjuvant, Metastatic, Early Versus Late

This subject takes us to the question of "when" to examine subjects in clinical trials. There is no great preclinical model to predict which setting works best for immune response in humans: early in disease or late. The general sense among immune therapy researchers is that starting early with lesser tumor load con-stitutes a better approach. There is evidence though that in some tumors, tumor microenvi-ronment is equally immunosuppressive between early and late stages [35]. Failure of most immunotherapy agents to achieve higher responses than initially seen, and complete fail-ure of major CV trials made researchers rethink. The challenge of getting good responses of a CV trial in metastatic stage is evident. Many suggested that the vaccine by itself in might not only be insufficient but could be detrimental as in Gliobastoma trial [36]. One proposed mechanism is

overexpression of ICI by tumors as PD-L1. Hence efforts are made to combine vaccines with check-point inhibitors in several clinical trials, but no major results from these are avail-able yet. The adjuvant setting is thought to be an appropriate clinical setting to test CVs as it optimizes the chances of an effective immune response when the tumor burden is the lowest. But, testing CVs in adjuvant settings has a chal-lenge with time of follow up and this is even true in some vaccines tested in Phase III clini-cal trials. While none of the CVs is approved in adjuvant setting, ICI anti-CTLA4 Ipilimumab is approved for use in Melanoma based on results of the EORTC 18071 trial. Even more exciting is the idea to test immunotherapy in the neoadjuvant setting. This approach is expected to give more insight on the mecha-nism of action or resistance by examining immune and tumor responses post-neoadjuvant treatments. A Phase I trial pre-sented at ESMO 2016 Congress showed neoad-juvant immunotherapy with the PD-1 inhibitor nivolumab was safe and feasible prior to sur-gery for early lung cancer [37]. Twelve of 15 resected patients (80%) had pathologic evi-dence of tumor regression, and 6 (40%) achieved major pathologic responses (MPR; <10% residual viable tumor), at the time of abstract submission. The PROSPER RCC trial will examine patients with nonmetastatic stage II or greater RCC to either neoadjuvant nivolu-mab followed by resection and further nivolu-mab, or to resection followed by observation. Questions remain though on the timing and sequence of therapy in each of these settings.

11.2.9 Statistical Challenges

The major challenge is due to a change in natural history of disease in response to immu-notherapy also known as kinetics of disease. This is completely different from chemotherapy as the clinical effect from immunotherapy is commonly delayed by months. Separation of Kaplan−Meier curves in different immunotherapy trials is often observed after 4−8 months or later following random assignment [38]. However, such kinetics is not universal among all immune therapy agents. The consequences from a statistical standpoint is that such a delay creates a gap or drop in power. This does not affect the Phase I part of the trial, but certainly affects Phase II and III. In a two-arm chemotherapy trial, the risk to develop an event in treated and untreated (placebo) is assumed to be constant and hence the hazard ratio to be constant or proportional over time. Log-rank test and Cox regression models used for statistical analysis in these trials assume that events occurring at all times are proportional. This assumption is not valid in immunotherapy as a delayed separation in survival curves contradicts proportional hazards. In immunotherapy, the hazard rates start equal then few months later, the hazard rates become unequal and the curves separate. For practical purposes, it is assumed for this discussion that the hazard rates after the delayed clinical effect eventually become proportional. If time to separation increases, loss of statistical power can be big [22]. Methods are needed to overcome such a hurdle which could make a whole trial useless. It is crucial to use nonproportional hazards assumption when a delayed clinical effect is expected. Moreover, repeat or interim size calculation, is a must in this condition. Lessons learned from early phases should be kept till late phases as well. Harmony between study assumptions, sample size, trial duration, and timing of the interim analysis is highly needed in immunotherapy trials.

11.3 CLINICAL EXPERIENCE WITH IMMUNOTHERAPY: NOVEL TOXICITY RISKS AND MTD

Most AEs associated with immunotherapy are due to a reactive T-cell response against normal tissue. These T cells when hyperactivated by immune therapeutic drugs lead to high levels of T-helper (CD4) cell cytokines or increased infiltration of cytolytic CD8 T cells into normal tissues. While checkpoint protein inhibition, vaccines, and adoptive cell therapy seem to activate more specific T cells (may cause specific organ damage), T-cell immune response is generally not tissue specific. Cytokines generate systemic effects and nonspecific T-cell responses are typically related to the dose and schedule (e.g., INF-α, IL-1, IL-2, and IL-15). In contrast, check-point inhibitors are more idiosyncratic in nature with unpredictable toxicities based on dose or schedule. The toxicity of agents targeting CTLA4 seem to be dose dependent whereas those targeting PD-1/PD-L1 are not clearly dose related. Some toxicities might be tissue specific (thyroid), lifelong, and require systemic and or prolonged therapy. As seen in some targeted therapies, a toxicity profile was found to correlate with therapy [39,40]. In this chapter, we limit the discussion in this chapter to CVs and ICIs.

11.3.1 Are Cancer Vaccines Safe?

Vaccines are not a single product administered into the human body and this is true also of CVs. They are made of different constituents: Antigen (true vaccine), Adjuvant, vehicle, and immunomodulators. Thus it is complex to understand the effects on the immune system from one vaccine to another. While some adjuvants induce T helper type 2 (TH2) response, others induce TH1 response or both. Similarly, vaccines can induce either or both types of immune responses. The toxicity of CVs is generally due to these constituents directly or due to cross reactivity with normal tissue expressing similar antigen to that found in vaccine itself. Tumor associated antigens are typically not shared with normal tissue and this could explain the low potential for CVs to cause major toxicity.

The safety of CVs in early phase clinical trials has been examined by Rahma et al. in 2014 [7]. They reviewed 239 Phase I, Phase I/II, and pilot therapeutic CV studies published between 1990 and 2011. Among a total of 4,952 patients assessed, a total of 162 grade three (3.37%) and 5 grade four treatment-related toxicities were reported. Of these toxicities, 60 were local reactions, 40 were constitutional symptoms, and 5 were related to the adjuvants used in the vaccines. They further subdivided toxicities based on vaccine type and found that highest vaccine-related toxicity rate among the synthetic vaccines was reported in the bacterial vector trials (a total of 7 events, 3.97 events per 100 patients). Local injection site reactions and constitutional symptoms such as myalgia and flu-like syndromes were the most common toxicities seen. Among the 22 dose-escalation trials that reported grade 3/4 systemic vaccine-related toxicities, only three trials reported DLTs. Of these three CV trials, two used live attenuated bacterial vectors (Listeria monocytogenes and Neisseria meningitides) and DLT was hypotension. The third used Allogenic HER2/neu + breast cancer cells (SC) with GM-CSF or BCG and DLT was nausea and vomiting. Types of CVs and antigens used in their development [41] are shown in Table 11.6.

Enhanced or aberrantly over-expressed self-proteins (e.g., human epidermal growth factor receptor, p53, and survivin) are commonly used as antigens. Vaccines directed against these self-proteins may only induce tumor-specific immunity. On the contrary, loss of tolerance against nonmalignant tissues expressing the targeted protein might happen. Vitiligo, for example, occurred after administration of melanoma vaccines directed against melanocyte differentiation antigens. Other antigens as epidermal growth factor receptor or HER2 used in cancer treatment vaccines did not affect normal skin or cardiac function. Possible explanations for this include lower expression in normal tissue than cancer or

TABLE 11.6   Types of Cancer Vaccines and Antigens Used in Their Development [41]

Types of Cancer Vaccines	Antigens Used in Cancer Vaccines
Peptides	Product of mutated genes
Live vectors, attenuated bacteria	Overexpression or aberrant expression
Cellular vaccines: tumor (autologous vs allogenic); dendritic cells (DCs)	Product of oncogenic viruses
Inert vectors targeting DCs	Oncofetal antigens
Dendritomas	Altered cell surface glycolipids and glycoproteins
DNA vaccines	Differentiation antigens
Antiideotype vaccines	
RNA nanoparticles	
Neo-antigens, NGS, and mutanome	
Mimitopes	

insufficient immunity to the vaccine. To overcome this challenge along with the immunosuppressive nature of disease, combination strategies are being tested. These combinations include the use of check-point inhibitors and other immune agents. Data so far from these combinations are encouraging for low and nonadditive toxicity potential.

Sipuleucel-T was the first approved treatment CV in 2010. It uses a prostatic acid phosphatase fusion to GM-CSF protein presented to in vitro matured dendritic cells and it had a favorable toxicity profile. The toxicities seen with sipuleucel-T included infusion reaction manifested within 24 hours of an injection, transient chills, fatigue, and fever commonly seen within 24—48 hours posttreatment. Back pain and chills are the most common grade 3—4 AEs which less than 4% in total.

Another vaccine like cancer treatment approved at the end of 2015 is T-VEC. It is derived from herpes simplex type 1 HSV1 by deleting 2 viral genes and modified by encoding the human gene for granulocyte-macrophage colony-stimulating factor. The most common AEs were grade 1 fever, constitutional symptoms, nausea, anorexia, and injection site reactions. One patient was reported to experience grade 2 fever, rigor, hypotension, tachycardia, and constitutional symptoms [42,43]. Overall, the toxicities were more intense in HSV-seronegative patients; an initial low-dose of T-VEC, leading to HSV seroconversion, followed by a series of higher dose injections was better tolerated.

In conclusion, cancer treatment vaccines seem to be safe alone or in combination but efficacy is lacking. Until adequate understanding of the deficiencies of previous vaccination attempts are known it will be difficult to make progress in this area. The use of vaccine candidates with intense monitoring of selected patients may be the best strategy to understand what steps are required to achieve tumor regressions.

11.3.2 Immune Check Point Inhibitors

Most immune therapy modalities remain in development phases. Aside from the one approved vaccine, there are only 3 families of check-point inhibitors with FDA approval (PD-1, PDL-1, and CTLA-4 antibodies). These include the PD-1 blocking antibodies (Pembrolizumab and Nivolumab), PDL-1 blocking antibodies (Atezolizumab), and CTLA-4 blocking antibodies (Ipilimumab). These agents are drastically different from chemotherapy in their side effect profile. Immune-related AEs have been the major side effect noted in a significant proportion of patients receiving checkpoint protein inhibitors. These side effects are typically delayed by few weeks from start of treatment and some might occur even a year after treatment has stopped [44]. Systems mostly involved are the gastrointestinal tract (colitis, diarrhea), lungs (pneumonitis), kidneys (nephritis), skin (dermatitis, rash), liver (hepatitis), endocrinopathies (thyroiditis), with variable frequency and severity based on agent and disease treated. For these reasons, it is recommended that all patients receiving these agents get metabolic panels, liver and thyroid function studies, and complete blood counts checked at each treatment and every 6–12 weeks for the first 6–12 months after finishing treatment. More testing might be needed in case symptoms as fatigue ensue (e.g., hypophysial pituitary axis (cortisol, adrenocorticotropic hormone ACTH) and testosterone)). Follow-up frequency may also increase depending on the AEs that patients might experience. Despite an early confusion among researchers on how to handle these side effects, guidelines on management of immune-related side AEs have been developed and education of patients to the need for early identification and treatment has dramatically improved outcomes. Corticosteroids can reverse nearly all manifestations of these drugs, but this therapy is generally reserved for grade 3–4 and prolonged grade 2 immune-related AEs. In cases refractory to steroids, an immune-suppressive agent is typically used as mycophenolate mofetil for liver toxicity and infliximab for steroid-refractory colitis. Infliximab use in immune-related hepatoxicity is contra-indicated, because of increased risk of hepatoxicity from the drug itself. Drug-related hepatitis is seen in 1%–2% of patients with checkpoint protein inhibitors. A major immune-related AE that could be fatal is cytokine release syndrome CRS. It is more frequent in CAR-T cells but not in ICIs. Moreover, toxicities in the past used to be dose dependent as agents used were mainly cytokines as interferon alfa (INF-α), tumor necrosis factor (TNF), and interleukins (IL-1, IL-2, IL-15, and IL-21).

This pattern is changed with some ICIs. Certainly, the dose and sequence of ICIs with each other or with other modalities of therapy might have a different toxicity level. Depending on the combination, this could be worse or similar to the single agents used. Therapy of immune related AEs in this case is relatively like that when each drug is used alone. A common principle learned with checkpoint inhibitors is that high suspicion, early diagnosis, and corrective use of corticosteroids or other immune suppressants for immune related toxicities can be lifesaving. Education of community practicing oncologists, has been a major recommendation in different immune therapy talks and conferences. Patients with prior autoimmune diseases or a history of viral hepatitis were routinely excluded from receiving ICI on trials, but recent data suggest that anti-CTLA4 ICI Ipilimumab can be given safely to those patients [45,46]. Certainly, caution should be taken in treating patients with recent or ongoing autoimmune conditions. At this point, we still have no validated biomarkers for the prediction of immunotherapy toxicity.

One major meta-analysis presented at ASCO 2016 annual meeting examined the rates of immune related toxicities in all ICI cancer clinical trials published on PubMed or presented at an ASCO meeting (only if not published on PubMed) during 2005–15. There were total of 104 studies (201 arms) that reported irAE and were reviewed. Eighty-one trials met the inclusion criteria (127 arms) for this meta-analysis. 116 (91%) arms used ICI monotherapy and 11 (9%) arms used combination of ICI to treat 11,400 pts. 122 (96%) arms included solid tumors. 102 (80%) arms were Phase I and Phase II (see Table 11.7 below). Higher percentage of patients with low grade irAE was observed with anti-CTLA-4 ICI followed by anti-PD-1 then anti-PD-L1 ICIs ($P < 0.0001$). ICI CTLA-4 had higher percentage of patient with high grade (≥ 3) irAE than others. There was no significant difference in high grade irAE between ICI PD-1 and PD-L1.

Hence, it is clear from this analysis as well as others, that grade 3 or above toxicities are much less compared to grade 3 toxicities seen with chemotherapies. The authors have not reported the rate of MTD in these trials. We highlight some of the toxicities seen with each subgroup of ICI below.

11.3.2.1 Toxicities With Anti-PD-1 Antibodies

The AE profiles of the two FDA approved anti—PD1 antibodies, nivolumab and

TABLE 11.7   Immune Checkpoint Inhibitors (ICI): A Meta-Analysis of Immune-Related Adverse Events (irAE) From Cancer Clinical Trials

ICI	Arms Met Inclusion Criteria	Evaluable Pts For irAE	Evaluable Pts For Response	% Pts With irAE, Any Grade	% Pts With irAE, Grade 3 +	% Pts With irAE Grade 5	Overall Response Rate-ORR
CTLA-4	56	4284	3160	54%	19%	1.4%	10.6%
PD-1	35	4074	3636	26%	3.8%*	0.8%	27.5%
PD-L1	25	2448	491	13.7%	5%*	1.1%	17.6%
PD-1 + CTLA-4	8	495	1242	NR+	NR	1.8%	47.8%
PD-L1 + CTLA-4	3	99	60	NR	NR	1.8%	28.6%
Total/P	127	11,400	8589	$P < 0.0001$	$P < 0.0001$	$P = 0.34$	$P < 0.0001$

*$p = 0.33$.
+ : not reported.

pembrolizumab are fairly similar. The most common drug-related AEs of any grade in this group are fatigue, pruritus, and rash. Percentage of all toxicities seen with nivolumab was not much changed at different dose levels ranging from 0.3 to 10 mg/kg. On the other hand, higher grade toxicities (grade 3–4 AEs) tended to increase with higher doses ($\geq$3 mg/kg) with a range of 5%–12%. On an average, about 70% of patients treated with nivolumab will develop some form of a treatment related toxicity. Most common toxicities (>5%) include fatigue, rash, pruritus, pneumonitis, diarrhea, infusion reaction, decreased appetite and hypothyroidism. High grade toxicities range from 0% to 19% and mainly include liver function abnormalities, pancreatitis, pneumonitis, colitis, diarrhea, rash, thrombocytopenia, fatigue, pyrexia and rarely interstitial nephritis and optic neuritis. Pembrolizumab has a similar profile with grade 3–4 AEs in the range of 10%–13% except for 1 study which showed a rate of 41% grade 3–4 toxicities [47].

11.3.2.2 Toxicities With Anti-PD-L1 Antibodies

There is a general impression that anti-PD-L1 antibodies are less toxic then anti-PD-1 antibodies. The data from meta-analysis shown in Table 11.7 confirms this impression. Atezolizumab, the most recently approved anti-PDL-1 antibody was studied as a single agent in patients with locally advanced and metastatic urothelial carcinoma. Any grade toxicity occurred in 69% of patients and most commonly Fatigue (30%), nausea (14%), decreased appetite (12%), pruritus (10%), pyrexia (9%), diarrhea (8%), rash (7%), arthralgia (7%), and vomiting (6%). Grade 3–4 immune-mediated AEs occurred in 16% of patients, and each toxicity was mostly 1%–2%. Immune-related toxicities were equally low at 5% and no treatment-related deaths occurred during the study [28]. Other studies showed a

similar toxicity profile as well [48,49].The other anti-PDL1 is Durvalumab, which has shown similar toxicity profile as well [50,51].

11.3.2.3 Toxicities With Anti-CTLA4 Antibodies

CTLA-4 directed Antibodies are relatively more toxic than Anti-PD1/PDL1 antibodies. Ipilimumab the first ICI approved for use in melanoma in 2011 has a toxicity profile that is dose related. In one study the rate of grade 3–4 drug-related serious AEs increased from 5% to 18% when the dose was increased from 3 to 10 mg/kg and was 0% at a dose of 0.3 mg/kg, with no deaths related to treatment [52]. In the initial trial that led to its FDA approval, Ipilimumab caused grade 3–5 immune-related AEs in 10%–15% of patients. In a large Phase II study of ipilimumab at 10 mg/kg, the rate of grade 3 to 4 immune-related AEs (irAEs) was 22% [53]. Toxicities with PD-1/PD-L1 agents may be slower to resolve than with ipilimumab, so long-term surveillance is advised. Most frequent irAE include rash, colitis (diarrhea), hepatitis, endocrinopathies with variable percentages and an interesting pattern [54]. Skin-related toxicities occur first; colitis appears next, after one to three doses; hepatitis and endocrinopathies occur last (8–12 weeks), often after the third or fourth dose of ipilimumab. The 2% risk of developing severe hepatitis increases dramatically when ipilimumab was combined with other agents (20% with dacarbazine [55], DLT with vemurafenib [56]). Endocrinopathies occur late and have been seen between weeks 12 and 24. The same phenomenon has been observed with nivolumab and pembrolizumab, with rashes and GI toxicity seen early and liver toxicity or endocrinopathies seen later.

In addition, other rare immune related conditions have been reported with these agents. These include cardiomyopathy, myocarditis, uveitis, conjunctivitis, episcleritis, encephalitis, Guillain-Barré syndrome, myasthenia gravis–like syndrome, autoimmune thrombo-cytopenia, leukopenia, bone marrow suppression and others.

11.3.3 How to Define Maximal Tolerated Dose in Early Immunotherapy Trials

The maximal tolerated dose (MTD) is conceptually the highest dose that most patients can tolerate, usually producing grade 3 or greater toxicity in less than 33% of patients. This is based on the dose-effect relationship traditionally seen with chemotherapy where more toxicity reflects more antitumoral effect. There is no evidence yet from the immunotherapy agents that any of them has a direct dose-effect relationship. The definition that applies to immunotherapy is really the minimally biologically active (also called minimum effective) dose that produces an "acceptable" level of toxicity. In traditional Phase I design, patients are pushed to a dose that produces a certain frequency of (medically unacceptable) reversible, DLT. DLT is typically defined by the investigators based on according to Common Terminology Criteria for Adverse Events developed by National Cancer Institute of the United States. In immunotherapy trials patients are permitted to experience toxicity that resolves within 4 weeks without being classified as dose limiting. Thus the time frame for accrual to studies can be altered.

The optimal biologic dose is defined as a dose that achieves a reliable immune response or impact on the disease under investigation. Potential parameters for biological activity include regulatory T-cell activity or immune response against target cells, molecular response (minimal residual disease) or any form of clinical activity. The need for a change from traditional design especially with CVs has been brought up early on by the Cancer Vaccine Clinical Trial Working Group. Usually there are no serious toxicity risks and no proof for a linear dose-potency relationship for CVs. The group concluded with these recommendations. There is no need for conventional dose-escalation to establish MTD. Dose and schedule are not determined through escalation based on toxicity. CV usually do not get metabolized and hence there is no need for conventional PK. Many CV are designed to address one tumor type and therefore there is no need for mixed tumor trials for target selection. Conventional short-term response criteria (e.g., RECIST) are not well applicable to CV and historical control comparisons on RR are not useful. Proof-of-principle endpoints should reflect biologic activity including immunogenicity. In the same conference at SITC, in 2013, Dr. Khleif et al. had similar conclusion recommending to omit MTD in CV trials except for bacterial vector vaccines based on their meta-analysis [7].

This brings us to the point that MTD should not always be used as an endpoint for Phase I clinical trial of immunotherapy. In targeted therapies alternatives to toxicity as a surrogate endpoint in Phase I clinical trials were explored, although no consensus has been reached. This is shown in a review of 60 Phase I trials of 31 single agents representative of the most common targets of interest at the time. Sixty percent of these trials still used toxicity, whereas only 13% used pharmacokinetic data as endpoints for selection of the RP2D [58]. Stepwise dose finding in which subject sampling plan is done in one stage has been explored in nonhuman studies [57]. Dr. Khleif et al. suggested in 2013 an OPED design which stands for One Patient Escalation Design. What the design suggests is that for drugs that are believed to have toxicities, a researcher might just stick to traditional 3 + 3 Phase I design to find MTD. If the vaccine is known to be safe, as a peptide vaccine, then immune active dose IAD from prior studies should be used as the RP2D. If there is no prior data and the vaccine is not expected to be toxic, then a modified Phase I design OPED is needed to find the IAD. So in this design, one patient is tested at time to reach an induced immune response IAD. If IAD is reached, expand up to seven patients, one patient at a time. If IAD is not reached in all seven, then start dose escalation in one new patient at a time to reach IAD again. The design might not be perfect, and it does not address the alternatives for ICI. Despite the fact that there is a general sense among all researchers that traditional design is not fit, majority continue to perform 3 + 3 design with toxicity as endpoint. There is a trend of combining Phase I/II or Phase II/III as a way to save time but this approach alone does not redefine MTD as it should be defined.

The I-Spy and MATCH trials have suggested that innovative designs are needed in the field of immunotherapy. The idea of providing ongoing treatment options for patients who do not achieve a complete or partial remission during treatment on an immunotherapy based regimen has resulted in such proposals as the FRACTION study. In this study patients are provided with the most active treatment regimen consisting of nivolumab and ipilimumab if untreated with these agents or nivolumab and an investigational agent if previously treated. The patient can then receive protocol defined therapy at the time of disease progression or failure to achieve an objective response at a defined time point. The study is accompanied by on treatment biopsies to investigate mechanisms of resistance and provide information that may identify patients responsive to the new combination.

11.4 RECOMMENDATIONS

We highly recommend a deeper understanding of biology behind the newly developed agents and their effect on human body and natural history of disease. Improved understanding of the biology of cancer has led to the identification of new molecular targets and the development of pharmacologic agents that hold promise for greater tumor selectivity than traditional cytotoxic agents. Immunotherapies certainly revolutionized the approach to cancer and it is considered one of the most impactful

discoveries of the century. The fact that these drugs behave different from traditional chemotherapy brings about a new world to discover. It is similar to the era when chemotherapies were first found. Many details are unveiled already, but we lack behind in fully understanding the human biology. There is certainly a huge combined effort between industry and academia to move this forward. These efforts are faced with multiple challenges as explained through this chapter. We mainly focused on early clinical trial design, which is an essential pillar to build an armory against cancer. There is a clear sense among the research community of these challenges reflected by increased publications rate in the field of immunotherapy, both preclinical and clinical.

As far as the clinical trial design is concerned, our recommendations are to have an early collaboration between research teams developing the protocol, design, and reviewing literature. An early consultation with statisticians is also crucial. We highlighted the fact that delayed responses by month could set off the power of the study as hazard rates are nonproportional anymore. The MTD remains controversial, in part because of difficulties in defining reliable alternatives as a true biologic activity. Validation efforts have been proposed to better address these issues by different working groups. Nevertheless, increased research efforts should be spent on the prospective evaluation and validation of novel biologic endpoints and innovative clinical designs so that promising immune therapy agents can be effectively developed to benefit the care of cancer patients. A need exists for improved definition of optimal biologic dose, schedule, dose, setting, and combination. In addition, more tolerable inclusion criteria as an ECOG extending to level 3, validating irRECIST through the FDA, spending more finance and effort on R&D all help push the wagon forward. Finally, allowing accelerated drug development through combined Phase I/II and Phase II/III clinical trial designs is a promising research area in the near future.

References

[1] Rickham P. Human experimentation. Code of ethics of the world medical association. Declaration of Helsinki. Br Med J 1964;2(5402):177.

[2] Massett HA, et al. Challenges facing early phase trials sponsored by the National Cancer Institute: an analysis of corrective action plans to improve accrual. Clin Cancer Res 2016;22(22):5408−16.

[3] Eisenhauer E, et al. New response evaluation criteria in solid tumours: revised RECIST guideline (version 1.1). Eur J Cancer 2009;45(2):228−47.

[4] Hunt JD, et al. Transfer and expression of the human interleukin-4 gene in carcinoma and stromal cell lines derived from lung cancer patients. J Immunother Emphasis Tumor Immunol 1993;14(4):314−21.

[5] Weber JS, Kähler KC, Hauschild A. Management of immune-related adverse events and kinetics of response with ipilimumab. J Clin Oncol 2012;30 (21):2691−7.

[6] Maude SL, et al. Managing cytokine release syndrome associated with novel T cell-engaging therapies. Cancer J 2014;20(2):119.

[7] Rahma OE, et al. Is the "3 + 3" dose-escalation phase I clinical trial design suitable for therapeutic cancer vaccine development? A recommendation for alternative design. Clin Cancer Res 2014;20(18):4758−67.

[8] Schadendorf D, et al. Pooled analysis of long-term survival data from phase II and phase III trials of ipilimumab in unresectable or metastatic melanoma. J Clin Oncol 2015;. p. JCO. 2014.56. 2736.

[9] Lowy DR, et al. Primary endpoints for future prophylactic human papillomavirus vaccine trials: towards infection and immunobridging. Lancet Oncol 2015;16 (5):e226−33.

[10] O'Quigley J, Pepe M, Fisher L. Continual reassessment method: a practical design for phase 1 clinical trials in cancer. Biometrics 1990;33−48.

[11] Manji A, et al. Evolution of clinical trial design in early drug development: systematic review of expansion cohort use in single-agent phase I cancer trials. J Clin Oncol 2013;31(33):4260−7.

[12] Conley BA, Doroshow JH. Molecular analysis for therapy choice: NCI MATCH. Semin Oncol 2014;41(3):297.

[13] Seghers AC, et al. Successful rechallenge in two patients with BRAF-V600-mutant melanoma who experienced previous progression during treatment with a selective BRAF inhibitor. Melanoma Res 2012;22(6):466−72.

[14] Ampie L, et al. Heat shock protein vaccines against glioblastoma: from bench to bedside. J Neurooncol 2015;123(3):441−8.

[15] Giuliano AR, et al. Efficacy of quadrivalent HPV vaccine against HPV infection and disease in males. N Engl J Med 2011;364(5):401−11.

[16] Hamid O, et al. Kinetics of response to ipilimumab (MDX-010) in patients with stage III/IV melanoma. In: ASCO annual meeting proceedings. 2007.

[17] van Baren N, et al. Tumoral and immunologic response after vaccination of melanoma patients with an ALVAC virus encoding MAGE antigens recognized by T cells. J Clin Oncol 2005;23(35):9008−21.

[18] Wolchok JD, et al. Guidelines for the evaluation of immune therapy activity in solid tumors: immune-related response criteria. Clin Cancer Res 2009;15 (23):7412−20.

[19] Nishino M. Pseudoprogression and measurement variability. J Clin Oncol 2016;34(28):3480−1.

[20] Kurra V, Pseudoprogression in cancer immunotherapy: Rates, time course and patient outcomes. In: 2016 ASCO annual meeting. 2016, J Clin Oncol 34, 2016 (suppl; abstr6580): Chicago.

[21] Hodi FS, et al. Evaluation of immune-related response criteria and RECISTv1. 1 in patients with advanced melanoma treated with pembrolizumab. J Clin Oncol 2016;JCO640391.

[22] Hoos A, et al. Improved endpoints for cancer immunotherapy trials. J Natl Cancer Inst 2010.

[23] Hoos A. Proposal of a clinical development paradigm for cancer immunotherapy: novel endpoints. In: Endpoints for immunotherapy studies: design and regulatory implications, American Society of Clinical Oncology (ASCO) Annual Meeting. 2008.

[24] Yuan J, et al. Novel technologies and emerging biomarkers for personalized cancer immunotherapy. J Immunother Cancer 2016;4(1):1−25.

[25] Hoos A, et al. A clinical development paradigm for cancer vaccines and related biologics. J Immunother 2007;30(1):1−15.

[26] Reck M, et al. Pembrolizumab versus chemotherapy for PD-L1−positive non−small-cell lung cancer. N Engl J Med 2016;375(19):1823−33.

[27] Herbst RS, et al. Pembrolizumab versus docetaxel for previously treated, PD-L1-positive, advanced non-small-cell lung cancer (KEYNOTE-010): a randomised controlled trial. Lancet 2016;387(10027):1540−50.

[28] Rosenberg JE, et al. Atezolizumab in patients with locally advanced and metastatic urothelial carcinoma who have progressed following treatment with platinum-based chemotherapy: a single-arm, multicentre, phase 2 trial. Lancet 2016;387 (10031):1909−20.

[29] Tang DN, et al. Increased frequency of ICOS + CD4 T cells as a pharmacodynamic biomarker for anti-CTLA-4 therapy. Cancer Immunol Res 2013;1(4):229−34.

[30] Gadgeel SM, Stevenson J, Langer CJ, Gandhi L, Borghaei H, Patnaik A, et al. Pembrolizumab (pembro) plus chemotherapy as front-line therapy for advanced NSCLC: KEYNOTE-021 cohorts A-C. In: ASCO 2016 annual meeting. 2016.

[31] Spigel D, Schrock A, Fabrizio D. Total mutation burden (TMB) in lung cancer (LC) and relationship with response to PD-1/PD-L1 targeted therapies. J Clin Oncol 2016;34(15_Suppl.):9017 May.

[32] Johnson D, et al. Hybrid capture-based next-generation sequencing (HC NGS) in melanoma to identify markers of response to anti-PD-1/PD-L1. Proc Am Soc Clin Oncol 2016.

[33] Rosenberg J, Petrylak D, Van Der Heijden M. PD-L1 expression, Cancer Genome Atlas (TCGA) subtype, and mutational load as independent predictors of response to atezolizumab (atezo) in metastatic urothelial carcinoma (mUC; IMvigor210). J Clin Oncol 2016;34.

[34] Le D, et al. Programmed death-1 blockade in mismatch repair deficient colorectal cancer. J Clin Oncol 2016;34.

[35] O'Toole A, et al. Tumour microenvironment of both early-and late-stage colorectal cancer is equally immunosuppressive. Br J Cancer 2014;111(5):927−32.

[36] Bloch O, et al. Newly diagnosed glioblastoma patients treated with an autologous heat shock protein peptide vaccine: PD-L1 expression and response to therapy. In: ASCO annual meeting proceedings. 2015.

[37] Forde P. Neoadjuvant anti-PD1, nivolumab, in early resectable non-small-cell lung cancer. In: ESMO 2016 meeting. Madrid; 2016.

[38] Finke LH, et al. Lessons from randomized phase III studies with active cancer immunotherapies—outcomes from the 2006 meeting of the Cancer Vaccine Consortium (CVC). Vaccine 2007;25:B97−109.

[39] Disis ML. Immunologic biomarkers as correlates of clinical response to cancer immunotherapy. Cancer Immunol Immunother 2011;60(3):433−42.

[40] Quaglino P, et al. Vitiligo is an independent favourable prognostic factor in stage III and IV metastatic melanoma patients: results from a single-institution hospital-based observational cohort study. Ann Oncol 2010;21(2):409−14.

[41] Van den Eynde BJ, van der Bruggen P. T cell defined tumor antigens. Curr Opin Immunol 1997;9(5):684−93.

[42] Ott PA, Hodi FS. Talimogene laherparepvec for the treatment of advanced melanoma. Clin Cancer Res 2016;22(13):3127−31.

[43] Hu JC, et al. A phase I study of OncoVEXGM-CSF, a second-generation oncolytic herpes simplex virus expressing granulocyte macrophage colony-stimulating factor. Clin Cancer Res 2006;12(22):6737−47.

[44] Sarnaik AA, et al. Extended dose ipilimumab with a peptide vaccine: immune correlates associated with clinical benefit in patients with resected high-risk stage IIIc/IV melanoma. Clin Cancer Res 2011;17(4):896−906.

[45] Kyi C, et al. Ipilimumab in patients with melanoma and autoimmune disease. J Immunother Cancer 2014;2(1):1.

[46] Ravi S, et al. Ipilimumab administration for advanced melanoma in patients with pre-existing Hepatitis B or C infection: a multicenter, retrospective case series. J Immunother Cancer 2014;2(1):1.

[47] Le DT, et al. PD-1 blockade in tumors with mismatch-repair deficiency. N Engl J Med 2015;372(26):2509−20.

[48] Herbst RS, et al. Predictive correlates of response to the anti-PD-L1 antibody MPDL3280A in cancer patients. Nature 2014;515(7528):563−7.

[49] Powles T, et al. MPDL3280A (anti-PD-L1) treatment leads to clinical activity in metastatic bladder cancer. Nature 2014;515(7528):558−62.

[50] Segal NH, et al. Preliminary data from a multi-arm expansion study of MEDI4736, an anti-PD-L1 antibody. In: ASCO annual meeting proceedings. 2014.

[51] Rizvi NA, et al. Safety and clinical activity of MEDI4736, an anti-programmed cell death-ligand 1 (PD-L1) antibody, in patients with non-small cell lung cancer (NSCLC). In: ASCO annual meeting proceedings. 2015.

[52] Wolchok JD, et al. Ipilimumab monotherapy in patients with pretreated advanced melanoma: a randomised, double-blind, multicentre, phase 2, dose-ranging study. Lancet Oncol 2010;11(2):155−64.

[53] O'Day S, et al. Efficacy and safety of ipilimumab monotherapy in patients with pretreated advanced melanoma: a multicenter single-arm phase II study. Ann Oncol 2010;21(8):1712−17.

[54] Hodi FS, et al. Improved survival with ipilimumab in patients with metastatic melanoma. N Engl J Med 2010;363(8):711−23.

[55] Robert C, et al. Ipilimumab plus dacarbazine for previously untreated metastatic melanoma. N Engl J Med 2011;364(26):2517−26.

[56] Ribas A, et al. Hepatotoxicity with combination of vemurafenib and ipilimumab. N Engl J Med 2013;368(14):1365−6.

[57] Polley MY, Cheung YK. Two-stage designs for dose-finding trials with a biologic endpoint using stepwise tests. Biometrics 2008;64(1):232−41.

Further Reading

Armand P, et al. Disabling immune tolerance by programmed death-1 blockade with pidilizumab after autologous hematopoietic stem-cell transplantation for diffuse large B-cell lymphoma: results of an international phase II trial. J Clin Oncol 2013;31(33):4199−206.

Cell-Based Therapies: A New Frontier of Personalized Medicine

Haneen Shalabi, Hahn Khuu, Terry J. Fry and Nirali N. Shah

National Institutes of Health, Bethesda, MD, United States

CONFLICT OF INTEREST: NONE

The content of this publication does not necessarily reflect the views of policies of the Department of Health and Human Services, nor does mention of trade names, commercial products, or organizations imply endorsement by the U.S. Government. The authors declare that the research was conducted in the absence of any commercial or financial relationships that could be construed as a potential conflict of interest.

12.1 INTRODUCTION

For decades, the mainstay of cancer therapy has relied on targeting rapidly dividing tumor cells with cytotoxic antineoplastic chemotherapy and/or radiation therapy, incorporating disease-specific surgical resection to debulk large tumor volumes when indicated. Relapsed or chemotherapy refractory disease, however, remains a problem and novel therapies are needed to overcome chemotherapy resistance. Additionally, the nonspecific targeting of standard antineoplastic therapies come with a host of broad toxicities, and limiting off tumor toxicity has long since been a goal in the development of advanced cancer therapeutics. Recent advancements in harnessing the immune system has led to the development of target-specific and other cell-based therapies which have revolutionized therapeutic strategies in a host of diseases and may limit side effects compared to conventional therapies, but nonetheless present with their own unique set of toxicities and must be systematically evaluated.

Based on the concept of redirecting the immune system to overcome chemotherapy resistance and revitalize an immune tolerant microenvironment that lacks the capacity to eliminate transformed cells [1–3], cell-based therapies incorporate a "personalized" approach in the treatment of cancer. Unlike standard drug trials where there are formulaic approaches to dose escalation, pharmacokinetic parameters to evaluate drug levels and well-established criteria to determine dose-limiting toxicity, the approach to testing cellular therapies in cancer patients require a highly complex infrastructure to develop and implement in clinical trials and an enhanced understanding of the extent of potential risks of cell-based therapies, particularly those involving gene modification. Accordingly, the focus of this chapter will be to provide a global overview of the many steps and challenges involved in the implementation of clinical trials utilizing such personalized approaches and to highlight the development and current state of the art and future directions of chimeric antigen receptor (CAR)-based therapies as one example of cellular therapy implementation.

12.2 GENERAL PRINCIPLES FOR CELL-BASED THERAPY MANUFACTURING

Whether the product is a natural killer (NK) cell culture expanded product, or a T-cell engineered to express a CAR for a specified antigen, or another cell-based therapeutic where the procedures, reagents, disposables, cell type, and culture conditions will vary, the overarching concepts are the same and accordingly, the overall process design to manufacture these products are similar and quality assurance principles apply to all manufacturing processes. Furthermore, biological drugs are regulated as both biological products and as drugs so both sets of regulations apply. Cellular therapy laboratories are considered manufacturers and therefore must follow current Good Manufacturing Practices (cGMPs) and/or meet other accreditation standards, such as those set by the Foundation for the Accreditation of Cellular Therapy (FACT-http://www.factwebsite.org/Standards/) which are employed to design, implement, and maintain compliance

of cell therapy production and extends well beyond the physical facility.

The purpose of good manufacturing practices is to ensure documentation for traceability of steps performed, personnel involved, equipment used, reagents and consumables used, assays performed and evaluate the environment where the cells are being produces, to ensure product safety, purity, and potency and encompass the entire manufacturing process. This section will outline some of the basic concepts of cellular therapy product manufacturing but is not intended to replace or be a substitute for institutional policies, processes, procedures or industry standards or government specific regulations.

12.2.1 Developing a Cellular Therapy Trial

The path toward a clinical trial involving an experimental drug (e.g., a small molecule) requires an investigational new drug (IND) application (see Chapter 5: The Challenges of Implementing Multiarmed Early Phase Oncology Clinical Trials). This involves submitting an application to a government agency seeking permission to perform an activity. The drug may be manufactured, for instance, by a commercial company, with its own regulatory and administrative infrastructure, but is generally a uniform product that is administered without much inherent variation in the product itself. The product is manufactured in sufficient quantity (i.e., lot or batch), required assays for product characterization, safety, and potency are performed and when all results are completed, the product is released for use as an off-the-shelf product.

In contrast, for a clinical trial involving a cellular therapy product, which is generally a custom-made product, often made from individual patients for personal use, the path forward in implementation is a bit more complex. Although uniform release criteria are used to allow for the infusion of cell products to ensure safety of the product itself, the inherent variability and patient specificity are nonetheless unique. INDs that include a cellular therapy product must have a section called the Chemistry, Manufacturing, and Controls (CMC) that is specific to the manufacture of the cellular therapy product, with more specific guidelines incorporated when gene therapy is involved.

There are specific items that must be included in the CMC, which include elements of the product manufacturing—including both components and materials (i.e., vector, cells, reagents, excipients) and procedures (i.e., vector production/purification, process timing, and storage), incorporate product testing (i.e., microbiological, purity, potency, viability) as well as product stability and final product release criteria testing. The CMC also includes items not directly involved with the manufacturing process such as, product tracking/labeling, description of the facility, cleaning procedures, preventive maintenance procedures, environmental monitoring procedures, and many other elements. The CMC will also incorporate any preclinical and clinical studies, including Pharmacology/Toxicology data—which may require performing additional studies to evaluate for off-tumor toxicity and other immunologic testing. The U.S. Food and Drug Administration (FDA), the regulatory agency that oversees INDs in the United States has a template for CMC submissions (https://www.fda.gov/BiologicsBloodVaccines/GuidanceCompliance RegulatoryInformation/Guidances/Cellularand GeneTherapy/ucm072587.htm) that provides additional guidance.

The description of the final product is the single most important item in the CMC. While it may seem obvious, and even easy, to describe a product that has been shown to have the intended effect in preclinical models, committing such a description to words can be a difficult task. The final product for infusion is the key process control point in the product manufacturing process. At that point, there will be several considerations. These may include, for instance, requiring clarity on whether the final product is cryopreserved and subsequently thawed for infusion. And if so, will the post-thawed product require further manipulation, such as washing? How long can the post-thaw product be stored, at defined storage conditions, before infusion? If the product will not be cryopreserved but infused fresh at the end of the manufacturing process, the previous question also must be posed, how long can the product be stored, at defined storage conditions, before infusion? Similarly, defining the final product for infusion will need to be done in a consistent matter and include specifically—the cell population of interest and incorporate what other cell populations may be present. Additionally, the excipients are present in the final product and what has been done to confirm that they are not being infused.

A Certificate of Analysis (COA) will accompany the final product and will generally list the product's cell count and transduced fraction, demarcate if any aliquots were cryopreserved, provide information on the product appearance and characterization in relation to % viable CD3 and % viable transduced T cells and delineate outcomes of the various safety testing parameters (e.g., sterility, gram stain, endotoxin, mycoplasma, bead detection, etc.). A sample COA is provided in Table 12.1.

Other issues pertinent to the final product are less apparent. For instance, compliance with labeling requirements can present challenges to the cellular therapy laboratory personnel. The vessel used as the container for the product will impact on how the product is labeled. The product's container may not have enough surface area to allow all required elements to be affixed to the container. Similarly, understanding the environment and the facility

TABLE 12.1   Sample Certificate of Analysis

Department of Transfusion Medicine, Cell Processing Section
FDA Registration # XXXX
Sample Certificate of Analysis
Autologous Anti-Target CAR Transduced T cells: DTM-FORM-XXXX

DIN: _____   Lymph **Ext:**_____   **Protocol # / IND #:** _____/_____
(Donation Identification Number)   (extension)
Principal Investigator: _____

Recipient ID: _____   **Recipient Weight:** _____kg

Product TNC content and label check

		Initials	Date
Viable anti-GD2 CAR transduced T cells cryopreserved	_____ x 10^6 /kg		
Viable total nucleated cells cryopreserved	_____ x10^6		
Number of aliquots cryopreserved	_____ aliquots		
Final product label is DTM-LABEL-5091 *T Cells, Apheresis, Genetically Modified, Cryopreserved For Autologous Use Only*	☐ label verified		

Product appearance and characterization

Test	Sample Date	Method	Limit	Result	Interpretation (Pass/Fail)	Initials/ Date
Appearance		Visual check	Normal = milky; no aggregates			
Viability		Trypan blue	≥ 70%			
% viable CD3+		Flow	≥ 80%			
% viable anti-TARGET CAR transduced T cells		Flow	≥15%			

Product safety testing

Assay/Determination	Sample Date	Acceptable Limit	Result	Interpretation (Pass/Fail)	Initials/ Date
Preliminary Sterility ☐ -24 ☐ -48 hours		No Growth			
* Final -___ hour Sterility		No Growth	*	*	*
* Final Product Sterility		No growth	*	*	*
Gram Stain		No organisms seen (NOS)			
Endotoxin		<5.0EU/mL			
Mycoplasma in process		Negative			
*Mycoplasma final product		Negative	*	*	*
Bead detection per 3x10^6 cells		< 100 beads			
RCR (PCR)		Negative			
*S+/L- Assay FN		Negative	*	*	*
Donor Eligibility		Autologous			

☐ Product meets release criteria   ☐ Product does **not** meet release criteria & requires PI notification

Comments:

Medical Review (initials/date):_____/_____   Record Review (initials/date):_____/_____

* Pending Assay-Final Results Reviewed (initials/date):_____/_____

COA-FORM-XXXX   Referenced in SOP-XXXX

where cells are to be produced is a critical element in moving forward with a cell therapy—based trial. These are some examples of issues that must be addressed in the process for product distribution.

Specific to cellular therapies that incorporate gene modification (e.g., CAR trials), there are additional considerations that must be taken into account when developing any cellular therapy trial. Due to the concern for the development of delayed or long-term adverse consequences to those subjects exposure to gene therapy (e.g., for instance, concern for the development of a secondary malignancy due to leukemogenic insertion of a viral vector), the FDA has provided specific guidelines for long term monitoring of such patients—that are adjusted based specifically on the risk related to the vector used and the anticipated persistence (e.g., adenoviral based vector may require a shorter period of observation than a lentiviral based vector). The guidance on Cellular and Gene Therapy can be found at: https://www.fda.gov/BiologicsBloodVaccines/GuidanceComplianceRegulatoryInformation/Guidances/CellularandGeneTherapy/default.htm. In certain cases, based on the specific vector and novelty of the trial, a protocol may need to be presented at the Recombinant DNA Advisory Committee for further review. Guidelines on this process can be found at: http://www.osp.od.nih.gov/office-biotechnology-activities/biomedical-technology-assessment/hgt/rac

These guidelines include both recommendations for routine timed surveillance of replication-competent retrovirus/lentivirus, and for monitoring for the persistence of the genetically engineered cells. Based on the requirements for long-term follow-up, some centers are developing specific long-term follow-up protocols that are complimentary to the cellular therapy treatment protocol to allow for a streamlined approach to the long-term monitoring of patients who have received genetically engineered cellular therapy.

12.2.2 Nuts and Bolts of Cell Processing

The cell processing laboratory is a specialized laboratory with restricted access. The personnel in the laboratory are trained to manufacture the product but also ensure compliance with applicable standards and regulations. The following will list some of the essential components needed to produce cell therapy.

12.2.2.1 Raw Material

The raw material, sometimes referred to as source material or starting material, usually refers to the source product of the cell from which manufacturing begins and from which the final product is derived. The starting material is generally a mononuclear cell suspension, collected by apheresis but may also be from whole blood, bone marrow aspirate, bone marrow harvest, or a peripheral blood progenitor cell collection. However, the cells are collected, the quality of the starting material is one of the most essential factors in the quality of the final product—but also the place where there is likely the most variability based on the product coming from each individual patient for dedicated use.

One of the greatest challenges in cellular therapy is specifically addressing the feasibility of collecting an adequate cell product, often derived from a patient with cancer, which will lead to a final product that meets established release criteria. Limitations in this regard may include either not having enough cells to begin with, potentially because of cumulative therapy, or having rapidly progressive disease. Consider for instance the following example of an autologous peripheral blood mononuclear cell collection from a patient with ALL for manufacture of CAR-T cells who had high level of circulating blasts. Although the apheresis resulted in a high cellular content, the product also had a high percentage of concomitant leukemia cells (91% of the collected product) which may impact the ability to grow and expand the CD3 cells, which are needed in a purified suspension for incubation with vector supernatant containing the receptor of interest. The high leukemic count in the apheresis product may affect the downstream processing steps to purify the CD3-positive cells.

In another example, where a CAR product could not be generated despite an adequate lymphocyte count revealed the inhibitory impact of contaminating myeloid cells on T cell growth and expansion, with which our institution is gaining growing experience [4]. Accounting for such factors and making changes in the cell processing steps can lead to further optimization of the final product, as has been demonstrated, for instance, by finding ways to optimize the apheresis product [5] or incorporating strategies to remove contaminating cells [6]. In all the circumstances, however, it is important to note that any change in product manufacturing also requires notification of the regulatory bodies to inform them that changes are being made.

Donor source is also an important consideration in the product manufacture, not in the technical sense, but will determine how the final product is labeled and will guide what is needed for the cells are cleared for infusion (Table 12.1). Should an allogeneic donor source be used; the donor must be cleared of any communicable diseases and undergo separate evaluations to be eligible to serve as a cell source.

12.2.2.2 Reagents

Sometimes referred to as excipients or ancillary materials, reagents used in the manufacturing process must be qualified for safety and suitability for infusion to patients. Many resources are available to the IND sponsor and the cellular therapy laboratory in qualifying the reagents needed. Reagents, whether culture media, buffer, cytokines, beads, or protein source, must be considered significant to

the safety of the product. If a reagent used in product manufacture may be harmful to the recipient, complete removal of reagent would need to be demonstrated.

One such example is with incorporation of lipopolysaccharide (LPS). LPS is a reagent used in some cell cultures. LPS is an endotoxin that must be completely removed from the final product prior to administration to the patient and the manufacturing process must show LPS is not present in the final product. Some reagents, on the other hand, may not be available in formulation suitable for infusion. For instance, vitamin B6 is available in many forms, including for both bench research experiments and for over-the-counter formulations for oral ingestion. If a reagent is available in approved for infusion formulation, though more expensive, choosing this formulation may save time and effort in qualifying a research-grade reagent. Reagents are sometimes categorized based on risk. For example, serum from an animal source, such as fetal bovine serum, is considered higher risk for transmission of infectious diseases. Normal saline packaged for infusion, on the other hand, is considered lowest risk. These important considerations need to be made upfront when designing a clinical trial utilizing cellular therapy.

12.2.2.3 Consumables

Consumables range from pipette tips to containers used in the manufacture of the cellular therapy product. Consumables may be single use custom kits to perform a specific procedure on specified equipment. Specific items may be incorporated into the CMC, and such an example may be use of a specific cell expansion bag made of a certain material that is used for its gas permeability. It would be important that this specific bag be used throughout an entire trial for production of a specific cell therapy to ensure consistency of a product.

12.2.2.4 Assays

A variety of assays are used to help in the characterization of the product. These assays may range from cell counts to flow cytometric analysis of surface or cytoplasmic content to PCR-based assays. Some of the assays are even used to ensure product safety (for instance, those performed at the time of product release for infusion as seen on the sample COA) (Table 12.1).

12.2.2.5 Facilities and Environmental Control

A description of facilities and the physical environment where the cellular therapy product is manufactured are a required part of the CMC. For example, most cell cultures are maintained in a controlled environment, such as an incubator, for which temperature, humidity level, and gas concentration can be determined and monitored. The same is true for the room air and the biologic safety cabinet where the air quality is controlled rigorously. The equipment maintenance records, validation records, cleaning records, maintenance of an aseptic environment, and usage records are requirements of GMP.

Important environmental considerations include understanding the unique needs of the separate cellular therapies. For instance, the nature of the starting material and whether production involves cell culture or a recombinant cell line may determine if multiple products can be made simultaneously in a single room or not. Similarly, understanding the actual process of manufacturing (closed or open system, steps required) is critically important when designing where and how the product will be developed.

12.2.2.6 Personnel

The concept of "It takes a village" certainly holds true for the development of cellular therapy. In addition to the cell processing team

responsible making the product, there is also the separate team performing the apheresis, the protocol team ensuring the implementation of study requirements and the clinical team providing ongoing patient care—among others. At each step, the teams need to have established expertise in the work they do, to optimize the cell product, allow for the safe testing of a product and having the skill set to take care of patients who may have side effects from cellular therapy. Accreditation standards include general requirements for personnel in an accredited blood bank or cellular therapy laboratory.

Medical directors of cellular therapy laboratories are, by definition physicians, although they may have different training backgrounds. Laboratory directors, while not required to be physicians, need to be knowledgeable in laboratory techniques, manage complex procedures, manage complex workflow, and a staff of technologists and technicians. Medical technologists or medical technicians, appropriately trained, are qualified to work in a cellular therapy laboratory but defining the degree of training needed may be less well defined. Procedures may be customized and the manufacturing process may require performing multiple complex procedures in a specified sequence to produce the desired product. Training a medical technologist may require many months, multiple repetitions to demonstrate proficiency, and enough through-put to maintain proficiency. Aside from staff directly involved in product manufacturing, other personnel are just as essential to the manufacturing process. GMPs include process controls, including but not limited to, document control, vendor qualification, reagent qualification, product labeling, and assay quality controls.

Within this complex web of teams, taking into account a heterogeneous patient population and perhaps a multitude of cellular therapies, effective communication and standardization of processes is integral to the successful implementation of early-phase testing in cell-based therapies. In this regard, it is strongly encouraged that clinicians testing the therapy have a basic understanding of the preclinical production steps and vice versa, so that each can inform the other about potential pitfalls and hurdles to effectively implement a clinical trial.

One of the most exciting examples of implementation of cell therapy is with the development of CAR therapy-based strategies. Using CAR-T cell therapies as one example, the next section will focus on outlining factors critical to trial design and highlight both the current state of the art and outcomes, and delineate the challenges and future directions in cell therapy. Although the scope within this chapter will be limited to CAR therapy-based strategies, the global concepts apply to any cell based therapy approach (e.g., NK cell therapy, tumor-infiltrating lymphocytes), with recognition that the specifics of the actual therapy are essential to implementation of any early-phase testing.

12.3 CAR T CELLS

Redirection of T cells, which rely on ex vivo manipulation to produce a tumor-specific therapy, have been efficacious as a targeted therapy. Prior to the development of CAR therapy, recombinant T cell receptor (TCR) lymphocytes were engineered to have high specificity against antigens expressed on tumor cells. A notable example of this is with the NY-ESO-1 reactive TCR for treatment of synovial sarcoma and melanoma which led impressive responses in heavily pretreated patients with these diseases [7,8]. Limitation to TCR-based therapies, however included the dependency on major histocompatibility complex (MHC) expression, requirement for human leukocyte antigen restriction that could limit patient eligibility, and toxicity which included the induction of manifestations mimicking autoimmunity (i.e., colitis, pericarditis) [9].

CAR T cells were first conceptualized in 1989 to recognize antigens in an MHC independent manner, creating hybrid receptor constructs that utilized antigen-binding domains from monoclonal antibodies, with the intracellular machinery of a T cell [1,10,11]. Over the last two decades, sophisticated new models of these CARs have been created. Simplistically, a CAR is comprised of an extracellular domain that is usually derived from a monoclonal antibody single chain variable fragment (scFv), a short linker between heavy and light chain, a transmembrane domain, and the intracellular T cell signaling domain [11–15].

Initially, first-generation CARs combined only the scFv antibody domain with the CD3-zeta endodomain of the T cell, however these CARs failed to generate potent antitumor effects [1]. Subsequent second- and third-generation constructs added one or two costimulatory signaling domains, which drive T cell activation, survival, expansion, and function [11,12]. Numerous costimulatory domains can be incorporated into CARs, including 4-1BB, CD28, OX40, DAP10, and ICOS and there has been no consensus reached on which, if any, are superior. Data from current clinical trials show that CD28 costimulation facilitates more rapid and higher peak T cell expansion [16,17], but also predisposes T cells to early exhaustion, which leads to poor long-term T cell persistence as a result of activation induced cell death [18]. 4-1BB costimulatory domains on the other hand are associated with a slower expansion rate, lower peak level, a diminished risk of T cell exhaustion and more prolonged persistence following adoptive transfer [19]. Third-generation CARs include two costimulatory domains and thus far, data is mixed as to whether this has greater efficacy than second-generation CARs [20,21].

12.3.1 Manufacturing and Administration of CAR T Cells

Differing practices regarding detailed production of CAR T cells occur at institutions worldwide. The general practice includes: (1) autologous collection of peripheral blood mononuclear cells, hence the "personalized" approach, (2) stimulation of T cells ex vivo using beads coated with anti-CD3/anti-CD28 monoclonal antibodies with IL2 support or other comparable T cell selection strategies (i.e., CD4/8 selection), (3) transduction of T cells using CAR genes introduced via lentiviral or retroviral methods, (4) expansion of CAR T cells, and finally (5) infusion of cells into patient. Total processing time generally varies from 10 to 21 days (Fig. 12.1).

In general, most patients receive lymphodepleting chemotherapy with cyclophosphamide (cy) and/or fludarabine (flu) prior to CAR cell infusion. This preparative chemotherapy is thought to decrease the number of endogenous

T cells, including T regulatory cells, which may otherwise suppress the in vivo expansion of the CAR T cells. Preclinical work has demonstrated that lymphopenia increased the availability of cytokines that drive T cell expansion, notably IL-7, and that increased availability of such factors lead to enhanced expansion and improved efficacy [22].

12.3.1.1 Antigen Selection

Hematologic malignancies have been a prime example of successful immunotherapy utilizing CAR T cells. In choosing antigens for directed therapy, one of the most important rules is to choose an antigen that is highly expressed on the target cell, with minimal expression on non-malignant tissue, thereby maximizing selectivity and minimizing off

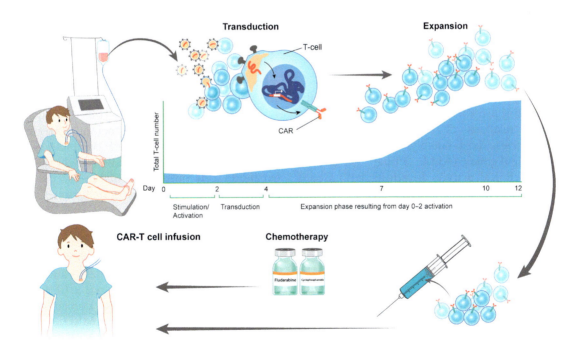

FIGURE 12.1   Illustration of CAR-T Product Development. Legend: Shown are the steps involved in the development of CAR-T cell product for individual patients. (1) Autologous collection of peripheral blood mononuclear cells, hence the "personalized" approach; (2) Stimulation of T cells ex vivo using beads coated with anti-CD3/anti-CD28 monoclonal antibodies with IL2 support or other comparable T cell selection strategies (i.e., CD4/8 selection); (3) Transduction of T cells using CAR genes introduced via lentiviral or retroviral methods; (4) Expansion of CAR T cells; and lastly (5) Infusion of cells into patient. Total processing time generally varies from 10 to 21 days.

tumor toxicity [14]. Using B cell ALL, there are multiple antigens for which CARs have been created that are restricted to B-lineage cells, specifically CD19, CD20, and CD22. Another potentially important feature of CAR antigen selection is finding the optimal epitope binding that will lead to an active CAR construct. Preclinical data from the CD22-targeted CAR design from the National Cancer Institute (NCI) tested multiple scFVs both distal and proximally bound, and showed that epitope selection mattered significantly to the function of the CAR, producing a much superior CAR killing response when bound proximally [20]. This highlights the importance of the CAR construct and choosing a construct which allows for the adequate spacing needed for ideal antibody: antigen engagement [20,23].

12.3.2 Experience from CAR T Cell Clinical Trials

In the last decade, several groups have published clinical results using CD19 CAR T cells to treat relapsed or refractory hematologic malignancies, most notably in acute lymphoblastic leukemia (ALL). Initial experience showed clinical activity in adults with B cell lymphoma and chronic lymphocytic leukemia [24,25]. Two pediatric patients with relapsed ALL went on to receive CD19 CAR T cell therapy, and an minimal residual disease (MRD) remission was attained [26]. Since then, studies across four major institutions have been published, with over 750 patients with B cell malignancies treated with CD19 CAR therapy [27].

Memorial Sloan Kettering Cancer Center recently reported on 51 patients that were treated with whom 50 were eligible for response assessment. They utilized the CD19-28z construct and patients received either cy alone (n = 42), or flu/cy (n = 9). Initially, they gave all patients a starting dose of 3 x 10^6 CAR T

cells/kg, however noted significant toxicity in patients with high burden disease. The protocol was amended to deliver 1 x 10^6 CAR T cells/kg to those with higher burden disease (> 5% blasts in bone marrow) and 3 x 10^6 CAR T cells/kg to those with minimal disease burden. Remarkably, 82% of patients treated in this study achieved a complete remission [28]. Utilizing a similar CD19-28z CAR construct, with a different CD19 scFv, investigators at the NCI performed a dose-escalation, incorporating a standard $3 + 3$ dose escalation design, intent-to-treat analysis on pediatric and young adult patients with relapsed and refractory ALL. 21 patients were enrolled in this cohort, and received a flu/cy regimen, and then were treated with either 1 x 10^6 CAR T cells/kg or 3 x 10^6 CAR T cells/kg. The maximum tolerated dose defined by this trial was 1 x 10^6 CAR T cells/kg. A 70% complete remission rate was achieved in this study [16].

Researchers at University of Pennsylvania and the Children's Hospital of Philadelphia reported their updated results of 59 children and young adults treated with 1–10 x 10^6 CAR T cells/kg using a CD19-4-1BB construct. A variety of lymphodeleting chemotherapy regimens were used, and a 93% complete remission rate based on those patients who had an expanded cell product available for use was reported [17,28]. At Fred Hutchinson Cancer Research Center (FHCRC), a CD19-4-1BB construct was also used, and they reported on their initial 30 adult patients with relapsed/refractory ALL. Cyclophosphamide based chemotherapy regimens were utilized, and doses from 2 x 10^5 CAR T cells/kg to 2 x 10^7 CAR T cells/kg were used. Ninety-four percent of evaluable patients achieved and MRD negative remission [29]. Despite using different scFv constructs, differing preparative regimens, and dosing plans, all these trials reproduced similar results yielding that CD19 CAR T cell therapy was highly active in patients with relapsed and refractory disease.

Numerous clinical and scientific insights have been gleaned from these studies. In general, it is uniformly accepted that in order to have antileukemia effect, the CAR T cells must expand in vivo. One study demonstrated a >1000-fold increase in the number of CAR T cells as compared to the initial administered dose but with variation in this number based on disease burden [26]. Additionally, persistence of CAR T cells is thought to be necessary for continued disease surveillance, however length of persistence is still debated [17]. In the trial performed at FHCRC, investigators noted when fludarabine was added to cyclophosphamide backbone, there was improved CAR T cell expansion, persistence, and better clinical outcome [29]. Another remarkable cornerstone of CAR therapy is the ability of these cells to traffic into the cerebrospinal fluid (CSF). In contrast to standard drug therapies which do not cross the blood−brain barrier or provide any clear antileukemia effect for CNS disease, that not only do CAR T cells effectively get into the CSF, they can clear leukemic disease [16,17].

12.3.2.1 Dose Selection

The relationship between CAR T cell dose and efficacy is less direct than that of a standard cytotoxic agent, however there does appear to be a biologic threshold dose needed for CAR T cell therapy to achieve a response. Phase I studies conducted across the country have tested varying dose escalation schemas to develop the maximum tolerated dose [16,17,19,29,30]. In most studies, the recommended dose of CD-19 CAR T cells is 1×10^6 cells/kg. In contrast to drug development where the pharmacokinetics/pharmacodynamics are generally more predictable with limited interpatient and intrapatient variation, CAR-T therapy shows a prime example of the significant range of variability that may occur despite infusion of a similar cell dose. Based on the disease burden, antigen stimulation, an environment primed to promote

expansion the degree of T cell expansion may be quite varied—leading to very different safety and toxicity parameters, making standard phase I dose escalation schemas a bit more difficult to implement and comprehend in the traditional sense.

12.3.2.2 Toxicity

Essential to the safe implementation of early-phase cellular therapies is the need for systematic evaluation of adverse events and toxicities—which may be unique and quite different from the experience with conventional therapies and other nonbiologics. The experience with CAR-T therapy is particularly notable in presenting with a distinguished toxicity profile that needs to be understood and treated to allow for the safe implementation of CAR therapy.

12.3.2.2.1 CYTOKINE RELEASE SYNDROME

Cytokine release syndrome (CRS) is a potentially life-threatening, systemic inflammatory response observed following administration of antibodies, and adoptive T cell therapy. Immune activation is the mainstay of this therapy, and as such, there has been an associated increase in a wide array of systemic proinflammatory cytokines, such as IL-6, C-reactive protein (CRP), ferritin, and IL-2, which coincided with peak-T cell expansion and destruction of ALL blasts [16,17]. Severity can vary from mild symptoms including fever, myalgia, and fatigue, to severe symptoms including but not limited to acute respiratory distress syndrome, hypotension, disseminated intravascular coagulation, and/or renal and liver toxicities [31]. Timing of symptom onset and CRS severity depends on the inducing agent and disease burden. In CAR therapy, it is currently debated whether the onset of CRS has a dependence on the costimulatory domain incorporated into the construct. In utilizing the CD28z domain, T lymphocyte expansion was seen around Day 3, corresponding to a rapid increase in CRP and

IL-6, with a concomitant decrease in cytokines usually by Day 10 [16]. Additionally, the baseline disease burden correlated with the severity of cytokine release syndrome, with those who had higher burden of disease experiencing more severe CRS [16,17,19].

Current guidelines for grading treatment related adverse events do not apply completely to complications that can be seen with adoptive cell therapy. A CRS grading system would allow for institutions to objectively assess and treat patients based on clinical severity. CRS has been categorized typically as mild or severe in CAR clinical trials, with one center defining diagnostic criteria for severe CRS (sCRS) to include prolonged fever, organ dysfunction, an increase in at least two cytokine profiles, and/or neurotoxicity [19]. A consensus algorithm was created to not only identify and grade CRS, but also to offer treatment recommendations at various time points during a patient's clinical course [31]. Such algorithms will require continual reassessment and modification as we learn more about CAR-therapy—related toxicities.

Mitigating strategies to reduce the severity of CRS have focused on limiting the peak levels of proinflammatory cytokines. IL-6, one of the major cytokines that drives CRS, has an FDA-approved antibody against the IL-6 receptor, tocilizumab, that most institutions are using to treat CRS [15,19,26,30,32]. It has been shown to rapidly improve symptoms associated with CRS, and not have a detrimental effect on the proliferation and efficacy of CAR T cells [16,17,32]. Most studies have moved tocilizumab into their protocol treatment algorithm for severe CRS. Additionally, corticosteroids have been used to ameliorate the systemic inflammatory response seen with CRS. Given the concern for steroids having a cytotoxic effect on T cells (and potentially CAR cells), that could diminish their antileukemia efficacy, steroid administration has often been used as second line therapy for sCRS [30] although

treatment paradigms from groups incorporating prophylactic interventions to limit CRS will be able to assess more clearly the role of steroids. Early detection and symptomatic management of CRS are vital in implementing current algorithms so that more significant toxicities do not arise.

12.3.2.2.2 B CELL APLASIA

The anticipated off-tumor toxicity associated with CD19 CAR is the destruction of nonmalignant B cells. B cell aplasia has correlated with the in vivo persistence of CAR T cells, and some institutions use this as a marker to detect continued activity of the CAR T cells [15,17]. The length of necessary B cell aplasia, i.e., CAR T cell persistence, for prolonged remission is unknown but there is a concern for relapse if early B cell regeneration is seen. Management for CAR-induced B cell aplasia includes monitoring serum immunoglobulins, and if less then 500 mg/dL to treat with intravenous immunoglobulin.

12.3.2.2.3 NEUROTOXICITY

Neurotoxicity is a major concern with CAR therapy and has been observed in a significant portion of patients treated with CAR therapy, approximately 30% in most series, and the mechanism of this is not fully understood [16,17,30]. Symptoms vary, from mild to severe, and can present clinically as confusion, aphasia, encephalopathy, and seizures to name a few. Most symptoms typically last 1—2 weeks and are reversible. Regardless of CNS status, CAR T cells traffic to the CSF, as shown in multiple studies with evidence of CNS leukemia clearance [16] and the relationship between neurotoxicity and CNS disease is uncertain, as neurotoxicity can occur in the presence or absence of CNS disease. The prevailing hypothesis regarding the pathophysiology of this syndrome is that it reflects nonspecific neurotoxic effects of cytokines and/or activated T cells, rather than a direct on-target effect of CAR T cells [15].

Recently, three deaths were reported as a result of severe neurotoxicity and cerebral edema in patients treated with CD19-CAR T cells. It is notable that the toxicity was limited to one specific trial and the initial deaths occurred following the addition of fludarabine chemotherapy to high dose cyclophosphamide administered as a single dose (60 mg/kg). Numerous other trials have incorporated cyclophosphamide and fludarabine using CD19-CAR T cells without similar toxicity. While not fully understood, the best plausible explanation for the fatal neurotoxicity observed in these cases is that it resulted from excessively rapid T cell expansion of a CD19 CAR with a CD28 costimulatory domain. Subsequently, even after removing the fludarabine, two additional deaths were noted in the same trial utilizing high dose cyclophosphamide alone. Given that more than 750 patients have been treated with these therapeutics, these events were unexpected and work is underway to understand the basis for this phenomenon. Development of prospective monitoring strategies, incorporation of antiseizure prophylaxis and an independent CAR-related neurologic toxicity grading, evaluation and management algorithm are all under consideration by those implementing CAR trials.

12.3.2.3 Limitations to CAR-T Response

Though not specifically discussed in this section, as mentioned earlier, a major limitation to CAR-T is the feasibility of being able to produce CAR T cells. The aforementioned studies are based primarily on outcomes of patients where CAR cells were able to be produced, but do not adequately take into account those patients for whom CAR-cells could not be made. In this regard, optimization of cell culture strategies to overcome inherent chemotherapy-induced lymphopenia or attain independence from the inhibitory effect of contaminating myeloid cells will be critical to making this therapy more widely available. Alternative strategies, may include, earlier collection of T cells in patients known to be at high risk for relapse who may need CAR therapy in the future and doing a T cell collection before they have more severe lymphopenia due successive chemotherapeutic attempts.

In those who do derive the optimal benefit from CAR therapy, although prolonged remissions have been seen (extending out as far as 4 years in ALL), relapse does remain a challenge with most of the relapsed occurring within 1 year of infusion. While approximately half of relapses occur due to decreased persistence of CAR T cells, or decreased function of T cells [16,33], a new mechanism of relapse with diminished expression or absent surface CD19 is also being identified [34].

In CD19 CAR T cell therapy, multiple studies have shown relapse of CD19 negative or dim ALL, resulting in a novel immune escape mechanism [16,17,26]. Investigation into the biology of these phenomena has begun to reveal a complex biology responsible for loss or downregulation of CD19 expression. There indeed appear to be two different pathways, antigen escape, and lineage switch. Antigen escape accounts for much of these cases, resulting in loss of surface CD19, while retaining other B-ALL characteristics. The CD19 isoform remains intracellular, however there is lack of the epitope that is targeted by all CD19 CAR T cells [35]. An alternative mechanism for loss of CD19 expression involves lineage switch of premature blasts resulting in clonal evolution to a more myeloid phenotype [36,37]. With persistent CD19 CAR immune pressure, cells with lineage plasticity can induce reprogramming resulting in relapse with aberrant hematopoietic lineages [37].

12.3.2.4 Future Directions

With the emergence of CD19 escape mechanisms, development of additional targets for B cell malignancies have begun. CD22 is a B-lineage differentiation antigen that is expressed on the surface of mature B cells, however is not expressed on pluripotent stem cells [38,39]. In one study, CD22 antigen expression was demonstrated in all patients with ALL (n = 163), making it a great antigen for targeted therapy [40]. Many treatment studies that target CD22 are currently underway, with promising results in early-phase trials [41,42]. Clinical testing of the first CAR to target CD22 is ongoing at the Pediatric Oncology Branch at the NCI. We recently reported on the first 16 patients in this dose–escalation trial. The study has shown it feasible to produce anti-CD22 CAR T cells in 15 of 16 patients enrolled, and the maximum tolerated dose achieved was 1×10^6 CAR T cells/kg. Patients available to enroll on the trial included CAR naïve patients, and previously CAR-treated patients most of which had CD19 negative leukemia. Additionally, at dose levels 2 and 3, 1×10^6 CAR T cells/kg and 3×10^6 CAR T cells/kg, a complete remission rate of 80% has been seen (ASH 2016). From this small series, CD22 CAR therapy has had comparable potency to CD19 CAR therapy, and importantly, those with relapse post CD19 CAR can be salvaged with this new construct, demonstrating the first evidence for salvage immunotherapy and opening the door for combinatorial antigen targeting strategies to reduce the risk of immune escape.

12.4 CONCLUSION

Due to the inherent complexity involved with the development of cellular therapy, the existing paradigm of early-phase drug development may not be sufficient for the testing of cell-based therapies. With the goal of providing a global overview of the technical aspects integral to the development of early-phase testing of cellular therapies through illustration of a prime example of cellular therapy in action, the complexity

inherent to cell-based therapies is evident. For a multifactorial host of reasons, including the personalized approach of custom made products, the need to assess the safety of the product being infused, and the potential for a unique side effect profile of cell therapy—including the concern for delayed effects of infusion of genetically engineered cells, implementation of cell-based therapy, particularly in early-phase testing is no easy task. As the field of cellular therapies grow, the approach to study design, an enhanced understanding of the limitations of standard phase I dose–escalation strategies and the ability to keep up with a rapidly evolving field, will require the ability to make dynamic changes based on growing knowledge of safety, toxicity, and efficacy will be needed to lead to the safe implementation of effective immunotherapeutic strategies in the armamentarium against cancer.

References

[1] Marr LA, Gilham DE, Campbell JD, Fraser AR. Immunology in the clinic review series; focus on cancer: double trouble for tumours: bi-functional and redirected T cells as effective cancer immunotherapies. Clin Exp Immunol 2012;167:216–25.
[2] Schreiber RD, Old LJ, Smyth MJ. Cancer immunoediting: integrating immunity's roles in cancer suppression and promotion. Science 2011;331:1565–70.
[3] Dunn GP, Old LJ, Schreiber RD. The three Es of cancer immunoediting. Annu Rev Immunol 2004;22:329–60.
[4] Stroncek DF, Ren J, Lee DW, Tran M, Frodigh SE, Sabatino M, et al. Myeloid cells in peripheral blood mononuclear cell concentrates inhibit the expansion of chimeric antigen receptor T cells. Cytotherapy 2016;18:893–901.
[5] Allen ES, Stroncek DF, Ren J, Eder AF, West KA, Fry TJ, et al. Autologous lymphapheresis for the production of chimeric antigen receptor T cells. Transfusion 2017;57(5):1133–41.
[6] Stroncek DF, Lee DW, Ren J, Sabatino M, Highfill S, Khuu H, et al. Elutriated lymphocytes for manufacturing chimeric antigen receptor T cells. J Transl Med 2017;15:59.
[7] Robbins PF, Kassim SH, Tran TL, Crystal JS, Morgan RA, Feldman SA, et al. A pilot trial using lymphocytes genetically engineered with an NY-ESO-1-reactive T-cell receptor: long-term follow-up and correlates with response. Clin Cancer Res 2015;21:1019–27.

[8] Robbins PF, Morgan RA, Feldman SA, Yang JC, Sherry RM, Dudley ME, et al. Tumor regression in patients with metastatic synovial cell sarcoma and melanoma using genetically engineered lymphocytes reactive with NY-ESO-1. J Clin Oncol 2011;29:917–24.

[9] Chmielewski M, Hombach AA, Abken H. Antigen-specific T-cell activation independently of the MHC: chimeric antigen receptor-redirected T cells. Front Immunol 2013;4:371.

[10] Gross G, Waks T, Eshhar Z. Expression of immunoglobulin-T-cell receptor chimeric molecules as functional receptors with antibody-type specificity. Proc Natl Acad Sci USA 1989;86:10024–8.

[11] Fry TJ, Mackall CL. T-cell adoptive immunotherapy for acute lymphoblastic leukemia. Hematology Am Soc Hematol Educ Program 2013;2013:348–53.

[12] Johnson LA, June CH. Driving gene-engineered T cell immunotherapy of cancer. Cell Res 2017;27:38–58.

[13] Kershaw MH, Westwood JA, Slaney CY, Darcy PK. Clinical application of genetically modified T cells in cancer therapy. Clin Transl Immunology 2014;3:e16.

[14] Shalabi H, Angiolillo A, Fry TJ. Beyond CD19: opportunities for future development of targeted immunotherapy in pediatric relapsed-refractory acute leukemia. Front Pediatr 2015;3:80.

[15] Tasian SK, Gardner RA. CD19-redirected chimeric antigen receptor-modified T cells: a promising immunotherapy for children and adults with B-cell acute lymphoblastic leukemia (ALL). Ther Adv Hematol 2015;6:228–41.

[16] Lee DW, Kochenderfer JN, Stetler-Stevenson M, Cui YK, Delbrook C, Feldman SA, et al. T cells expressing CD19 chimeric antigen receptors for acute lymphoblastic leukaemia in children and young adults: a phase 1 dose-escalation trial. Lancet 2015;385:517–28.

[17] Maude SL, Frey N, Shaw PA, Aplenc R, Barrett DM, Bunin NJ, et al. Chimeric antigen receptor T cells for sustained remissions in leukemia. N Engl J Med 2014;371:1507–17.

[18] Long AH, Haso WM, Shern JF, Wanhainen KM, Murgai M, Ingaramo M, et al. 4-1BB costimulation ameliorates T cell exhaustion induced by tonic signaling of chimeric antigen receptors. Nat Med 2015;21:581–90.

[19] Brentjens RJ, Davila ML, Riviere I, Park J, Wang X, Cowell LG, et al. CD19-targeted T cells rapidly induce molecular remissions in adults with chemotherapy-refractory acute lymphoblastic leukemia. Sci Transl Med 2013;5 177ra38.

[20] Haso W, Lee DW, Shah NN, Stetler-Stevenson M, Yuan CM, Pastan IH, et al. Anti-CD22-chimeric antigen receptors targeting B-cell precursor acute lymphoblastic leukemia. Blood 2013;121:1165–74.

[21] Zhong XS, Matsushita M, Plotkin J, Riviere I, Sadelain M. Chimeric antigen receptors combining 4-1BB and CD28 signaling domains augment PI3kinase/AKT/Bcl-XL activation and CD8 + T cell-mediated tumor eradication. Mol Ther 2010;18:413–20.

[22] Mackall CL, Fry TJ, Gress RE. Harnessing the biology of IL-7 for therapeutic application. Nat Rev Immunol 2011;11:330–42.

[23] James SE, Greenberg PD, Jensen MC, Lin Y, Wang J, Till BG, et al. Antigen sensitivity of CD22-specific chimeric TCR is modulated by target epitope distance from the cell membrane. J Immunol 2008;180:7028–38.

[24] Kochenderfer JN, Yu Z, Frasheri D, Restifo NP, Rosenberg SA. Adoptive transfer of syngeneic T cells transduced with a chimeric antigen receptor that recognizes murine CD19 can eradicate lymphoma and normal B cells. Blood 2010;116:3875–86.

[25] Porter DL, Levine BL, Kalos M, Bagg A, June CH. Chimeric antigen receptor-modified T cells in chronic lymphoid leukemia. N Engl J Med 2011;365:725–33.

[26] Grupp SA, Kalos M, Barrett D, Aplenc R, Porter DL, Rheingold SR, et al. Chimeric antigen receptor-modified T cells for acute lymphoid leukemia. N Engl J Med 2013;368:1509–18.

[27] Hay KA, Turtle CJ. Chimeric antigen receptor (CAR) T cells: lessons learned from targeting of CD19 in B-cell malignancies. Drugs. 2017;77(3):237–45.

[28] Geyer MB, Brentjens RJ. Review: current clinical applications of chimeric antigen receptor (CAR) modified T cells. Cytotherapy 2016;18:1393–409.

[29] Turtle CJ, Hanafi LA, Berger C, Gooley TA, Cherian S, Hudecek M, et al. CD19 CAR-T cells of defined CD4 + :CD8 + composition in adult B cell ALL patients. J Clin Invest 2016;126:2123–38.

[30] Davila ML, Riviere I, Wang X, Bartido S, Park J, Curran K, et al. Efficacy and toxicity management of 19-28z CAR T cell therapy in B cell acute lymphoblastic leukemia. Sci Transl Med 2014;6 224ra25.

[31] Lee DW, Gardner R, Porter DL, Louis CU, Ahmed N, Jensen M, et al. Current concepts in the diagnosis and management of cytokine release syndrome. Blood 2014;124:188–95.

[32] Frey NV, Porter DL. Cytokine release syndrome with novel therapeutics for acute lymphoblastic leukemia. Hematology Am Soc Hematol Educ Program 2016;2016:567–72.

[33] Maude SL, Teachey DT, Porter DL, Grupp SA. CD19-targeted chimeric antigen receptor T-cell therapy for acute lymphoblastic leukemia. Blood 2015;125:4017–23.

[34] Topp MS, Kufer P, Gokbuget N, Goebeler M, Klinger M, Neumann S, et al. Targeted therapy with the T-cell-engaging antibody blinatumomab of chemotherapy-refractory minimal residual disease in B-lineage acute lymphoblastic leukemia patients results in high response rate and prolonged leukemia-free survival. J Clin Oncol 2011;29:2493−8.

[35] Sotillo E, Barrett DM, Black KL, Bagashev A, Oldridge D, Wu G, et al. Convergence of acquired mutations and alternative splicing of CD19 enables resistance to CART-19 immunotherapy. Cancer Discov 2015;5:1282−95.

[36] Gardner R, Wu D, Cherian S, Fang M, Hanafi LA, Finney O, et al. Acquisition of a CD19-negative myeloid phenotype allows immune escape of MLL-rearranged B-ALL from CD19 CAR-T-cell therapy. Blood 2016;127:2406−10.

[37] Jacoby E, Nguyen SM, Fountaine TJ, Welp K, Gryder B, Qin H, et al. CD19 CAR immune pressure induces B-precursor acute lymphoblastic leukaemia lineage switch exposing inherent leukaemic plasticity. Nat Commun 2016;7:12320.

[38] Bendall SC, Davis KL, Amir EL, Tadmor AD, Simonds MD, Chen EF, et al. Single-cell trajectory detection uncovers progression and regulatory coordination in human B cell development. Cell 2014;157:714−25.

[39] Tedder TF, Poe JC, Haas KM. CD22: a multifunctional receptor that regulates B lymphocyte survival and signal transduction. Adv Immunol 2005;88:1−50.

[40] Shah NN, Stevenson MS, Yuan CM, Richards K, Delbrook C, Kreitman RJ, et al. Characterization of CD22 expression in acute lymphoblastic leukemia. Pediatr Blood Cancer 2015;62:964−9.

[41] Kantarjian H, Thomas D, Jorgensen J, Kebriaei P, Jabbour E, Rytting M, et al. Results of inotuzumab ozogamicin, a CD22 monoclonal antibody, in refractory and relapsed acute lymphocytic leukemia. Cancer 2013,119.2728−36.

[42] Raetz EA, Cairo MS, Borowitz MJ, Blaney SM, Krailo MD, Leil TA, Children's Oncology Group Pilot Stydy, et al. Chemoimmunotherapy reinduction with epratuzumab in children with acute lymphoblastic leukemia in marrow relapse: a Children's Oncology Group Pilot Study. J Clin Oncol 2008;26:3756−62.

Further Reading

Algar E. A review of the Wilms' tumor 1 gene (WT1) and its role in hematopoiesis and leukemia. J Hematother Stem Cell Res 2002;11:589−99.

Hsu FJ, Benike C, Fagnoni F, Liles TM, Czerwinski D, Taidi B, et al. Vaccination of patients with B-cell lymphoma using autologous antigen-pulsed dendritic cells. Nat Med 1996;2:52−8.

Mackall CL, Merchant MS, Fry TJ. Immune-based therapies for childhood cancer. Nat Rev Clin Oncol 2014;11:693−703.

Miwa H, Beran M, Saunders GF. Expression of the Wilms' tumor gene (WT1) in human leukemias. Leukemia 1992;6:405−9.

Ni M, Hoffmann JM, Schmitt M, Schmitt A. Progress of dendritic cell-based cancer vaccines for patients with hematological malignancies. Expert Opin Biol Ther 2016;16:1113−23.

Rosenberg SA, Yang JC, Restifo NP. Cancer immunotherapy: moving beyond current vaccines. Nat Med 2004;10:909−15.

Schuster SJ, Neelapu SS, Gause BL, Janik JE, Muggia FM, Gockerman JP, et al. Vaccination with patient-specific tumor-derived antigen in first remission improves disease-free survival in follicular lymphoma. J Clin Oncol 2011;29:2787−94.

Shah NN, Loeb DM, Khuu H, Stroncek D, Ariyo T, Raffeld M, et al. Induction of immune response after allogeneic Wilms' tumor 1 dendritic cell vaccination and donor lymphocyte infusion in patients with hematologic malignancies and post-transplantation relapse. Biol Blood Marrow Transplant 2016;22:2149−54.

Shortman K, Naik SH. Steady-state and inflammatory dendritic-cell development. Nat Rev Immunol 2007;7:19−30.

Steinman RM. The dendritic cell system and its role in immunogenicity. Annu Rev Immunol 1991;9:271−96.

Timmerman JM, Czerwinski DK, Davis TA, Hsu FJ, Benike C, Hao ZM, et al. Idiotype-pulsed dendritic cell vaccination for B-cell lymphoma: clinical and immune responses in 35 patients. Blood 2002;99:1517−26.

Tjoa BA, Lodge PA, Salgaller ML, Boynton AL, Murphy GP. Dendritic cell-based immunotherapy for prostate cancer. CA Cancer J Clin 1999;49(117−28):65.

Tjoa BA, Simmons SJ, Bowes VA, Ragde H, Rogers M, Elgamal A, et al. Evaluation of phase I/II clinical trials in prostate cancer with dendritic cells and PSMA peptides. Prostate 1998;36:39−44.

Van Tendeloo VF, Van De Velde, Van Driessche A, Cools N, Anguille S, Ladell K, et al. Induction of complete and molecular remissions in acute myeloid leukemia by Wilms' tumor 1 antigen-targeted dendritic cell vaccination. Proc Natl Acad Sci USA 2010;107:13824−9.

Veglia F, Gabrilovich DI. Dendritic cells in cancer: the role revisited. Curr Opin Immunol 2017;45:43−51.

The following additional references are provided for additional information on cellular and gene therapy clinical trials.

- Cellular & Gene Therapy Guidance: https://www.fda.gov/BiologicsBloodVaccines/

GuidanceComplianceRegulatoryInformation/ Guidances/CellularandGeneTherapy/default.htm

- Considerations for the Design of Early-Phase Clinical Trials of Cellular and Gene Therapy Products (Guidance for Industry): https://www.fda.gov/downloads/BiologicsBloodVaccines/

GuidanceComplianceRegulatoryInformation/ Guidances/CellularandGeneTherapy/UCM359073.pdf

- NIH Office of Science Policy; NIH Guidelines for Research Involving Recombinant or Synthetic Nucleic Acid Molecules (Biosafety): http://osp.od.nih.gov/office-biotechnology-activities/biosafety/nih-guidelines

Incorporating Patient-Reported Outcomes Into Early-Phase Trials

Alice P. Chen, Sandra A. Mitchell, Lori M. Minasian and Diane C. St. Germain

National Cancer Institute, Bethesda, MD, United States

13.1 INTRODUCTION

Understanding the impact of cancer treatment from the patient's perspective has long been recognized as critical. The patient's perspective on their health status and treatment experiences has been captured in health-related quality of life (HRQOL) assessments in phase 3 cancer clinical trials [1]. With this approach the patient's overall experiences of the investigational regimen or the standard treatment regimen are compared, in the context of regimen efficacy.

Early-phase cancer clinical trials are designed to evaluate the safety and tolerability of new therapies, determine the optimal dose and schedule, and explore for a signal of efficacy. Increasingly, early-phase trials set the stage for accelerated approval by the U.S. Food and Drug Administration (FDA) [2]. Many of the agents evaluated in early-phase trials do not have well-defined toxicity profiles, patients have complicated baseline symptoms, and, frequently, patients receive only a limited number of treatment cycles. The need to include the patient's

perspective in early-phase trials is even more important now with an increase in the number of oral agents available for cancer treatment. Often the oral molecularly targeted agents are administered for prolonged duration and may have chronic symptomatic adverse events (AEs) that can interfere with adherence and prompt elective treatment discontinuation [3,4].

The inclusion of patient-reported outcome (PRO) endpoints in phase 3 trials has provided valuable insight into the effects of cancer therapy on symptoms, functioning, and HRQOL, and determinations of treatment benefit. To date, early-phase clinical trials have typically not included PRO measures. Shifts in the landscape of early cancer drug development, however, now encourage the consideration of PROs in early-phase cancer clinical trials. In this chapter, we briefly trace the history of the inclusion of PROs in cancer clinical trials, highlight selected PRO measures, and outline important considerations when measuring, analyzing, and reporting PROs in early-phase clinical trials. We also highlight best practices to ensure that the investment in collecting and analyzing PRO data yields scientifically and clinically valid results that aid in interpreting overall trial outcomes.

13.2 INCLUSION OF PATIENT-REPORTED OUTCOMES IN CANCER CLINICAL TRIALS

Although the terms quality of life (QOL) and HRQOL are often used interchangeably, they are two distinct concepts. QOL reflects general well-being, life satisfaction, and happiness, while the term HRQOL narrows the focus to the effects of health, illness, and treatment on QOL domains that include health status, physical functioning, symptoms, psychosocial adjustment, and well-being [5]. By design, HRQOL measures typically evaluate multiple domains (e.g., physical function, emotional well-being, social function, and symptoms) and yield a summary score that can be compared over time within an individual, and between arms of a trial. The summary score reflects in aggregate a patient's perception of the effects of their disease and its treatment on the solicited health domains (e.g., symptoms, physical function, social function).

An initial framework for incorporating HRQOL endpoints into National Cancer Institute (NCI)-sponsored cancer clinical trials was identified in a 1990 workshop [6] when cancer treatment trials compared surgery with nonsurgical treatment on the endpoints of survival and organ preservation (e.g., laryngeal preservation in head and neck cancer, limb sparing in sarcoma). In this context, the patient's perception of their functional outcomes was needed to gauge treatment benefit.

Both QOL and HRQOL are PROs (see Fig. 13.1). PROs are defined as, "any report of the status of a patient's health condition that comes directly from the patient, without interpretation of the patient's response by a clinician or anyone else" [7]. Many cancer clinical trials include as secondary endpoints

PRO measures of disease and treatment effects such as symptom burden, self-assessed health status, and HRQOL [8]. PROs can enhance our understanding of the clinical benefit and tolerability of treatment, as well as the patient experience. PROs can be particularly useful when the results of a trial are equivocal, informing the patient and clinician which treatment has less symptomatic toxicity or produces a more desirable effect on HRQOL, thereby facilitating treatment decision-making [9].

13.2.1 Central Patient-Reported Outcome Concepts for Early-Phase Cancer Clinical Trials

The traditional approach of drug development through phase 1, phase 2, and phase 3 trials has been evolving into a more seamless paradigm [2]. Because of the increased interest in expediting the cancer drug development and approval process, the sequential trial phases that lead up to approval are becoming blurred. Agents may receive accelerated or priority approval based on results from single arm trials [10].

With the blurring of the phases of trials in drug development the incorporation of PROs into early-phase clinical trials has assumed greater importance. The inclusion of PROs in early-phase clinical trials should be designed to fit the endpoints of early-phase trials, such as identifying the incidence, severity, and resolution of new toxicities. The capture of symptomatic AEs using a PRO allows for the identification of treatment-emergent AEs that could be prospectively assessed in the expansion cohort if a potential signal for efficacy was demonstrated.

Typically, data generated during the conduct of an early-phase trial are assessed and the trial design potentially modified. New AEs are identified and then prospectively captured

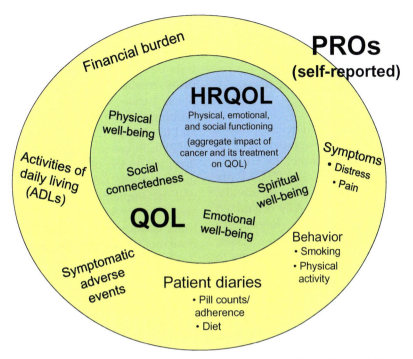

FIGURE 13.1 PROs, QOL, and HRQOL. *PRO*: patient-reported outcome. A Patient-Reported Outcome is any report of the status of one's health, well-being, behavior or human experience (e.g. perceptions, cognitions, judgements) that is gathered directly from a person, without interpretation of that report by a clinician, observer, or anyone else; *QOL*: quality of life. A person's perception or evaluation of their current level of well-being, life satisfaction, and happiness; *HRQOL*: health-related quality of life. A multidimensional concept that reflects the impact of health, illness, and treatment on domains that include symptoms, well-being, and physical, mental, emotional, and social functioning. HRQOL is a subset of QOL.

in patients subsequently accrued to the trial. Thus the collection of symptomatic AEs should allow for the flexibility to add new symptomatic AEs for prospective surveillance during the study, based on the development of treatment-emergent events. Standard HRQOL measures have a fixed set of questions that are not typically modified over the course of the trial and, thus, may not be optimal for the early-phase trial context.

In phase 2 trials the goal is to determine biologic activity in specific disease cohorts. If there is a signal for efficacy, even in a subset of patients, then there is an opportunity to evaluate chronic dosing in those patients who demonstrate tumor response or at least stable disease. Many molecularly targeted therapies and immunotherapies

have AEs that are low grade, develop gradually, and may become persistent and/or intolerable with sustained treatment. Additionally, some AEs may be heralded by seemingly low-grade or innocuous experiences that are not always identified or reported.

Thus incorporating PROs into early-phase cancer clinical trials in a way that informs the primary endpoints of safety and efficacy may add valuable information. These data can be integrated into the study design to inform dose and schedule to improve tolerability, to refine comparisons of two or more treatment regimens, and to predict survival [11–13]. PRO measures to capture symptomatic AEs, functional status, and disease-specific symptoms are described later in this chapter.

13.3 SYMPTOMATIC ADVERSE EVENTS

13.3.1 Adverse Event Reporting: Common Toxicity Criteria for Adverse Events

The standard lexicon for clinician grading and reporting of AEs in NCI-sponsored clinical trials is the Common Terminology Criteria for Adverse Events (CTCAE). The CTCAE are used in many clinical trials worldwide. Containing approximately 800 AEs organized across Medical Dictionary for Regulatory Activities (MedDRA) System Organ Classes, the CTCAE utilize a 5-point grading system to assess the severity of an AE (Table 13.1). Attribution, itself, is not a part of the library of terms in CTCAE.

The CTCAE grading criteria serve many functions within an early-phase clinical trial. Most important among these are the assessment of toxicity in the development of an agent and regulatory reporting of AEs. By providing standardized criteria for assigning a grade, the CTCAE allow for comparison of risks and benefits of a single agent, as well as comparison of different agents. Additionally, trial-specific criteria include CTCAE grades of toxicities from prior treatment to determine eligibility. In phase 1 trials, CTCAE are used to define dose-limiting toxicity and maximum tolerated dose, and to identify the recommended phase 2 dose (RP2D). In cancer clinical trials, dose modifications are based on CTCAE grading. Typically, in therapeutic cancer trials, dose modification will be implemented if Grade ≥ 3 toxicity is seen. For prevention trials or nontherapeutic trials, Grades 1 and 2 toxicities may also prompt dose modification or discontinuation.

The CTCAE criteria are designed for clinician grading of AEs based on the patient's history, physical examination, and diagnostic testing. The grading criteria are reported in aggregate based on the worst severity experienced by the patient over the course of a cycle. This approach was designed to efficiently characterize cytotoxic chemotherapy AEs, which typically will demonstrate their worst severity in the first or second cycle.

TABLE 13.1   CTCAE Grades and PRO-CTCAE Scores

CTCAE Grade	Description
0	No adverse event (or within normal limits)
1	Mild; asymptomatic or mild symptoms; clinical or diagnostic observations only; intervention not indicated
2	Moderate; minimal, local, or noninvasive intervention (e.g., packing, cautery) indicated; limiting age-appropriate instrumental activities of daily living (ADL)
3	Severe or medically significant but not immediately life-threatening; hospitalization or prolongation of hospitalization indicated; disabling; limiting self-care ADL
4	Life-threatening consequences; urgent intervention indicated
5	Death related to adverse event

Example:

CTCAE					
Adverse Event	Grade				
	1	2	3	4	5
Mucositis oral	Asymptomatic or mild symptoms; intervention not indicated	Moderate pain; not interfering with oral intake; modified diet indicated	Severe pain; interfering with oral intake	Life-threatening consequences; urgent intervention indicated	-

PRO-CTCAE

Please think back over the past 7 days:
What was the severity of your MOUTH OR THROAT SORES at their WORST?
None / Mild / Moderate / Severe / Very severe
How much did MOUTH OR THROAT SORES interfere with your usual or daily activities?
Not at all / A little bit / Somewhat / Quite a bit / Very much

Attribute	PRO-CTCAE Scores				
	0	1	2	3	4
Frequency	Never	Rarely	Occasionally	Frequently	Almost Constantly
Severity	None	Mild	Moderate	Severe	Very Severe
Interference	Not at all	A little bit	Somewhat	Quite a bit	Very much
Present/Absent	Absent	Present	None	None	None

CTCAE: Common Terminology Criteria for Adverse Events; PRO-CTCAE: patient-reported outcome version of the CTCAE.

Some novel agents may have low-grade toxicities seen in the first or second cycle that become more bothersome or intolerable over a longer period of chronic exposure. Although the evaluation of acute toxicity in the first cycle will provide an estimation of the tolerable dose, it does not reflect the cumulative side effects of treatment or necessarily indicate the dose that will be tolerable over the longer term [3,14,15]. Chronic, lower grade, but bothersome symptomatic adverse effects associated with many of the new orally administered agents have been implicated as contributing to elective treatment discontinuations or patient nonadherence to therapy [4,16—18]. There is a need to further understand the chronic dosing of anticancer therapy to improve its tolerability [13]. One approach to better appreciate the symptomatic toxicity of treatment is the inclusion of PROs to capture the frequency, severity, and interference of specific AEs. Analyzing the level of severity of a symptomatic AE together with the associated functional interference may ultimately provide an improved approach to identifying a more tolerable dosing schedule over time.

13.3.1.1 Patient-Reported Outcome-Common Toxicity Criteria for Adverse Events

The NCI patient-reported outcome version of the CTCAE (PRO-CTCAE; https://health-caredelivery.cancer.gov/pro-ctcae/) [19] is a publicly available PRO measurement system developed to capture the frequency, severity, and interference with daily activities associated with a wide range of symptomatic AEs in patients receiving cancer treatment. The PRO-CTCAE item library contains 78 symptomatic AEs with 124 individual questions which were derived from AE terms in CTCAE version 4.0. PRO-CTCAE is designed to be complementary to, and used in conjunction with, the CTCAE, bridging the gap between the clinician's concern for medical safety and the patient's concern about the impact of side effects on day-to-day functioning [20]. Thus data generated from the use of PRO-CTCAE reflect the patient perspective of treatment tolerability.

PRO-CTCAE symptom attributes include frequency (e.g., "In the last 7 days, how often did you have nausea?"), severity (e.g., "In the last 7 days, what was the severity of your pain?"), interference with daily activities (e.g., "how much did fatigue interfere with your usual or daily activities?"), and presence/absence/amount (e.g., "In the last 7 days, did you have any bed sores?"). As shown in Table 13.1, PRO-CTCAE scores range from 0 to 4, corresponding to the response choices. The reference period for each question is the past 7 days [21].

CTCAE and PRO-CTCAE item structures are shown in Table 13.1. Whether PRO-CTCAE questions address symptom frequency, severity, and/or interference with daily activities depends on the symptom under consideration [20]. For example, PRO-CTCAE symptom terms such as pain, anxiety, and depression are addressed using three attributes (frequency, severity, and interference), whereas others include one or two attributes—fatigue (severity, interference), nausea (severity, frequency), vomiting (severity, frequency), radiation skin reaction (severity), and difficulty swallowing (severity). CTCAE criteria for clinician grading of symptomatic AEs typically include a combination of these attributes. PRO-CTCAE can be collected using electronic- and paper-based methods of data collection. An analysis of PRO-CTCAE data collected via the internet, hand-held computer, interactive voice-response system, and paper-demonstrated good correlations [22]. Electronic administration of PRO-CTCAE can reduce patient burden via use of conditional branching, in which additional questions are not asked if the symptomatic AE is reported as absent.

The PRO-CTCAE adult version is validated for use in individuals 18 years or older, but can be used in adolescents as young as 16 years [23]. A pediatric version and a parent-proxy version of PRO-CTCAE for children and adolescents with cancer (ages 7–17) are undergoing testing. There is no proxy measure available for PRO-CTCAE (e.g., for adults with cognitive deficits). By 2018 it is anticipated that PRO-CTCAE will be available in more than 20 languages, thereby supporting the global conduct of cancer clinical trials.

The PRO-CTCAE item library has demonstrated favorable measurement properties including content validity, construct validity, reliability, and responsiveness using both qualitative and quantitative techniques [24–26]. This is important as measures intended for patient self-reporting of symptomatic AEs must possess the content validity and item structure to allow ascertainment of the full range of patient-reportable treatment toxicities.

It is important to note that PRO-CTCAE *scores* do not correspond to CTCAE *grades*. CTCAE and PRO-CTCAE were not developed for direct comparison. Rather, they were designed to be complementary strategies for capturing symptomatic AEs.

Differences between CTCAE and PRO-CTCAE reporting should not be over-interpreted. Disagreement between PRO-CTCAE and CTCAE toxicity assessments may not represent "under-ascertainment" by clinicians or "over-reporting" by patients. These are two unique sources of information, and clinicians and patients are reporting on the toxicity using two different rating systems and may also perceive the toxicities differently. For example, a clinician may grade vomiting by CTCAE criteria as a *Grade 2* (3–5 episodes separated by 5 min in a 24-h period); but to the patient, four daily episodes of vomiting constitute a very severe symptom with a severity *score of 4*. Most symptoms in PRO-CTCAE do not have corresponding CTCAE grades higher than CTCAE Grade 3. For example, CTCAE Grades 4 and 5 are rarely

applicable to symptomatic toxicities such as fatigue, tinnitus, hoarseness, or xerostomia. Thus a PRO-CTCAE patient-report of "severe" or "very severe" may not correspond to CTCAE Grade 4 (life threatening) toxicity. Indeed a life-threatening AE requiring urgent intervention would not be expected to be reported by patients. Other factors may account for differences between patient and clinician report. Patients may under-report symptoms to their clinicians due to time constraints, or a desire to avoid an appearance that they are complaining and/or avoid being removed from a study protocol or receiving a lower dose of treatment if they report toxicities. In some instances, clinicians and patients are also reporting on slightly different phenomena (e.g., sadness via PRO-CTCAE vs depression via CTCAE).

13.3.2 Functional Status

Functional status has long been captured through clinician reporting of performance status using Karnofsky or Eastern Cooperative Oncology Group (ECOG) clinician-reported performance status [27]. Performance status has been an eligibility criterion in early-phase trials to assure that recruited patients are sufficiently able to tolerate therapy and thereby allow an appropriate evaluation of the investigational agent or regimen.

13.3.2.1 Patient-Reported Outcomes Measurement Information System

Functional status has been identified by the FDA as a core PRO domain to be considered for inclusion in cancer clinical trials [28]. One tool for measuring functional status is the Patient-Reported Outcomes Measurement Information System (PROMIS), which offers a robust and efficient PRO evaluation of this construct [29]. Developed through a National Institutes of Health (NIH) consortium, PROMIS is comprised of more than 60 item banks that measure child and adult health across a variety of domains of physical, mental, and social health and well-being (http://www.nihpromis.com). The item banks measure several domains that are relevant to cancer clinical trials, including physical function; symptoms such as pain, sleep disturbance, depression, anxiety, and fatigue; as well as the ability to participate in social roles and activities. The domain framework for PROMIS is presented in Fig. 13.2.

PROMIS is not disease-specific, but rather is designed for use in both research and clinical practice to assess health outcomes across medical conditions. PROMIS uses modern measurement theory (specifically, item response theory (IRT)) as the basis for item development, survey construction and administration (including computer adaptive testing (CAT)), validation, scoring, and interpretation.

PROMIS item banks are constructed and validated using IRT. IRT is based on the idea that each PRO question or item contained in the item bank has a unique ability to discriminate between respondents at a given severity level. Thus some items within the item bank may be excellent at discriminating respondents with a low level of physical function, for example, "Are you able to get in and out of bed?," while others may be able to discriminate among respondents with a high level of physical function, for example, "Are you able to run or jog 5 miles?"

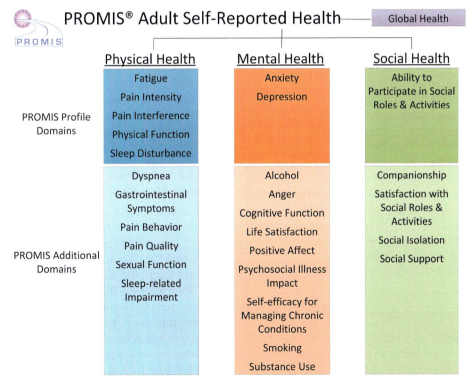

FIGURE 13.2 PROMIS domain framework, adult self-reported health measures. © 2008−2017 PROMIS Health Organization and PROMIS Cooperative Group. Reprinted with permission. Source: *http://www.healthmeasures.net/explore-measurement-systems/promis/intro-to-promis.*

CAT administration significantly enhances measurement precision and efficiency. The fundamental underlying principle of CAT is that to measure a phenomenon precisely and efficiently, the questions that are posed initially should allow for a preliminary estimate of the phenomenon of interest (e.g., physical function, pain, fatigue). Each successive question serves to measure that phenomenon within a narrower range, based on the patient's response to a previous question, thereby achieving greater precision.

The PROMIS measures are psychometrically sound and can be used across both acute and chronic medical conditions. Reference values for the various PROMIS domains have been determined for both healthy and clinical populations [30]. The measurement properties of PROMIS item banks, including mode invariance and responsiveness to change, have been extensively explored, including evaluation in samples of patients undergoing cancer treatment [31–35].

Interest in using PROMIS measures to measure HRQOL endpoints in cancer clinical trials is expanding [29]. A number of studies currently in development or in progress are using PROMIS measures as their PRO endpoint. As experience with using PROMIS in cancer clinical trials evolves, so too will the understanding of the practical aspects of including PROMIS in early-phase cancer trials—such as the advantages and limitations of the PROMIS short forms versus the CAT technology versions, and the feasibility and infrastructure considerations with respect to data collection [36].

13.3.3 Disease-Related Symptoms

A variety of disease-related symptom measures are available as a component of many of the well-validated HRQOL instruments, such as those developed by the European Organisation for Research and Treatment of Cancer (EORTC), the Functional Assessment of

Cancer Illness Therapy (FACIT) measurement system, and the National Comprehensive Cancer Network (NCCN). These disease-specific measures contain questions that reflect both disease- and treatment-related side effects. These validated instruments are intended to compare responses between arms and may be useful in randomized phase 2 studies.

Criteria for reviewing disease-related symptom measures for possible inclusion in an early-phase trial include that the measure contains items appropriate to the population of interest, has been used previously in the population of interest, and reflects the particular symptom dimension or attribute of interest (e.g., symptom frequency, severity, interference, distress, or bother) [37]. The measure should also be valid, reliable, brief, and easy to score. Options for measurement of disease-related symptoms based on consensus by expert panels or through systematic reviews include the Edmonton Symptom Assessment Scale (ESAS), MD Anderson Symptom Inventory (MDASI), Memorial Symptom Assessment Scale (MSAS), the Symptom Distress Scale, PRO-CTCAE, EORTC QLQ C-30 core instrument and its modules, and selected domains within PROMIS (e.g., fatigue, pain, sleep disturbance) [38–43].

13.3.3.1 Selecting a Patient-Reported Outcome Measure

When selecting a PRO measure, several conceptual, psychometric, administrative, and interpretive considerations must be addressed to ensure that the data are gathered efficiently, accurately represent the patient's experience, and provide information that is useful for clinical decision-making (Table 13.2).

It is important to consider the conceptual distinction between measures/items that assess the *status* of an aspect of HRQOL (e.g., how much fatigue do you have?) versus a measure/item that asks the respondent to make an *evaluation* of that state (e.g., how satisfied are you with your current level of functioning?) [44,45].

TABLE 13.2   Implementation Considerations for Patient-Reported Outcome Measures

	Implementation Considerations
Conceptual	• Is the patient-reported outcome measure relevant to the target population, illness, and treatment of interest? • Is the recall period (e.g., within the past day, week, month) optimal for the measure and for the phenomenon being measured? • Is the objective individual diagnosis or group-level comparison?
Psychometric	• Have the psychometric properties (validity and reliability) been examined in the target population? • Is there evidence of linguistic equivalence and cultural relevance for language translations? • Do the response choices allow for sufficient variability in the outcome? • In cognitively impaired or pediatric populations, has use of the measure for proxy-ratings been evaluated?
Administrative	• Is the language and literacy level appropriate for the target population? • What resources are required for data collection—e.g., pencil and paper versus web based? • Are there clear guidelines for scoring? • Is the respondent burden reasonable? • Is use of the measure conditional upon securing permission or payment of licensing fees?
Interpretive	• Are age- and gender-matched norms and diagnostic cut scores available? • Are ceiling or floor effects a concern in the target population? • Has a minimally important clinical difference been determined to aid interpretation of clinically meaningful change? • Are processes established to alert clinicians when diagnostic criteria for distress or other actionable response to a questionnaire item (e.g., suicidal ideation) is revealed by the PRO measure?

This distinction is important because some PRO measures are composed predominantly of status questions, while other PRO measures are primarily comprised of evaluation questions. Answers to these two types of questions (status and evaluation) must be interpreted quite differently, and may explain why there has been variability observed in the predictors of HRQOL both within and across populations.

PRO measures can also be distinguished as generic versus condition specific. Generic measures offer the advantage of comparisons with the general population and can be used across disease or treatment groups [46]. Generic measures tend to be broad and may therefore be so general that they fail to address the issues of greatest concern. On the other hand, condition-specific measures focus on concerns specific to an illness or treatment and may be more responsive to change. However, comparisons across populations may be problematic, and reference values for condition-specific measures are typically not available to facilitate interpretation.

There is general agreement that both generic and condition-specific instruments should be considered for use. Guidance concerning best practices when selecting, administering, and interpreting PRO measures is available [47–49].

Advances in the development of item banks, CAT, and digital formats for PRO data collection continue at a rapid pace [50,51] and may ultimately improve the precision with which PROs are measured, reduce investigator and study participant burden, and enhance comparability among outcome measures.

13.4 STUDY DESIGN, ANALYSIS, INTERPRETATION, AND REPORTING OF EARLY-PHASE TRIALS THAT INCLUDE PATIENT-REPORTED OUTCOMES

Selecting which PRO instrument best fits the need of a trial depends on the study objectives and the patient population. It is important for the investigator to first identify what domain or domains (symptomatic AEs, physical function, or others) they wish to measure based on their underlying hypothesis. A PRO is chosen based on its measurement properties (validity, reliability, ability to detect change), interpretability, and pragmatic considerations (feasibility, respondent burden).

With respect to PRO-CTCAE, the symptomatic AEs and time points of measurement should be specified in a manner similar to that used to define the AE surveillance plan for the trial more broadly. To identify those symptomatic AEs likely to be associated with the regimens in the trial, the study team reviews published data, as well as data from earlier-phase trials or animal models, if available, and incorporates information about the known or anticipated on- and off-target effects of agents in a similar mechanistic class [52].

The timing of PRO-CTCAE assessments should also consider that the optimal recall period for PRO-CTCAE items is the past 7 days [21]. In clinical trials that employ paper-and-pencil PRO-CTCAE or in-clinic-only PRO-CTCAE administration, and where there are concerns about temporal breaks in reporting, a longer recall period (e.g. the past month) or supplementary methods of reporting (e.g., paper diaries) may have to be implemented. Concerns about temporal breaks in reporting may be less pertinent in study contexts where symptomatic toxicities are anticipated to be stable, or to be changing only subtly—e.g., with chronically administered oral therapies, or during long-term follow-up after treatment completion when toxicities are expected to have stabilized.

The rationale for the PRO-CTCAE items chosen and for the time points of assessment should be summarized in the AE reporting sections of the protocol and in any associated publications. Trial designs should allow for the capture of unsolicited symptomatic AEs. Allowing for write-ins that may capture unexpected symptomatic AEs provides a valuable safeguard against ascertainment bias. Write-ins can be handled more feasibly when electronic reporting is employed and in small clinical trials. Feasible strategies to capture and analyze free-text data in larger trials need to be tested.

Any protocol that includes a PRO should explicitly indicate whether PRO results are to be shared with clinicians. Additional guidance and standard elements to be addressed when developing study protocols that include PROs have been articulated [53].

Protocols that include a PRO should explicitly describe the thresholds for alerts (e.g., severe symptoms, notable decline in physical functioning), the procedures for monitoring PRO responses, and the actions to be taken and required documentation by site and central study staff, when a PRO report warrants clinical intervention [54,55]. All PRO data collection tools should clearly indicate to the patient that they should discuss their symptoms and health status with their clinician.

Missing data and data quality are important considerations that require explicit planning and ongoing monitoring since missing PRO data clouds trial-level interpretations, particularly with respect to symptomatic toxicity. Every effort should be made to avoid data being missing at the baseline and at the off-treatment. Reasons for missing data should be captured. Instances where the patient is too sick to complete PRO reporting should be documented as "not available," rather than missing, for the purposes of metrics of data quality.

Attribution of patient-reports as treatment related, versus a symptom attributable to disease or to another comorbid condition, is a consideration that requires continued study. Attribution to treatment may be particularly challenging with respect to symptoms such as weight loss, anorexia, fatigue, or even shortness of breath. While systematic capture of the presence and severity of symptoms at baseline may contribute to isolating treatment-emergent symptoms, disentangling treatment toxicity attributable to the anticancer therapy under study, from the side effects of therapy for comorbidities, and from disease-related symptoms of disease progression, will continue to be extremely challenging.

Adjudication of attribution at the trial level and in the context of available clinical data is ultimately required to reach a definitive conclusion about the relationship between a symptom report and the treatment under study. Some symptoms such as skin rash, peripheral neuropathy, and muscle/joint pain may be easier to attribute due to the timing of their onset following treatment initiation.

Subgroup analysis of the profile of AEs in those with disease progression may also help clarify attribution. Similarly, continued surveillance after treatment discontinuation might identify the offset of AEs with treatment discontinuation versus persistence or worsening that would be expected with disease-related symptoms. However, as therapy is often discontinued due to disease progression and declining performance status, the difficulties of continuing to capture PRO data in that circumstance may make such an approach infeasible in many study contexts.

Scoring, analysis, and interpretation of a PRO measure is often complex, and collaboration between trial lists and PRO researchers is strongly encouraged. Inclusion of a PRO researcher on the study team from the earliest stages of trial design is important to ensure that inclusion of the PRO yields information that is robust, interpretable, and meaningful. There are many different approaches that can be considered in analyzing PROs in trials, including longitudinal analyses, graphical analyses, responder analysis, and descriptive analyses [48,56–59]. Efforts are ongoing to provide standards for the analysis of PRO endpoints in cancer clinical trials [60]. For toxicity assessments, innovative approaches

such as longitudinal assessments of toxicity over time, bar charts/histograms, and cumulative toxicities are also being explored [61–64]. PRO-CTCAE scores should be presented in conjunction with CTCAE grades for the corresponding time points. In any PRO analysis the proportion of missing data should also be summarized to aid interpretation. Additional principles and best practices for the design, conduct, and interpretation of trials using PROs are outlined in Table 13.3.

13.4.1 Value of Including Patient-Reported Symptomatic Adverse Events in Early-Phase Drug Development Studies

In phase 1 trials, PRO-CTCAE can be used to thoroughly explore the profile of symptomatic toxicities. This knowledge sets the stage for more focused and efficient toxicity evaluations in phase 2 trials and beyond, and may also help to define the supportive care that should be included as part of the standard of care within later-phase trials. PRO-CTCAE may also have value in confirming the tolerable dose over time in phase 1 trials [65]. PROs can also be used to identify meaningfully different subgroups within the sample, and to explain treatment drop-out and missing data.

Surveillance for symptomatic treatment toxicity using PRO-CTCAE has the potential to enhance the efficiency, reliability, and comprehensiveness of AE data capture. PRO-CTCAE systematically characterizes baseline symptoms at study entry, supporting a more accurate and efficient attribution of symptomatic AEs at the study level [66]. PRO-CTCAE permits identification in real-time of AEs that may escape detection because they occur between visits, and captures the offset or resolution of symptomatic AEs, something that is often missed in our current approach and may be particularly informative in early drug development studies.

TABLE 13.3   Considerations for PRO-CTCAE Study Design, Survey Administration, and Data Analysis

Adverse events section of the protocol	• PRO-CTCAE items correspond to the CTCAE toxicities of interest and reflect comparable timeframes to permit concurrent interpretation.
	• PRO-CTCAE assessments are included in the main protocol schedule of assessments.
	• Protocol specifies how (e.g., pencil and paper, tablet) and where (e.g., clinic, home) PRO-CTCAE assessments will be captured.
	• Approach to capturing and analyzing unsolicited (unexpected) symptomatic AEs, if used, is described.
	• Procedures for data collection and management to minimize and monitor missing data (e.g., central data quality monitoring, reminders for missed surveys, site reminders) are described.
	• Use of PRO-CTCAE is limited to describing in aggregate the safety and tolerability of a therapy or regimen, and protocol states explicitly that clinician CTCAE grades are to be used when making clinical decisions about trial eligibility, dose delays, dose reductions, or treatment discontinuation.
PRO-CTCAE survey administration	• PRO-CTCAE data collection tools should include explicit instructions reminding the respondent that they should discuss their symptoms and health status with their clinician.
	• Study protocol should specify the allowable grace period for completing a scheduled PRO-CTCAE assessment before it will be considered missing.
	• Electronic data capture provides efficiency and flexibility for survey scheduling and administration, reduces the need for manual data entry, and permits centralized, real-time monitoring of missing data and patient or site reminders for overdue surveys.
PRO-CTCAE data analytic plan	• Complements and extends the analytic plan for CTCAE.
	• Specifies the approach to descriptive or graphical analysis, including the use of approaches that capitalize on the longitudinal data structure and accommodate baseline values (e.g., time-to-event analyses, area under the curve).

CTCAE: Common Terminology Criteria for Adverse Events; PRO-CTCAE: patient-reported outcome version of the CTCAE.
Based on information from: Mitchell et al. Patient-reported outcomes version of the Common Terminology Criteria for Adverse Events: principles for use in cancer clinical trials. Under review with Journal of Clinical Oncology.

PRO-CTCAE may also strengthen our capture of persistent and delayed late treatment effects, creating a more complete and precise understanding of the toxicity profile of treatment, and permitting more nuanced interpretation of the relationships among treatment, treatment-related toxicities, and the early and later HRQOL outcomes that increasingly are included as secondary endpoints in cancer clinical trials [67].

In later phases of drug development the emphasis shifts from tolerable dose and the associated toxicity profile, to comparing the effectiveness of two or more treatment approaches. Precise characterization of the profile of patient-reported treatment toxicities, including mild or moderate symptomatic toxicities, may be particularly important in these contexts when disease-modifying therapies are administered for extended periods. Patient adherence may be negatively affected by persistent mild adverse treatment effects, which may result in early treatment discontinuation.

One of the other gaps in AE reporting that PRO-CTCAE can fill is that of documenting the resolution of AEs. This is something that is often informal/imprecise, unless a decision about protocol-directed management of the AE is involved. Yet knowing the duration and resolution of an AE during therapy and follow-up is important to manage toxicity and provide patients with anticipatory guidance.

13.5 CONCLUSION

Treatment tolerability is an important endpoint when drawing conclusions about therapeutic effectiveness, and accurately gauging the toxicity profile of new agents is essential in cancer drug development. There are a variety of ways in which the inclusion of patient reporting of symptomatic AEs can enhance the accuracy, precision, validity, and efficiency of AE reporting in early-phase cancer clinical trials.

Adverse event reporting is particularly important in early-phase drug development. In this context, samples are typically small, and toxicity may be the primary endpoint, or the goal may be to gauge preliminary signals about relative benefits versus risk. In early-phase trials the toxicity assessment often focuses on the first cycle of treatment to determine the tolerable dose.

While the inclusion of PROs in early-phase trials has the potential to yield information that is valuable to clinicians, patients, regulators and other decision-makers, challenges in collecting, interpreting, and disseminating PRO data remain.

The use of PROs, especially PRO-CTCAE, in early-phase trials can provide data to inform the design of later-phase trials, identifying the symptomatic toxicities that should be monitored and managed, and informing the selection of primary or secondary PRO endpoints that aid the interpretation of efficacy outcomes.

Acknowledgments

The authors would like to thank Ann O'Mara, Andrea Denicoff, Gwen Moulton, and Rebecca Enos for the support they provided in the development of this chapter.

References

[1] O'Mara AM, Denicoff AM. Health related quality of life in NCI-sponsored cancer treatment trials. Semin Oncol Nurs 2010;26:68–78.

[2] Prowell TM, Theoret MR, Pazdur R. Seamless oncology-drug development. N Engl J Med 2016;374:2001–3.

[3] Edgerly M, Fojo T. Is there room for improvement in adverse event reporting in the era of targeted therapies? J Natl Cancer Inst 2008;100:240–2.

[4] Verbrugghe M, Verhaeghe S, Lauwaert K, Beeckman D, Van Hecke A. Determinants and associated factors influencing medication adherence and persistence to oral anticancer drugs: a systematic review. Cancer Treat Rev 2013;39:610–21.

[5] Ferrans CE. Definitions and conceptual models of quality of life. In: Lipscomb J, Gotay CC, Snyder C, editors. Outcomes assessment in cancer: measures, methods, and applications. Cambridge: Cambridge University Press; 2005.

[6] Nayfield SG, Ganz PA, Moinpour CM, Cella DF, Hailey BJ. Report from a National Cancer Institute (USA) workshop on quality of life assessment in cancer clinical trials. Qual Life Res 1992;1:203–10.

[7] USDHHS. Guidance for industry: patient-reported outcome measures: use in medical product development to support labeling claims. U.S. Department of Health and Human Services. Food and Drug Administration; 2009 [online] Available from: <http://www.fda.gov/downloads/Drugs/GuidanceComplianceRegulatoryInformation/Guidances/UCM193282.pdf>; [accessed 14.03.17].

[8] Secord AA, Coleman RL, Havrilesky LJ, Abernethy AP, Samsa GP, Cella D. Patient-reported outcomes as end points and outcome indicators in solid tumours. Nat Rev Clin Oncol 2015;12:358–70.

[9] Au HJ, Ringash J, Brundage M, Palmer M, Richardson H, Meyer RM. Added value of health-related quality of life measurement in cancer clinical trials: the experience of the NCIC CTG. Expert Rev Pharmacoecon Outcomes Res 2010;10:119–28.

[10] Gnanasakthy A, DeMuro C, Clark M, Haydysch E, Ma E, Bonthapally V. Patient-reported outcomes labeling for products approved by the office of hematology and oncology products of the US Food and Drug Administration (2010–2014). J Clin Oncol 2016;34:1928–34.

[11] Hareendran A, Gnanasakthy A, Winnette R, Revicki D. Capturing patients' perspectives of treatment in clinical trials/drug development. Contemp Clin Trials 2012;33:23–8.

[12] Kluetz PG, Chingos DT, Basch EM, Mitchell SA. Patient-reported outcomes in cancer clinical trials: measuring symptomatic adverse events with the National Cancer Institute's Patient-Reported Outcomes Version of the Common Terminology Criteria for Adverse Events (PRO-CTCAE). Am Soc Clin Oncol Educ Book 2016;35:67–73.

[13] Minasian L, Rosen O, Auclair D, Rahman A, Pazdur R, Schilsky RL. Optimizing dosing of oncology drugs. Clin Pharmacol Ther 2014;96:572–9.

[14] Postel-Vinay S, Collette L, Paoletti X, Rizzo E, Massard C, Olmos D, et al. Towards new methods for the determination of dose limiting toxicities and the assessment of the recommended dose for further studies of molecularly targeted agents-dose-Limiting Toxicity and Toxicity Assessment Recommendation Group for Early Trials of Targeted therapies, an European Organisation for Research and Treatment of Cancer-led study. Eur J Cancer 2014;50:2040–9.

[15] Postel-Vinay S, Gomez-Roca C, Molife LR, Anghan B, Levy A, Judson I, et al. Phase I trials of molecularly targeted agents: should we pay more attention to late toxicities? J Clin Oncol. 2011;29:1728–35.

[16] Creel PA. Optimizing patient adherence to targeted therapies in renal cell carcinoma. Clin J Oncol Nurs 2014;18:694–700.

[17] Lee HS, Lee JY, Ah YM, Kim HS, Im SA, Noh DY, et al. Low adherence to upfront and extended adjuvant letrozole therapy among early breast cancer patients in a clinical practice setting. Oncology 2014;86:340–9.

[18] Meggetto O, Maunsell E, Chlebowski R, Goss P, Tu D, Richardson H. Factors associated with early discontinuation of study treatment in the mammary prevention. 3. Breast cancer chemoprevention trial. J Clin Oncol 2017; Jco2016688895.

[19] National Cancer Institute. Patient-Reported Outcomes version of the Common Terminology Criteria for Adverse Events (PRO-CTCAE™) [Online]; 2017. Available from: <https://healthcaredelivery.cancer.gov/pro-ctcae/>. [accessed December 2017].

[20] Basch E, Reeve BB, Mitchell SA, Clauser SB, Minasian LM, Dueck AC, et al. Development of the National Cancer Institute's patient-reported outcomes version of the Common Terminology Criteria for Adverse Events (PRO-CTCAE). J Natl Cancer Inst 2014;106. Available from: http://dx.doi.org/10.1093/jnci/dju244.

[21] Mendoza TR, Dueck AC, Bennett AV, Mitchell SA, Reeve BB, Atkinson TM, et al. Evaluation of different recall periods for the US National Cancer Institutes PRO-CTCAE. Clin Trials 2017;14(3):255–63. Available from: https://doi.org/10.1177/1740774517698645 PMID: 28545337.

[22] Bennett AV, Dueck AC, Mitchell SA, Mendoza TR, Reeve BB, Atkinson TM, et al. Mode equivalence and acceptability of tablet computer-, interactive voice response system-, and paper-based administration of the U.S. National Cancer Institute's Patient-Reported Outcomes version of the Common Terminology Criteria for Adverse Events (PRO-CTCAE). Health Qual Life Outcomes 2016;14:24.

[23] Reeve BB, McFatrich M, Pinheiro LC, Freyer DR, Basch EM, Baker JN, et al. Cognitive interview-based validation of the patient-reported outcomes version of the common terminology criteria for adverse events in adolescents with cancer. J Pain Sympt Manage 2017;53 (4):759–66. Available from: https://doi.org/10.1016/j.jpainsymman.2016.11.006; PMID: 2806234.

[24] Dueck AC, Mendoza TR, Mitchell SA, Reeve BB, Castro KM, Rogak LJ, et al. Validity and reliability of the US National Cancer Institute's Patient-Reported Outcomes Version of the Common Terminology Criteria for Adverse Events (PRO-CTCAE). JAMA Oncol 2015;1:1051–9.

[25] Hagelstein V, Ortland I, Wilmer A, Mitchell SA, Jaehde U. Validation of the German patient-reported outcomes version of the common terminology criteria for adverse events (PRO-CTCAE). Ann Oncol 2016;27:2294–9.

[26] Hay JL, Atkinson TM, Reeve BB, Mitchell SA, Mendoza TR, Willis G, et al. Cognitive interviewing of the US National Cancer Institute's Patient-Reported Outcomes version of the Common Terminology Criteria for Adverse Events (PRO-CTCAE). Qual Life Res 2014;23:257–69.

[27] Yates JW, Chalmer B, McKegney FP. Evaluation of patients with advanced cancer using the Karnofsky performance status. Cancer 1980;45:2220–4.

[28] Kluetz PG, Slagle A, Papadopoulos EJ, Johnson LL, Donoghue M, Kwitkowski VE, et al. Focusing on core patient-reported outcomes in cancer clinical trials: symptomatic adverse events, physical function, and disease-related symptoms. Clin Cancer Res 2016;22:1553–8.

[29] Cella D, Stone AA. Health-related quality of life measurement in oncology: advances and opportunities. Am Psychol 2015;70:175–85.

[30] Jensen RE, Potosky AL, Reeve BB, Hahn E, Cella D, Fries J, et al. Validation of the PROMIS physical function measures in a diverse US population-based cohort of cancer patients. Qual Life Res 2015;24(10):2333–44.

[31] Cella D, Riley W, Stone A, Rothrock N, Reeve B, Yount S, et al. The Patient-Reported Outcomes Measurement Information System (PROMIS) developed and tested its first wave of adult self-reported health outcome item banks: 2005–2008. J Clin Epidemiol 2010;63:1179–94.

[32] Jensen RE, Moinpour CM, Potosky AL, Lobo T, Hahn EA, Hays RD, et al. Responsiveness of 8 Patient-Reported Outcomes Measurement Information System (PROMIS) measures in a large, community-based cancer study cohort. Cancer 2017;123:327–35.

[33] Liu H, Cella D, Gershon R, Shen J, Morales LS, Riley W, et al. Representativeness of the patient-reported outcomes measurement information system internet panel. J Clin Epidemiol 2010;63:1169–78.

[34] Rothrock NE, Hays RD, Spritzer K, Yount SE, Riley W, Cella D. Relative to the general US population, chronic diseases are associated with poorer health-related quality of life as measured by the Patient-Reported Outcomes Measurement Information System (PROMIS). J Clin Epidemiol 2010;63:1195–204.

[35] Bjorner JB, Rose M, Gandek B, Stone AA, Junghaenel DU, Ware Jr. JE. Method of administration of PROMIS scales did not significantly impact score level, reliability, or validity. J Clin Epidemiol 2014;67:108–13.

[36] Bingham 3rd CO, Bartlett SJ, Merkel PA, Mielenz TJ, Pilkonis PA, Edmundson L, et al. Using patient-reported outcomes and PROMIS in research and clinical applications: experiences from the PCORI pilot projects. Qual Life Res 2016;25:2109–16.

[37] Cooley ME, Siefert ML. Assessment of multiple co-occurring cancer symptoms in the clinical setting. Semin Oncol Nurs 2016;32:361–72.

[38] Aktas A, Walsh D, Kirkova J. The psychometric properties of cancer multisymptom assessment instruments: a clinical review. Support Care Cancer 2015;23:2189–202.

[39] Cleeland CS, Sloan JA, Cella D, Chen C, Dueck AC, Janjan NA, et al. Recommendations for including multiple symptoms as endpoints in cancer clinical trials: a report from the ASCPRO (Assessing the Symptoms of Cancer Using Patient-Reported Outcomes) Multisymptom Task Force. Cancer 2012;119 (2):411–20.

[40] Cleeland CS, Zhao F, Chang VT, Sloan JA, O'Mara AM, Gilman PB, et al. The symptom burden of cancer: evidence for a core set of cancer-related and treatment-related symptoms from the Eastern Cooperative Oncology Group Symptom Outcomes and Practice Patterns study. Cancer 2013;119:4333–40.

[41] Gilbert A, Sebag-Montefiore D, Davidson S, Velikova G. Use of patient-reported outcomes to measure symptoms and health related quality of life in the clinic. Gynecol Oncol 2015;136:429–39.

[42] Basch E, Abernethy AP, Mullins CD, Reeve BB, Smith ML, Coons SJ, et al. Recommendations for incorporating patient-reported outcomes into clinical comparative effectiveness research in adult oncology. J Clin Oncol 2012;30:4249–55.

[43] Reeve BB, Mitchell SA, Dueck AC, Basch E, Cella D, Reilly CM, et al. Recommended patient-reported core set of symptoms to measure in adult cancer treatment trials. J Natl Cancer Inst 2014;106. Available from: http://dx.doi.org/10.1093/jnci/dju129.

[44] Ferrans CE. Differences in what quality-of-life instruments measure. J Natl Cancer Inst Monogr 2007;37:22–6.

[45] Ferrans CE. Advances in measuring quality-of-life outcomes in cancer care. Semin Oncol Nurs 2010;26:2–11.

[46] Coons SJ, Rao S, Keininger DL, Hays RD. A comparative review of generic quality-of-life instruments. PharmacoEconomics 2000;17:13–35.

[47] Mokkink LB, Prinsen CA, Bouter LM, Vet HC, Terwee CB. The COnsensus-based Standards for the selection of health Measurement INstruments (COSMIN) and how to select an outcome measurement instrument. Braz J Phys Ther 2016;20:105–13.

[48] Reeve BB, Wyrwich KW, Wu AW, Velikova G, Terwee CB, Snyder CF, et al. ISOQOL recommends minimum standards for patient-reported outcome measures used in patient-centered outcomes and comparative effectiveness research. Qual Life Res 2013;22:1889–905.

[49] Terwee CB, Mokkink LB, Knol DL, Ostelo RW, Bouter LM, de Vet HC. Rating the methodological quality in systematic reviews of studies on measurement properties: a scoring system for the COSMIN checklist. Qual Life Res 2012;21:651–7.

[50] Jensen RE, Rothrock NE, DeWitt EM, Spiegel B, Tucker CA, Crane HM, et al. The role of technical advances in the adoption and integration of patient-reported outcomes in clinical care. Med Care 2015;53:153–9.

[51] Jensen RE, Snyder CF, Abernethy AP, Basch E, Potosky AL, Roberts AC, et al. Review of electronic patient-reported outcomes systems used in cancer clinical care. J Oncol Pract 2014;10:e215–22.

[52] Cella D, Wagner L. Re-personalizing precision medicine: is there a role for patient-reported outcomes? J Commun Support Oncol 2015;13:275–7.

[53] Calvert M, Kyte D, Duffy H, Gheorghe A, Mercieca-Bebber R, Ives J, et al. Patient-reported outcome (PRO) assessment in clinical trials: a systematic review of guidance for trial protocol writers. PLoS One 2014;9: e110216.

[54] Kyte D, Draper H, Calvert M. Patient-reported outcome alerts: ethical and logistical considerations in clinical trials. JAMA 2013;310:1229–30.

[55] Kyte D, Ives J, Draper H, Calvert M. Management of patient-reported outcome (PRO) alerts in clinical trials: a cross sectional survey. PLoS One 2016;11:e0144658.

[56] Coyne KS, Wyrwich KW. ISPOR task force for clinical outcomes assessment: clinical outcome assessments:

conceptual foundation-report of the ISPOR clinical outcomes assessment – emerging good practices for outcomes research task force. Value Health 2015;18:739–40.

[57] McLeod LD, Cappelleri JC, Hays RD. Best (but oft-forgotten) practices: expressing and interpreting associations and effect sizes in clinical outcome assessments. Am J Clin Nutr 2016;103:685–93.

[58] Wyrwich KW, Norquist JM, Lenderking WR, Acaster S. Methods for interpreting change over time in patient-reported outcome measures. Qual Life Res 2013;22:475–83.

[59] Bonnetain F, Fiteni F, Efficace F, Anota A. Statistical challenges in the analysis of health-related quality of life in cancer clinical trials. J Clin Oncol 2016;34:1953–6.

[60] Bottomley A, Pe M, Sloan J, Basch E, Bonnetain F, Calvert M, et al. Analysing data from patient-reported outcome and quality of life endpoints for cancer clinical trials: a start in setting international standards. Lancet Oncol 2016;17:e510–14.

[61] Cappelleri JC, Bushmakin AG. Interpretation of patient-reported outcomes. Stat Methods Med Res 2014;23:460–83.

[62] Lee SM, Backenroth D, Cheung YK, Hershman DL, Vulih D, Anderson B, et al. Case example of dose optimization using data from bortezomib dose-finding clinical trials. J Clin Oncol 2016;34:1395–401.

[63] Basch EM, Pugh SL, Dueck AC, Mitchell SA, Berk L, Fogh S, et al. Feasibility of patient reporting of symptomatic adverse events via the Patient-Reported Outcomes version of the Common Terminology Criteria for Adverse Events (PRO-CTCAE) in a chemoradiotherapy cooperative group multicenter clinical trial. Int J Radiat Oncol Biol Phys 2017;98 (2):409–18. Available from: https://doi.org/10.1016/j.ijrobp.2017.02.002; PMID: 28463161.

[64] Thanarajasingam G, Atherton PJ, Novotny PJ, Loprinzi CL, Sloan JA, Grothey A. Longitudinal adverse event assessment in oncology clinical trials: the toxicity over time (ToxT) analysis of alliance trials NCCTG N9741 and 979254. Lancet Oncol 2016;17:663–70.

[65] Le Tourneau C, Razak AR, Gan HK, Pop S, Dieras V, Tresca P, et al. Heterogeneity in the definition of dose-limiting toxicity in phase I cancer clinical trials of molecularly targeted agents: a review of the literature. Eur J Cancer 2011;47:1468–75.

[66] Hillman SL, Mandrekar SJ, Bot B, DeMatteo RP, Perez EA, Ballman KV, et al. Evaluation of the value of attribution in the interpretation of adverse event data: a North Central Cancer Treatment Group and American College of Surgeons Oncology Group investigation. J Clin Oncol 2010;28:3002–7.

[67] Smith AW, Mitchell SA, KDeAguiar C, Moy C, Riley WT, Wagster MV, et al. News from the NIH: person-centered outcomes measurement: NIH-supported measurement systems to evaluate self-assessed health, functional performance, and symptomatic toxicity. Transl Behav Med 2016;6:470–4.

Index

Note: Page numbers followed by "*f*," "*t*," and "*b*" refer to figures, tables, and boxes, respectively.

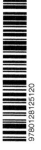